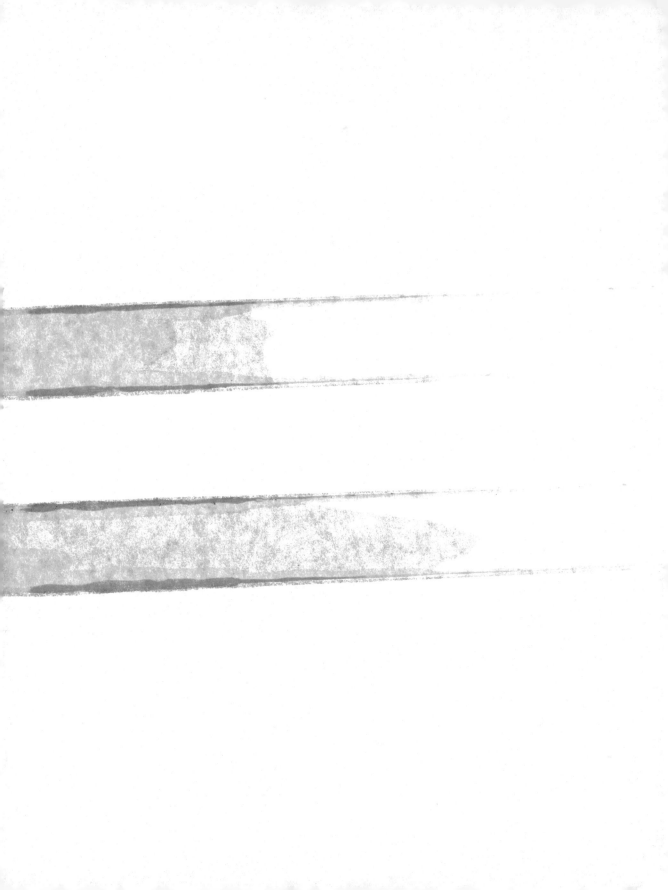

Anxious Eaters,
Anxious Mealtimes

Anxious Eaters, Anxious Mealtimes

Practical and Compassionate Strategies
for Mealtime Peace

Marsha Dunn Klein, OTR/L, MEd, FAOTA

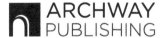

Archway Publishing books may be ordered through booksellers or by contacting:

Archway Publishing
1663 Liberty Drive
Bloomington, IN 47403
www.archwaypublishing.com
1 (888) 242-5904

Interior Art by Jennifer Ferguson and Chris Sternberg

ISBN: 978-1-4808-8003-0 (sc)
ISBN: 978-1-4808-8004-7 (e)

Library of Congress Control Number: 2019908821

Print information available on the last page.

Archway Publishing rev. date: 7/25/2019

Praise for the Book

To any parent who has felt the pressure to *get her child to eat*, this book is a treasure. Marsha champions a whole new mindset. Page by page she breaks down the process of introducing new flavors, textures, and foods into micro-steps that feel doable, comfortable, and natural. Her kind, compassionate approach will transform mealtime anxiety into joyful possibilities and lasting change. This gem of a book will restore your hope.

Laura Wesp, Teddy's Mom

This accessible book is a goldmine for parents and professionals. Marsha Dunn Klein teaches parents that there IS a route to positive mealtimes and that, with sensitivity to (and respect for) children, we can help them learn to explore new foods, tolerate novelty and build their eating confidence. Marsha has a wonderful way of expressing important concepts like "change happens" and "mealtime peace." She writes with huge compassion and without judgement, always seeing things from the perspective of the many, many families she has worked with.

Jo Cormack, MA, Therapist and Feeding Specialist, Emotionally Aware Eating

I have always loved the work of Marsha Dunn Klein in her the Get Permission Approach because it's given me such practical ways to help families. I highly recommend this book for parents and practitioners who are feeling stuck and need new ideas to help them support the anxious eaters in their lives. This is the book every feeding therapist needs! Marsha understands the struggles of families with anxious eaters and offers kind and thoughtful advice. Her wisdom and experience will be a welcome addition to any family welcoming a picky eater to their table.

Karen Dilfer, MS, OTR/L, Pediatric Occupational Therapist

This book will give you the hope, insight, strength and tools to help you and your child succeed at mealtime. One of the greatest gifts Marsha gives us is that there are a thousand ways to get there- if one way isn't working we can try another! We won't give up!

Lauri Ziemba, Brady's Mom

This book is a wonderful tool in our "toolbox" for helping children with Pediatric Feeding Disorder. Ms. Dunn Klein understands that these children suffer from some physical or skill-based deficit that has impeded their ability to trust that eating will be safe or comfortable. For many of these children, they have had months if not years of trying to eat, while experiencing pain and discomfort, or pressure. Over repeated experiences, children with Pediatric Feeding Disorder learn to avoid eating. Perhaps the original problem with eating is long gone; but they continue to avoid foods – sometimes new foods, sometimes familiar foods in a different setting or prepared in a different way. By understanding the reasons behind the anxious behaviors, both the professional and the parent can appropriately help these children learn the skills for eating. Ms. Dunn Klein explains the various skills necessary for eating – across several physical and developmental domains. Rather than trying to "fix the child's behavior," Ms Dunn Klein helps the adults recognize why mealtimes have become so challenging, and how to help their child and family enjoying eating and mealtimes once again. She illustrates key points throughout the book with stories of clients, helping both parents and professionals to recognize their own struggles while at the same time helping parents understand their child's behaviors are not unique. I believe every parent, at one point or another, would benefit from understanding how to help their child move from saying "NO" to enjoying the wonderful array of foods we have available. From working with these children, I know that these anxious eaters are found in every country, across the age ranges of early toddlers to adult. It is so refreshing to have a skilled, experienced therapist who has successfully worked with these children provide her insight and her expertise. This is a roadmap, a guide book, towards once again enjoying mealtimes with our children. Thank you, Marsha – from all of us!

Erin Sundseth Ross, Ph.D., CCC-SLP Pediatric Speech Pathologist

Marsha Dunn Klein is a well-known and well-respected expert in the field of treating children with feeding challenges because of her unique ability to explain how to help these children in down-to-earth, parent friendly language. Both Feeding Therapists and Parents/Caregivers alike will find the information in <u>Anxious Eaters, Anxious Mealtimes</u> easy to understand, and the practical strategies in this book are a welcomed addition to the field. I am certain that Ms. Dunn Klein's book will help teach parents, teachers, caregivers and therapists alike how to sensitively change the way in which their children eat for the better for their lives.

Dr. Kay A. Toomey, Pediatric Psychologist, SOS Approach

Finally, a brilliant book full of practical and commonsense information that will help parents and therapists build healthy and enjoyable mealtimes with their children and patients!

Shannon Goldwater, Founder Feeding Matters

Navigating how to help a family struggling with mealtimes and feeling the pressure to add nutritional foods to their anxious eater's diet can be overwhelming. Marsha provides foundational concepts and practical strategies that will assist in decreasing stress and bringing joy back to mealtimes!

BreAnne Robison, MS, OTR/L, Mealtime Connections

Anxious Eaters, Anxious Mealtimes is a must-read for every professional doing feeding therapy with children.

Katya Rowell, MD, coauthor, <u>Helping Your Child with Extreme Picky Eating:</u> *A Step-by-Step Guide for Overcoming Selective Eating, Food Aversion, and Feeding Disorders and Conquer Picky Eating for Teens*

Marsha Dunn Klein gets it. In this book she speaks directly to parents in their rightful roles as leaders of family mealtimes. She offers them practical and proven techniques that not only will help their anxious eaters expand their horizons, but does so in a way that nurtures family interaction and protects the child's lifelong relationship with food.

Jennifer Berry, MS. OT/L, Pediatric Occupational Therapist, Founder, Thrive with Spectrum Pediatrics

Marsha's approach to working with children who are extremely cautious and nervous around food is a master's class in responsive feeding. She helps to remind clinician and parent alike that at the center of therapy is celebrating a child for who the child is, not her feeding challenge. Marsha's approach teaches us how to take a step back from the pressure of quantity and the next bite and teaches us how to break the next bite down into smaller *asks* that everyone involved in the therapy session, therapist, parent, and child, can achieve and celebrate.

Mandy Guendelsberger Carlsen, OTR/L, Co-Founder Mealtime Connections

This book is a must have for all feeding therapists. Marsha provides guidance and well thought out strategies to traverse the slippery road of anxious eaters. I am a seasoned therapist but am always looking for new and better ways to help my clients which I have found in this book. I love Marsha's techniques of *rehearsals* and *stretching* to prepare a child and help them feel more comfortable. I have seen wonderful results with my anxious picky eaters by using these strategies.

Krisi Brackett, MS, SLP-CCC, UNC Hospital Pediatric Feeding Team

Marsha has done it again. This is a great resource for anyone dealing with pediatric feeding disorders. It reads like an ongoing conversation with a true feeding expert. Stressed little eaters now have a voice. Add this one to your library!

Cheri Fraker, CCC/SLP, Speech Language Pathologist, co-author,
<u>Food Chaining: The Proven 6-Step Plan to Stop Picky Eating,</u>
<u>Solve Feeding Problems and Expand Your Child's Diet</u>

Marsha Klein is a brilliant feeding therapist who has transformed the lives of many families in my own practice. Now she offers us a wonderful book that enables both parents and professionals to make use of her 50 years of experience. it is thorough, practical and readable, it should be on the shelf of every feeding professional as well as any parent who has a child with feeding problems.

Sanford C. Newmark MD, Osher Center for Integrative Medicine, author
<u>ADHD Without Drugs: A Guide to Natural Care of Children with ADHD</u>

I was delighted to read Marsha's book because it reflects experiences one encounters on the long road to feeding a child with feeding challenges. She understands that feeding is a dance. It is a relationship, a partnership based on trust. Marsha understands that any feeding relationship is based on the partnership of three groups of people - the expert on the child (parent), the child, and the expert on feeding techniques (feeding professional). Many people forget each group is an integral part of the team and must work together to help the child develop and thrive. Marsha gets it and this roadmap illustrates it. Her decades of experience and knowledge, guided by her love of children and the families who care for them is evident, and I cannot say enough good things about Marsha or this book. I can only hope that parents, who may have lost hope, or feeding professionals, who struggle with challenges posed by certain children, read this book and recommend others do the same. Like any expert, one needs tools, techniques, and encouragement, and this book provides them.

C's Mom

Marsha Dunn Klein has written a wonderfully detailed book with specific, creative and fun strategies to bring even the most worried eaters back to the family table. Marsha demonstrates compassion and concern for all family members and understands how to start from where the family and child are now. This book fills a much-needed gap in the literature well beyond the typical advice for managing picky eating behavior. A must-have on every pediatric dietitian resource list.

Melissa Davis, MS, RDN, Registered Dietitian

Marsha has a wealth of knowledge and experience with families and children who are anxious eaters. In this book, Marsha provides insight as well as practical strategies for these feeding challenges.

Catherine Riley MD, Developmental Pediatrician

I am thrilled to have this book to reference and to recommend! Marsha blends her years of therapeutic experience together with parent and child perspectives to help give insight into the complicated world of picky and anxious eaters. This book provides a road map for analyzing the relevant factors and helping the child learn to take baby steps toward finding fun and enjoyment in eating. Parents and therapists will find an abundance of practical tips paired with relatable examples and a sense of humor.

E. Rose Langston, MS, OTR/L, Pediatric Occupational Therapist, Pediatric Possibilities

I love this book! Marsha has healing words for parents and therapists of children who struggle with food or whose mealtimes have become fractured with anxiety, fear or stress. Instead of only theories and "don't dos," she gives practical words and strategies to help find a way forward for children and those who care for them, their eating and their futures. This will definitely go in my library for both parents who need hope and other therapists who want to provide rest and a direction to their patients and families.

Heidi Liefer Moreland, MS, CCC-SLP, Pediatric Speech pathologist, Clinical Coordinator at Thrive with Spectrum Pediatrics

Anxiety is a big concern in our modern world which is likely related to our current busy (on-the-go) lives. I was born into a farm family who toiled in the fields. Meals were important breaks for interaction, relaxation, and eating local foods without distractions. This is not the case today. In this book, Marsha helps parents and professionals understand how anxiety impacts eating and drinking habits and skills. She supports families and professionals (who work with them) move forward to create easy, heathy, and enjoyable mealtimes. Thank you, Marsha for all you have done over the years for all of us.

Diane Bahr, MS, CCC-SLP, Speech Language Pathologist, author <u>Nobody Ever Told Me (Or My Mother)That! Everything From Bottles and Breathing to Healthy Speech Development</u> and <u>How to Feed Your Baby and Toddler Right.</u>

The feeling we all want at mealtime is connection - with the food we love and the people we eat with. *Anxious Eaters* offers practical strategies and ideas that will reconnect you and your child at the table! It provides guidance and thought-provoking insights to consider when feeding children who are worried about eating. Overall, this book teaches compassion while empowering the reader to support anxious eaters, find mealtime peace, and help children reach positive food discoveries. Most importantly, it takes the blame off of children (and the adults who feed them) and gives your family a fresh start.

Dawn Winkelmann, M.S, CCC-SLP, speech language pathologist and pediatric feeding specialist, co-author of <u>Making Mealtime ezpz</u>.

I love this book! Such a multitude of wonderful ideas and thought-provoking questions to help therapists consider their practice and work with parents. I know all of these wonderful strategies will be used with the children in my therapy program!

Jenny McGlothlin, MS, CCC/SLP, CLC Feeding Therapist and Author of <u>Helping Your Child with Extreme Picky Eating</u> & <u>Conquer Picky Eating for Teens and Adults</u>

Acknowledgements

There are so many people who shared in this vision and helped this book become a reality.

First, I need to thank the children and families who have taught me about anxious eating. They are the teachers I celebrate every day!

There are so many people to thank. Several parents, in particular, helped in remarkable ways. Laura Wesp is mother of Teddy, a darling child who is learning to try new foods. She helped me realize this book needed to get into the hands of parents. She went above and beyond to personally take on the challenge of insuring that I get this book done! She painstakingly read and re-read versions to insure I sensitively included the parent voice. Her attention to detail is amazing and her empathy for other struggling parents is unending. Throughout this book, you will hear Laura's voice sharing her personal experiences on her journey.

Lauri Ziemba and her son, Brady were the initial inspiration for me to write this book. They told me this book **needed** to be written and challenged me to write it. Lauri offered her heartfelt thoughts about the deep and personal ways these issues affect families. She reminded me that sometimes parents just do not feel playful or optimistic or patient and this can be an overwhelming journey. And that parents need to feel supported (and not judged, no matter what)! Her eight-year-old son, Brady, wants to enjoy food. He wants to try new foods. But trying new foods and enjoying new foods are both still quite a challenge for him. He wanted to help, so he has made videos to share his experiences about new food trying with other kids. Brady's sister, Wednesday Aparisi, is the amazing artist who painted the grasshopper picture on the back cover and helped Brady make his Brady's Tasting Tips videos! https://www.youtube.com/watch?v=xWiP_MU7frk&feature=youtu.be

Parents Jake and Garrett Barnes for inspiration and input along my journey as a feeding therapist. Thanks to Kind Dad and Marta for their stories.

Shannon Goldwater took her triplets all around the country to find feeding support for them. Along the way, she founded the non-profit, Feeding Matters, to further advances in Pediatric Feeding Disorder by accelerating identification, igniting research and promoting collaborative care for children and families. She has always lovingly challenged therapists around her to be their best, to listen and to hear parents. Thank you, Shannon.

Suzanne Evans Morris, PhD wrote the foreword for which I am so grateful, but mostly, I have to thank her for the powerful influence she has been on my life. She helped inspire my love of feeding and I appreciate her mentorship as I entered this field many decades ago. I appreciate her as a colleague as I have gone on to find my own voice in this field, and I appreciate her friendship.

Karen Dilfer, OTR/L needs an award for the number of times she read and re-read drafts of this book. She gets the way I think about feeding and "Gets Permission!" I appreciate her compassion for families and her enthusiasm for sharing this information. BreAnne Robison, OTR/L also "Gets Permission" and shares a passion for feeding children. She read and re-read drafts and gave her loving feedback throughout. They both are helping me spread Get Permission thoughts about feeding.

Thank you to friends and colleagues in the feeding world who have taken the time to read various drafts and provide feedback along the way. Diane Bahr, Krisi Brackett, Jennifer Berry, Jo Cormack, Melissa Davis, Cheri Fraker, and Joni Kiser, Rose Langston, Anna M. Lutz, Jenny McGlothlin, Heidi Liefer Moreland, Sanford Newmark, Catherine Reilly, Erin Sundseth Ross, Katja Rowell, Kay Toomey, and Dawn Winkelmann.

I must thank my colleagues at Mealtime Connections, the pediatric feeding clinic in Tucson where I used to be a partner, before *semi-retirement*. Co-owners, Kim Edwards and Mandy Carlsen and the amazing team of therapists at Mealtime Connections shared my learning playground about children and families as the Get Permission Approach evolved into what it is today. Thank you for sharing the compassion and energy for helping our families

I thank Tom Spitz for the cover photography and his support of our vision. I thank Jenn Ferguson for the painstaking hours she spent with art and graphic design cheerfully meeting every unreasonable deadline. (And thank you Chris Stenberg for doing some of the original art.) My deepest appreciation and love to Don who has always believed in me! And my two sons, Jason and Brennan who taught me about feeding my own children.

About the Author

Marsha Dunn Klein OTR/L, MED, FAOTA is a pediatric occupational therapist with close to five decades of experience lovingly feeding children. She received her bachelor's degree in occupational therapy from Boston University, Sargent College in 1971 and then a Masters of Education degree in Special Education from the University of Arizona in 1975. She has been a clinician, author, and educator throughout her career. She has co-authored a number of books on feeding including <u>Pre-Feeding Skills, First and Second Editions</u>, <u>Mealtime Participation Guide</u> and <u>Homemade Blended Formula</u> with Suzanne Evans Morris and <u>Feeding and Nutrition for the Child with Special Needs</u> with Tracy Delaney. She is trained in neurodevelopmental therapy. She has been awarded Fellow of the American Occupational Therapy Association.

Marsha has a passion for feeding children and sharing knowledge. She presents locally, regionally, nationally and internationally and loves sharing her responsive and loving approach to pediatric feeding challenges in her Get Permission Approach to Pediatric Feeding Challenges course series. Marsha and her family love to travel and explore foods globally. She considers herself a food celebrator.

About the Foreword

Suzanne Evans Morris, PhD, CCC-SLP, and Marsha have collaborated about feeding for decades. She is a speech-language pathologist with New Visions. Suzanne is a pioneer in the treatment of feeding and pre-speech disorders. She has presented extensively both nationally and internationally sharing her feeding passion, knowledge and inspiration on the global stage. She has studied the Neurodevelopmental Treatment approach in England, Switzerland and the United States. Suzanne has published Pre-Feeding Skills, First and Second Editions, Mealtime Participation Guide and Homemade Blended Formula with Marsha as well as other extensive writings about pediatric feeding. She has spent a career inspiring multiple generations of young feeding therapists. We thank and celebrate her for her contributions to children, families, and the global pediatric therapy community!

Contents

Foreword

Marsha Dunn Klein and I share deep perspectives about infants and children who experience difficulties with feeding and mealtimes. At the core of these perspectives is the belief that one of the highest values of mealtimes is the enjoyment of food and the internal desire and regulation of eating and drinking. *Anxious Eaters – Anxious Mealtimes* addresses the dual perspective that when children feel anxious about aspects of food and eating, the entire mealtime can become a negative space of reverberating anxiety for everyone. As the mealtime anxiety of others increases, children become more worried and less comfortable with the meal. It becomes a reverberating cycle of negativity.

These children have always been a part of our Western culture of food and eating. At the same time the number of children whose anxiety contributes to their discomfort with eating and mealtimes appears to be increasing. Their underlying fear of new foods, unfamiliar presentation of familiar foods, or variations of any aspect of the mealtime results in a refusal to eat or in a highly structured ritual around eating and drinking. This severely limits their choice of foods and the situations in which they are comfortable eating. Many of these children have underlying physical, sensory or emotional roots that support the internal choices they have made to restrict their diet to foods that they believe are comfortable and acceptable to them.

Many children who are anxious eaters develop their deep-seated worry because they are not comfortable in their physical, mental and emotional bodies. Food and the act of eating are associated with physical, sensory or gastrointestinal discomfort. They may learn to associate the nausea, pain, sensory discomfort, lack of physical coordination or control with food and mealtimes. As they notice this connection, they often decide that specific foods or whole categories of food – or even all foods – are dangerous. They may stop eating, take in only enough food to reduce hunger, or discover a limited number of foods that feel safe and comfortable. Many of the symptoms of physical and emotional stress are very subtle or invisible to the adults who are feeding them. Their adults consider the child's unusual eating patterns through their own worry, pushing them to eat more, try the vegetables they have prepared, or eat a healthier diet.

Parents may not fully understand their child's current or remembered discomfort associated with food and eating. In addition, children have appetite levels that differ, based on genetic patterns. Some children have a very low appetite or interest in food based on their genetic makeup. Yet, many physicians and dietitians still push parents to increase the volume or caloric value of the foods they offer the child. Children's attempts to comply with the pressure of their adults often goes against the internal messages from their own body, telling them when to start or stop eating. The fear and anxiety of both the adult and child may increase. The resulting stress can increase the child's desire to erect protective barriers to feel safe and in control. It may increase the adult's tendency to push against these barriers and use direct or indirect pressure to get their child to eat in a different way.

The wisdom of earlier thinkers in our culture is always available to support the insights of our current writers and thinkers. In addition to specific physiological and environmental contributions to children's eating patterns, eating choices at different ages can be influenced by the historical and cultural patterns of humankind. A primary goal of our species is to perpetuate the genes of the current population. Historically, individuals who made choices based on the avoidance of potentially deadly negative consequences, survived. Those who were initially drawn toward a positive event, frequently died. For example, in Paleolithic cultures those adults who paid attention to the slight movement of the grass that suggested the presence of a tiger or venomous snake were more likely to survive than those who were attracted initially by a bush of delicious berries. Those who responded quickly to the negative event were more likely to pass on their genes to future generations. As a result, the brain developed with a strong negativity bias. We are hard wired for fear and caution in order to protect our species. The brain's negativity bias has been passed down through thousands of generations. It is present today for most people. We can receive dozens of positive comments about our work and a single negative comment. However, we tend to give intense attention to the negative feedback. This is what we remember. Our initial response to many unfamiliar or unexpected events often is a feeling of vulnerability and being threatened. Negative events have a stronger emotional response and are rapidly stored in memory. The psychologist, Rick Hanson PhD, has written extensively about the role of the negativity bias in our lives. He describes the brain as being "like Velcro for negative experiences and like Teflon for positive ones."[*] The underlying brain wiring, however, is different for different

---

[*] Hanson, Rick. (2013) *Hardwiring Happiness: The New Brain Science of Contentment, Calm, and Confidence.* Harmony Books (Random House), p.41

 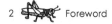

children and adults. Some people are more sensitive and respond to potentially negative events very intensely. Others have a tendency to initially perceive new situations with milder negativity and switch to a neutral or positive feeling relatively quickly.

In addition to a general negativity bias in life, a reluctant or negative bias toward new foods has been described in older toddlers and young children. A child during the Hunter-Gatherer period of history needed protection from aspects of curiosity that could be deadly. It is probable that, like today's young children, they were curious about new objects and put many things in their mouths. This potentially included new plants and brightly colored berries. This led toward poisoning and death for those who tried to mouth or eat these intriguing new foods. Some children in a tribe were more cautious than others. Their negativity bias may have been stronger. They were more reluctant, and watched adults more closely to find out what was safe. With the exposure of observing their parents and having small tastes, they gradually accepted the new food. These cautious children were more likely to survive into adulthood and pass on their cautious-genes to today's children. This period of food reluctance and refusal of new foods has been labeled "neophobia." It is seen a large number of young children as they expand their relationship with food.

A strong negativity bias describes most of our children who are anxious around food and mealtimes. Some research, however, has shown that this bias is diminished when the amount of positive information and interaction is at least five times greater than the negative information or experience.

Anxious Eaters, Anxious Mealtimes describes a highly successful approach to children who are worried and anxious about new foods and mealtime experiences. Marsha Dunn Klein understands these challenges and is able to take a compassionate and reflective position that supports both the child and parent. She knows that the most important elements are rooted in the feeding relationship that connects the therapist, child and parent in a trusting bond. This connection supports the release of fear and moves toward a positive relationship with food and mealtimes. She listens to the individual verbal and nonverbal feedback of children and their parents, and trusts that they are doing the very best that they know how. She understands the sensory nature of food and the sensorimotor skills that are needed to feel both comfortable and successful in taking tiny steps toward change in children's relationship with food. She recognizes that many children have difficulty changing their approach to eating by themselves because they don't know how to negotiate the sensory processing hurdles that they face. She knows that some of these challenges lie in current sensory processing dysfunction, while others exist primarily in the fear memory of the child or parent. Fear coexists with imagined danger, based on the negativity bias and early life experiences. It is just as powerful as the inner decision to avoid or reduce a current physical or sensory discomfort. In creating the appropriate balance between negative bias and positive associations, frequent positive experiences and successes tip the balance toward change. This is the underlying approach described in the book.

Anxious Eaters – Anxious Mealtimes offers many suggestions that help children develop a different relationship with food. These are based on tiny steps of change leading toward success. Marsha describes this as a process of tiptoeing through a variety of sensory progressions that blend subtly and smoothly into each other. Each sensory continuum is sequenced in a flow that has both a structural order and an intuitive application to the specific child and parent. This is a book that is both practical and philosophical. It addresses the questions and needs of both parents and professionals. Ultimately, it provides a successful pathway towards guiding the cautious, anxious child toward experiencing curiosity, discovery and joy in the process of eating and sharing mealtimes

Suzanne Evans Morris, PhD

Introduction

If you have picked up this book you probably know a child, or children who are anxious eaters. These children are *worried* about eating, pretty "picky" and eat a very narrow diet with very specific foods. They may only eat one brand of macaroni and cheese and may like their waffles round. They may like any food with a crunch, but no wet foods. Their preferred cheese is a particular string cheese, but only white, not yellow! They may like fast food nuggets from only one restaurant and they must be fresh and warm. They may drink milk, but only from their special cup and apple juice from the green box. Their yogurt may need to be one flavor, brand, color and must be eaten directly out of that container, not a bowl! They may have no vegetables or fruits in sight. Your attempts to introduce new foods, different foods, healthier foods, are met with resistance and maybe even tears. There is lots of worry about foods! Parents of these anxious eaters describe their children as **well beyond** typical *picky*.

Some children are anxious about ANY type of *change* at mealtimes. They might become upset when their mother cuts their familiar toast into a different shape. They may reject yogurt if it has been served in a bowl, and not out of the container. Other anxious eaters are really worried about new foods. Every anxious eater experiences their own specific kind of worry. While worry can be seen as the common thread, different children worry about different aspects of eating and mealtimes.

Many of you have already read everything you could find. You are looking for answers. Many of the popular books, parent blogs, and headlines tell you to just relax, to bring your child back to the table and just offer the food your family is eating. Just have that food around and he will eventually try it. Just relax and take away the pressure. And so many of you have tried all those things. You have tried serving family meals, invited your child to the table, had nice mealtime conversation. AND you tell us your child STILL does not try anything new. You tell us if you did not remind, cajole, coerce, bribe, threaten or force your child to eat, he would only eat his favorite crackers. And that it is BECAUSE you love your child and you worry about him that you remind, cajole, coerce, bribe, threaten, or force him to eat. You are told not to pressure! You tell us it is not fair for us to take away the only strategy you have without giving you a new plan, new ideas. Eliminating pressure and having positive mealtimes together are good ideas and an important starting point, but maybe YOUR child needs more. Maybe we need to look at the Big Picture differently for your child.

You may be a parent or you may be a professional. This book is written for both of you. I wanted parents and feeding therapists to have the same information. As feeding partners, we all need to be on the same page, with a philosophy that can help us get to the common goal of helping children who are struggling to eat. The challenge with inviting both parents and professionals to read this book is that it becomes an encyclopedia of ideas, too many for some and not enough for others. I have tried to share a variety of ideas along a continuum of varying degrees of mealtime worry. Some ideas work for some children and other ideas work for others. I hope readers pick and choose what works for them and the children they love.

The seeds for the foundation philosophy of this book are found in the books I have co-authored with Suzanne Evans Morris. Pre-feeding Skills, First and Second Editions, have been books that have influenced feeding therapists and teams for decades. They are based on the belief that feeding is a relationship based on trust, a mealtime dance of communication between the child and parent. I have further described these ideas in the Get Permission Approach courses that describes a sensitive, responsive dialogue between child and parent that helps us discover which foods your child LOVES? We look at how can we help children find enjoyment of their foods, confidence in their skills and internal motivation to eat enough to grow and thrive.

At the core of my beliefs about eating is that it is a relationship between parents and their children. Parents nurture both through the calories of food and also through the love with which they offer that nourishment. In a real way, mealtimes nourish both bodies and souls. This philosophy is reflected in the title of this book. When children are anxious eaters, mealtimes can lose their balance. We parents worry when our children are not able to eat the good foods we offer. In our worry, we try HARDER, and in their worry, they push back harder, hence "anxious mealtimes." Children eat three to five meals a day. That is twenty-one to thirty-five meals a week! That is a lot of opportunities to enjoy mealtimes together, or to be worried about meals together. Many parents tell us they do not enjoy meals, or no longer enjoy cooking. They are preparing more than one meal each night. The new foods they make with the hope of expanding their child's diet are often rejected. Food is wasted. The stress about the mealtime, the food and the interactions can lead to stress not only between the anxious eater and parents, but also between parents. Siblings also feel the constant anxiety of their parents and brothers and sisters.

In a career that is inching close to five decades, I have met parent after parent who is struggling with the worry, stress, guilt, anger and hopelessness of trying to feed their really anxious eater. I would like to acknowledge right from the start that I understand this is hard work. It is hard work for parents and hard work for children. My bottom line belief is that parents are doing the best they can *and* children are doing the best they can. Parents *want* to help their children eat and grow. I believe that generally children *want* to eat and when they do not, cannot, will not eat, it is our grownup job to try to understand why. What are they trying to communicate with us? What are they telling us about how they feel, how their body works, why they are not enjoying meals? Are we being responsive to their concerns? It is my hope that in this book I can provide some clues about how the mealtime ended up with this worry and what might be done to get back to mealtime peace.

One of the concerns I hear regularly from parents is that progress for these very worried eaters is so slow. "My child has been working on the same goal for a year and still has not added a new food!" We need to find ways that parents can see change and see that light at the end of the tunnel, or at least see the pathway to that tunnel! It is way too discouraging to have a goal of adding ten new foods to a diet and, a year later, the goal is the same. Something is **not** working. It is not working for parents and not working for children. Something must change. Hopefully this book offers ideas that can help with that change.

One of the themes of this book is finding ways to help your child get from **here to there** along a continuum of tiny, tiptoe steps. What is working and what is not working **now**? What would it take to find a comfortable, happy and peaceful **now**? We will always start at a familiar and safe starting point. From there, how can we guide your child through tiny, achievable steps toward the **there**, the goal? Those tiny steps are different for each and every child, for each and every family.

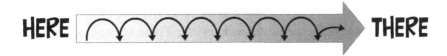

But as we think of **here to there** for children, we also will think about **here to there** for grownups. Grownups need little steps too. To get from a **now** of worry, struggle, and maybe even a mealtime battleground, to a mealtime without worry will require change. Einstein is widely credited with giving us the definition of insanity, though it could have been others. The concept is so meaningful, though, regardless of who actually was the author. The quote is that "the definition of insanity is doing the same thing over and over again but expecting different results." Yes! To get different results for your child *something* needs to change. For mealtimes to improve, for therapy to improve, we need to do something different, a different presentation, a different approach, a different offer, a different food, a different attitude, a different set of tiny steps. Something. We know we cannot continue to do the same thing we are doing and expect things to get better. Hopefully this book provides ideas for those tiny steps from **here to there** that help get those different results.

You will also notice throughout this book that I am always looking for hope, hope for children and hope for parents. When therapists or doctors say *Johnny does not do this*, and *cannot do that* and *will not do this*, parents can get very discouraged. I prefer what I call, the **YET terminology**. (How about, *Johnny is not* **yet** *able to chew hard foods*, or *Johnny does not* **yet** *enjoy that texture?* **Yet** gives hope. It reminds us that Johnny is on a continuum of tiny steps from **here to there**. He is not **yet** there but is on the way. We all need hope! I have been describing this concept to therapists for years in my courses as a way of writing hopeful evaluations without all those negatives about all the things children **cannot** do. I am thrilled the educational research and writings of Carol Dweck, PhD has made these concepts mainstream from her book, <u>Mindset, the New Psychology of Success</u>[1] and her "Power of Yet," Ted Talk ™.[2] What she calls the "growth mindset" truly works well with my approach to new food trying and anxious eaters.

We will come back to four principles throughout this book. 1.) We will look together at how to help families get to a starting place of **mealtime peace** from the often stressful and worried place of NOW. Once parents and children trust mealtime will again be inviting, less pressured and more peaceful, we will want to help children learn to experience change in their mealtimes without tipping them over into their worried place. 2.) We will teach them **change happens** and it's okay. 3.) On these important foundations of mealtime peace and change happens, we can help children learn comfortable strategies for **new food trying**. These strategies can be learned away from the peaceful mealtime and brought back to the mealtime once they are comfortable and established. 4.) And finally, every invitation to the table, every change that happens, every new food trying strategy will all be offered and supported **at each child's pace requiring both parent and child success**.

Throughout the book I will share my ideas through examples and stories both from my experiences and also from families who live this. Families and children have always been our best teachers if we take the time to really listen. Some amazing parents have taken the time to share their insights from their long anxious eater journey with us. You will see from the experiences shared in the book that I value parent feedback. I believe parents are the center of their child's feeding team. Feeding therapists have ideas from their years of experience, but parents know their child and MUST be heard. It is sad for me when I meet a family who has lost their parent instinct when a well-meaning feeding team has pressured them to go in directions that just did not fit their child, their family or their parent instinct. There will be lots of ways to get from **here to there**, but first we need to find ways for each child and each family to feel celebrated!

I have written this book as a conversation accessible to parents and professionals. Anxious eaters are boys and anxious eaters are girls. They are infants, toddlers and older children. (They are adults too). The focus of this book is on children, though many of the basic ideas will work well with adults. Instead of referring to all these children as *they* or *them* or *the child*, I have alternated *he* and *she* throughout. Because I am speaking to both parents and professionals, I will describe the children in this book as *your child*. *Your child* fits for each parent reading it and can also fit for the therapist thinking about the child on their caseload. Your child. I will also refer to feeders as *parents*. By *parents* I mean anyone feeding or eating with that child. *Parents* can be caregivers, and grandparents, babysitters, or the feeding therapists and team members. It is the person who is trying to help your child enjoy food.

Of course, the ideas shared within this book are just ideas. They are not meant to be given as medical advice and **must** be adapted for each child and each family. There can be underlying factors contributing to a child's reluctance to eat. It goes without saying that those need to be explored with appropriate medical and professional alongside any ideas shared in this book

Many of you have heard of the Grasshopper Story. In fact, I have been called that Grasshopper Therapist. ☺ The book is guided by the Grasshopper Story which you will read early on in the book. This story is based on an experience my family had trying grasshoppers in Mexico. The experience gave me some powerful insight on the plight of worried eaters. I will encourage you to think of new foods as *grasshoppers* to help in your **here to there** thinking about your child's eating worries. Think of what support you might need to have to try to eat grasshoppers and you will already have a framework for offering new foods to the worried eaters you know.

I encourage you to read through the whole book. It offers hope and suggestions that you and your team can use to surround these children with love and guide them into new mealtime skills. The ideas will need to be individualized for each child. No suggestion fits everyone. Some are great ideas but need to be adapted and others will just not work for the specific child you have in mind. But, read on. I want to help you find perspective on these issues of mealtime. I want to help you consider the mealtime challenges within the big picture of your whole child. I want to help you get back to celebrating your child every day and every meal for all that he is beyond these eating challenges. I want to help you find hope.

Let's begin,
Marsha

Dear Parent,

You have picked up this book because you have concerns about the anxious eater you love, your child who eats a narrow diet, wants the same foods, the same brands, the same presentation and maybe even the same cups or plates! Your child who does not want foods to touch, who cannot eat his fish crackers broken, or who does not have a fruit or vegetable in sight. Your child who may not even be able to eat at the same table as the family! You are probably struggling to figure out how to help your child eat a more nutritious diet and how you can help him or her learn to try new foods without tears and anger. You are likely worn out and have so many questions. I am glad you found this book because there is lots of information and understanding here. I know this is hard.

I knew **both** parents and feeding therapists would read this book. The challenge for me was that parents have told me they are desperate for information about their child, their situation, their mealtimes. Feeding therapists have told me that want information that is broader that can work for lots of children they know with a great array of different challenges. I know these anxious eaters to have themes that are similar while at the same time each child is so very unique in their sensitivities about foods and mealtimes. In other words, there will end up being way more information presented here than you may need for *your* child. I have tried to offer both in-depth information while also providing summaries and *Dear Parent* letters and questions to help you focus on the Big Picture information on your child.

Throughout this book, I want to suggest some new ways of approaching mealtimes and new food trying so that you might try some different strategies. I cannot ask you to try harder, because you already are trying so hard. But I might suggest you try *differently*. You are likely feeling exhaustion, discouragement, burn out, but the tips I am suggesting in the following pages and chapters will hopefully bring more peaceful mealtimes and more insight into the journey.

I recommend you read the book as an overview of ideas and pick the ones that work for you. I will not tell you the exact way to get from where you are to where you want to be because I do not know *your* child. But I will give you the framework to get there. I will provide lots of examples, so many of which will ring very true to you. You will probably identify with many of the stories and examples I share.

I do also recommend you work with a feeding team that can evaluate your child. I will describe the complicated process of eating and all the multitude of influences on eating. The feeding team can help you look at factors for your child that influence on his (or her) eating worry. I cannot make specific medical recommendations for your child. I do not know your child. This book is intended to give general ideas and recommendations, not take the place of the medical evaluation and support your child might need. Since this is a hard road, a slow process, I wish for you to have help beyond this book. I wish for you to have support from professionals who understand your child specifically and your journey. Your child will make the most progress, I believe, when you and your team work together, when you are on the same page of understanding your child. I hope this book helps you get to that same page.

Yes, this is a slow journey and is a hard one for parents and children. But I am hoping to offer hope of change in little tiny succeed-able steps through practical helpful tips to start improving your family mealtimes. Hope. Instead of saying "your child only eats six foods," I will be more likely to say, "your child enjoys six foods and does not **YET** like seven." We are going to look at the **YET** of your child's eating and try to figure out together how to get to hope.

I believe children who are very anxious about eating are doing the best they can, given their wiring and their experiences. I believe you have been doing the best you can to try to help your child. It is my hope to dissipate the anger and frustration, the pressure and worry and to provide some positive strategies that give your child the opportunity to develop the curiosity and motivation to explore more foods and improve the narrow diet. I also believe your child would try all those new foods if he/she could, but the worry about change is so great that he can't. Your child may have created a world where he just cannot allow change in his diet. Change may be the enemy of his mealtime. Let us look at change through a different lens.

Shall we start our journey?
Marsha

Dear Feeding Professional,

You have picked up this book because you know anxious eaters, too. The challenges these children have are big and affect every member of the family. When children do not eat, parents struggle to feed them. When children are anxious, worried eaters, mealtimes become stressed. It is my hope that we, the professionals families come to for help, can find ways to lovingly support both children and parents find calm, find progress and reasons to celebrate.

Parents want help. As I wrote this book I knew both parents and professionals would find it. I offer lots of information and at the risk that it could be overwhelming for some families. But, I believe information is important. I have tried to address a variety of situations and theories but also address parents directly with questions and summaries throughout in Dear Parent boxes. These may also be helpful questions for you to consider as you get to know families.

I encourage parents to read this book as compliment to what is happening in feeding therapy. So many parents tell me this is an overwhelming and slow journey and they WANT HELP. We can help them together. This book is absolutely not intended to replace feeding therapy and medical team evaluation. I believe children eat when they can, when it feels good, so when children do not eat, we must try to figure out why. Since feeding is so complicated, it often takes a whole team to figure things out. But we can never lose sight of the fact that the parent is at the center of that team. THEY know their child. THEY know their family. THEY know what is possible and what is not in THEIR home. We must listen!

I believe in my heart that parents and children are doing the best they can, given their experiences and wiring. I hope you believe that too. As eight-year-old Brady tells us, *it is okay, go slow, help them*. He was addressing parents in relation to their children but he couldn't he just as easily be addressing us in relation to families? Best wishes as you read on. Hopefully you will find some new ideas to compliment your feeding therapy strategies.

Best,
Marsha

Dear Parent,

By the very fact that you're holding this book, we have much in common. We are traveling together on this journey of feeding with all of its ups and downs.

Marsha has given me the privilege of sharing some of our successes throughout this book, and I am so grateful for the opportunity to pass along any tidbits that could possibly help another sweet child. Sharing them has been a joy. But, as you read these stories, insights, and suggestions, please hold them in perspective. They are the happy victories along a challenging and often discouraging road. For every success there are also moments of utter discouragement. I have become quite familiar with the floor of my closet. The last thing I would want to do is overwhelm you with ideas or project the impression that every day is smooth sailing in our home. There are definitely valleys when I question why I'm pouring in the effort. And yet, there are the small victories that offer glimmers that progress is indeed real! We spend most of our time in the in between, just living out our lives day-by-day, one meal or snack at a time. We are not making big steps forward, but just continuing to build positive associations with food little by little — a strawberry here or a bread stick there. If I could encourage you in any way, I would gently suggest that you go at your own pace. Listen to your child. Trust your Momma heart (or Dad heart as the case may be!) When you take care of yourself, you will have something joyful to spill over onto your family.

There may be days when all you can muster is a fast food drive through. Embrace it! Be thankful for those nuggets. They may provide just the respite you need to carry on and be more creative tomorrow. Accept that this is a marathon. As those victories come — and they surely will — hold onto them. Cherish them. Write them down or post them on Instagram. They will be sources of encouragement.

I've had a lot of practice and have been so very fortunate to have had amazing guidance and advice throughout my parenting journey. In some way or another, I've had a professional assist me with feeding my children for nearly fifteen years, whether it's a dietitian to help expand food choices or a gastroenterologist to assist with medical management of a chronic illness.

I am indebted to Marsha for helping me re-find my voice as a Mom. Our son had serious medical issues as a result of a GI motility disorder. A wonderful team of gastroenterologists, dietitians, and therapists cared for him and I followed their advice to a "T" just hoping to make my baby better and well. I trusted them completely. But, somewhere along the away, I stopped following my intuition hoping against hope that they had the magic solution to make him well. Marsha helped me wake up to the fact that I am his Momma and that I know him best. I may not be a feeding expert, but I am certainly an expert in my child. Once I started trusting my instincts and following a path that felt happy and joyful to me, the feeding journey became easier. His medical complications have not resolved, and nor has his progress been quick. But the journey has certainly been a lot more pleasant for everyone. We found an approach that was sustainable and for that I am incredibly thankful to Marsha.

Marsha has supported me and offered hope and direction throughout our journey. I love that she is doing the same for you in the pages of this book. It has long been my heart to expand access to the techniques and strategies of the best therapists. Not every family lives near or has time to pursue weekly feeding therapy. How wonderful that Marsha has shared both the practical strategies she's used in her career and the guiding principles upon which they are based. Her ideas can be transformative, and yet they are not out of reach of a loving caregiver. We can all establish mealtime peace and tip toe toward change. When Marsha started talking to me about those concepts, they sounded so appealing, but I couldn't see the end goal. It was hard to imagine that those itty-bitty baby steps could really add up. But they do!

Very sincerely,
Laura Wesp

Dear Feeding Team Professional,

I'm not sure there are words great enough to express the vital role you play in the success (or failure) of feeding therapy. I am a mother of triplets who all relied on feeding tubes for over a decade to survive. During the first three years of their lives, our family spent over a year living in and out of various feeding programs across the United States. We were desperate for help and solutions that would work for our family. In addition, my children also had outpatient therapy services five days a week for the first five years of their lives. Along the way, I have learned a tremendous amount about myself, my children, and the incredible therapists who have been instrumental (and not so instrumental) to our children's success.

As a direct result of my children's own suffering, I found my own passion by founding the non-profit organization Feeding Matters. Our mission is furthering advances in Pediatric Feeding Disorder ("PFD") by accelerating identification, igniting research, and promoting collaborative care for children and families. I believe one of the most powerful ways we can work toward meeting our mission is by empowering parents and professionals who are dedicated to helping every child meet their maximum feeding potential. What a better way to learn than to consider what others before us have learned along the way (and many times the hard way)!

From a parent please consider:

Parents voices must MATTER above all else. Ultimately you are treating the family and not just the patient, because it is the family that is responsible for carrying out the treatment you suggest. Doctors and therapists always listen, but does what we say actually MATTER? A family's voice and intuition must not be ignored even if does not make sense or does not seem plausible to you. What works for one child may not work for another, which is why every family and child is unique. No one understands more than a parent what their child is experiencing.

Help parents identify exactly what about feeding their child is their greatest challenge. Do they dread something? For example, for me that was having one or more of my children cough, choke, gag, vomit, or retch every time they came to the kitchen table (even if they were going to be tube fed and not asked to try any food). When therapists initially asked me what I wanted to work on most, I would immediately say to get them off the tube. Since that scenario is very different for each child, perhaps a better question would have been: I'd like you to think about your daily routine with your child and identify one thing that, if improved, would greatly improve your day? Focusing on whatever that is for each family is the ONLY place to start!

Don't let your knowledge and training undermine the power of common sense. Looking back, I cannot believe how often common sense is thrown out the window. For example, what makes anyone think that a child would ever be internally motivated to eat if every time they did it made them feel sick, choke, gag, or vomit? Would any human being be motivated to do something that made them feel sick, caused discomfort, and/or made them anxious? Probably not, and in most instances, we might start to develop strong behaviors to avoid that experience. Common sense tells us we should identify and start with something that the patient enjoys and the family agrees might work -- and build on that! Often times parents need help understanding and remembering this.

Understand that you likely won't have all the solutions or answers to every family's needs, and that's OK. Parents value and appreciate knowing that they are not alone. They often feel like a failure and want you to "fix their child." I believe therapists have the best of intentions, but if you push a child beyond his or her skill limit or ask parents to do unrealistic things, you are setting everyone up for failure. What is realistic to you might not be realistic for the family. When you don't know the answer, the most reassuring response is "I don't know, but I will work with you and your other providers to find a solution."

Remember that feeding a child is not something parents ever get to take a break from, because children have to be nourished several times a day every day of their life, no-matter-what. This is why it is so important for parents to enjoy feeding their child. Families are often under a tremendous amount of pressure and feeding their child can consume them. Remind them that they are extraordinary, they are not alone, and this is not their fault!!

Best,
Shannon Goldwater,
www.feedingmatters.org

Who are Anxious Eaters?

"Picky, to me, implies choice and some of these
kids just don't have any options."
Lauri Ziemba

~ David (three-year-old) eats seven foods including round waffles (a particular brand), yogurt (if it is vanilla, and a particular brand), chicken nuggets (fresh from a particular fast food chain), apple juice (from a certain green box).

~ Mariah (five-year-old) eats six to eight containers of yogurt (must be pink and Mom must feed her). She drinks whole milk (from a certain cup) and apple juice (a particular brand).

~ Rod (two-year-old) used to eat most baby food presented and lately has dropped all but the fruit groups and wants them only in pureed form (from certain colored pouches, just from Mom only).

~ Juaquin (six-year-old) eats pizza, (only cheese pizza from a particular restaurant), and most any kind of cracker, (blue) sport drink and water, and most anything (presented between flour tortillas in a quesadilla form).

~ Henri (five-year-old) eats (plain) spaghetti, apples, (if they are peeled and quartered), most crackers, (two) breakfast cereals, (two kinds of) grated cheese, nuggets (fast food as well as dinosaur shaped) and peanut butter sandwiches on a (certain bread), with a (certain) peanut butter, (crusts off) and then cut in triangles, (NOT squares).

~ Tiffany eats (two kinds of) cereal, (a particular kind of) macaroni and cheese (one brand and one shape), many crackers, cookies and chips, and a (particular toddler) spaghetti dinner (in the container, room temperature), whole milk, and any kind of homemade pancakes.

~ Justin (four-year-old) eats corn dogs, hot dogs, chicken nuggets and drinks (one particular) juice in the box and little (round) crackers with peanut butter.

~ Benji (ten-year-old) eats a particular variety of foods, but is unable to eat mixed textures, eats no unfamiliar foods, and refuses most vegetables.

~ Willard (fourteen-year-old) eats separately from his friends at school because he does not like to see them talking with food in their mouth. The chaos of the school cafeteria is too much. He eats alone and eats his same few foods.

The List

Do any of these descriptions sound familiar? To understand the complexity of these mealtime challenges and how children got there, we need more details. We can start by looking together at your child's food list. As parents of a very picky, worried eater you *know* about **THE LIST**, right? These are that narrow list of foods your child will actually eat on a regular basis, the foods you can count on them eating. The foods they exist on! Let us look at this *List*.

What are your child's **favored** foods, usual foods, preferred foods? These are the foods your child eats every day, or most meals. These are the foods you buy in bulk and stress about if you run out. These are the foods your child eats to energize his day, every day! (We used to call these "safe" foods but are trying to be more sensitive about the words we use. If only some foods are *"safe,"* does that mean all the others are not *safe*? With the layers of issues in eating for these children, we do best to avoid words that further add to the worry).

What are the **sometimes** foods? You know these foods. They may be eaten now and then. But you cannot count on your child to *always* eat them when offered. Frustratingly, you can never quite figure out when or why you might get a *yes* or a *no*.

Next, what about the **used to** foods? These are foods that *used to be* on your child's *List* but that your child no longer eats. These foods may have been enjoyed when your child was younger but are absolutely off the *List* now! Or they may be foods she ate last week, but now are pushed away. (It is helpful to think about these foods, because sometimes they are a good starting point in finding foods to add back on their *List*). And then, we ask about **goal** foods, what foods would you like your child to be able to eat?

The Food *List*

Favored Foods
Sometimes Foods
Used to Foods
Goal Foods

In this book, we are going to call your child's specific foods, their *List*. Their personal, very important, unique-to-them, *List*. These *List* foods help us look together at your child's diet and mealtime worries and help us in find hints about how to help. A most important part of this *List* is to understand the *qualifiers*. Let us look at them.

When describing your child's *List* foods, try it in this specific way. Consider if someone else were to babysit for your child and offer a meal, what would they need to know about the particular food on the favored *List* in order for your child to be willing or interested in eating it? You cannot usually just say *yogurt*, right? If you say *my child eats yogurt*, they would need to know the details, the qualifiers. Qualifiers include the specific information that they would need to know about that food to serve it? Does your child need that food presented in a certain way? Certain bowl, shape, temperature, brand, color, flavor, texture or presentation? What are the important specifics, the qualifiers, that would make the meal successful, comfortable, happy? We then might write down the *List* something like this:

Sam's Food *List*

Yogurt (certain brand, whipped, vanilla flavor with Sam opening it himself.)

Pizza (Cheese pizza from a particular restaurant cooled almost to room temperature).

Milk (whole milk in the blue cup).

Water (bottled water, room temperature opened in front of Sam)

Waffles (round, one brand, not too cooked, butter only)

Eggs (scrambled dry, salt but no pepper, no brown flecks)

Cheese (mozzarella white cheese sticks, opened but plastic still on, not orange or multicolored cheese sticks)

Crackers (four specific brands, not broken)

Cereals (one brand, dry, in the Truck bowl, with no milk)

Chips (one brand of Nacho Chips)

Sam's diet

Let's look at Sam's diet and see what we know. His diet is narrow. No fruits, no vegetables, no meats. There is not much color change except for the pizza, most other foods are a brown or white variation. We know Sam can chew as he can manage nacho chips, pizza, and dry cracker and cereal. He may well need some help with refined chewing. We do not know that yet because his *List* is small and he is not choosing foods requiring more complicated grinding like meats and apples or hard carrots, but he certainly has some basic skills. Within the skills Sam does have, he COULD eat other foods that require only those skills.

If Sam likes yogurt, he does have the skills to eat other yogurts or smooth food but doesn't. He has the skills to eat a cereal, so he has the skills to eat other cereals, but doesn't. He has the skills to eat waffles, but why only one shape and brand? And what is that truck bowl or blue cup all about? It is not that he only eats one texture food because he *can* eat wet yogurt from a spoon as well as finger food chips, cereal and pizza. He has an appetite for these foods. He likes these foods. And when he eats these foods he is not picky and has a good appetite for them. He is only picky when ANYTHING ELSE AT ALL IS OFFERED. The biggest challenge for Sam seems to be that he MUST have his food the SAME. *Give me THESE foods and I am fine.* **Change my foods and I become UPSET. Change is very, very hard for me!**

Parentheses diet

When the diet can be described as a *List* of specific foods with parentheses qualifiers after each, we affectionately call this *List* the **parenthesis diet**. The parentheses are for the qualifiers. The qualifiers are important and can make all the difference in whether or not the food is enjoyed or tried at all! These qualifiers reflect the need for **same**. *THIS IS WHAT I LIKE. THESE ARE THE FOODS I CAN EAT. <u>DO NOT CHANGE THEM!</u>*

The choices these children make seem to have a personal logic to them. They may make no logical sense to others. Why can you ONLY drink milk from *that* cup? Why does it have to be *that* brand? What difference does it make that the waffle is ROUND? Why only THIS brand of Mac and Cheese? Don't they all taste the same? Though the reasons may not be clear to us, your child is very clear about his **same**, right? And the qualifier is very, very, VERY important. Parent tell us they want to get this right but feel like they are walking on eggshells! If they unintentionally get it wrong, it can ruin the meal. You know. You have probably been there. Children with this level of qualifiers can become highly stressed, worried, anxious, with ANY presentation of food that is different from their image of *their* food. The parentheses suggest that the **need for same and the worry about change is the top issue** keeping the diet restricted.

The Parentheses Diet

Ex. Food (   )

Food (   )

Food (   )

Food (   )

Food (   )

Food (   )

Food (   )

Food (   )

Food (   )

Food (   )

Every child and every diet is different and unique to your child and your family. *Lists* are different in number and degree of qualifiers and parentheses vary. Some children qualify every single food in the most rigid way. Others have qualifiers in some foods but do allow for some variation in others. Some food *Lists* are very short with one or two or even six foods and others eat more. However, there are certain trends and characteristic threads we see as we specifically look at these *parentheses diets*. Some common characteristics include:

Limited number of foods

A characteristic of these parentheses diets is a limited number of **favored foods** and a tendency toward a narrowing of the diet. The **used to foods** *List* can be quite long. Some parents say their child was worried right from the start and had a tough time transitioning from breast feeding to anything else. Others describe a one or two-year-old that seemed to be progressing naturally with age appropriate foods, only to start seriously eliminating foods and food groups as a toddler. Others describe the hyper-vigilance with any introduction of new food sensations, textures, colors, brands and flavors. *The List*, for their child is short and specific. And still others regularly just plain stop eating a food they have eaten for a long time! It is no longer on their *List*.

Elimination of complete food groups

Many children never added fruits or vegetables to their diet or promptly eliminated them as worry over change in their diet began. Some only have milk and yogurt or a specialized formula. Others have one meat and it is a fast food, processed variety (from one particular restaurant). When entire food group elimination occurs, parents understandably have increased concern about nutrition!

Color similarities

Some parents describe their child's preferred *List* of foods as the brown, beige, yellow/white diet with predominately foods such as cereals, crackers, waffles, pancakes, chicken nuggets, and white yogurt and milk. Maybe a specific brand of macaroni and cheese. There are often no colorful fruit or vegetable rainbows, often no reds, blues and greens.

Flavor similarities

Children can become very specific about flavors, wanting only one flavor (and one brand) of apple juice, or one flavor of yogurt. One parent described trying to expand her shopping possibilities by dumping out a whole box of a favored "O" cereal and substituting the generic brand of "O" cereal only to have the box completely rejected (thrown) as not *their* food. Some parents tell us their complete frustration when a brand unexpectedly changes their recipe and the child *knows* and rejects it! Parents wonder how did they *know?* The child's highly sophisticated senses of smell and taste can identify the slightest flavor change. This often leads to brand specificity. As one parent recently described, her child was brand *loyal*. Maybe we could go so far as to say brand *dependent*.

Texture similarities

Many children want one texture, such as smooth puree only or crunchy only. Others only drink their nutrition (one flavor and from a can). One child only ate baby food, baby food apricots, 36 jars a day! Another would eat *any* food at all (if it was fed to him in a puree form). Others seem to eat almost any snack food, cookie, cereal or cracker, (as long as it crunches).

For children who do not like change, familiarity and consistency of food texture is important so they know just what to expect. A box of macaroni and cheese has no surprises. It usually feels (and chews) predictably each time it is served. There are no random vegetable lumps or parsley flecks or seeds to surprise their tongue. A specific brand of frozen waffles can be counted on to feel similar and familiar as it is being chewed. (Contrast these textures with the mixed textures and sensory surprises of Grandma's casserole or a salad!)

And texture matters with touching food too. Many children are very sensitive to touching different foods with their hands. They pull away and want others to do all the food touching. The touch sensitivity matters! Would you **eat** a food that you couldn't, wouldn't even touch?

Presentation specificity

Presentation matters for many of these children. It may matter who feeds them! Feeders can become all mixed up in the ritual and routine of the presentation. Feeders often must not change. Or it matters that Mom feeds them one way and Dad feeds the another. It may matter what cup that favored juice is in. It may matter what shape the food is presented in. (That sandwich must be cut in triangles!) It may matter that the pasta be plain and not touch nearby foods. It may matter that there be no visible little brown flecks in the waffle. It may matter that the macaroni be spiral and not elbow. The look and the presentation matter. They can really, *really* matter!

Mouth skills may matter, or not

Parentheses diets can give us clues about the oral motor skills of the child. For some children one of the factors in the narrow diet may be inexperience with more complicated food textures, so a child may prefer liquids or smooth purees. Perhaps they never progressed to more complicated chewing because they never allowed change from liquid. But now they only know liquid and have liquid drinking skills but no experience at all with chewable textures. Others can navigate any crunchy texture if the cracker or cookie or puff snack is melt-able, dissolvable with saliva and easily chewed. This is beginning chewing and does not require a more complex rotary, grinding kind of chew pattern. This may have been the limiting factor in early diet narrowing but may end up as inexperience with more difficult textures. But remember that within the textures the child does have, these children narrow their changes even when they do have the developmental or motor mouth skills to eat variation.

The strong need for *no change* may influence the child's texture preferences as development of more mature feeding skills requires food experiences to stimulate that growth. However, we have a group of children who do drink liquids, who do chew crunchy foods, who do eat (red) apples, and chicken nuggets and one brand of vanilla yogurt. In other words, they do have a variety of eating skills. They can drink liquids. They can eat puree. They can eat crunchy. They can eat ground meat. They can eat a specific apple. They have the oral skills to eat this variety, but they still have a narrow diet. They have basic skills. Like Sam, with the skills they do have they would be able to eat many different foods, more and different liquids, more purees, more ground meats and easy to chew waffles and pancakes and other fruits and vegetables. But they don't, won't eat other foods. In this situation, the oral skills may not be age appropriate due to inexperience, but with the skills the child already has the diet should be greater. And it is *not*, and that seems to be due to the worry about **change**. In this case the oral skills may not be the immediate limiting factor. Yes, they probably could use work, but our support may need to focus on helping them with **change** first.

Beware of surprises

It is clear that worry about change is a factor in eating for so many of these children. However, well-meaning grownups, family and therapists, may also have unintentionally contributed to the cycle of worry and distrust of new foods. Children remember that time when we snuck in a new ingredient in those homemade waffles or told them it was the same yogurt (but it was not). They remember when the peanut butter sandwich was a surprise new peanut butter. Those *sensory surprises* leave an impression. Though we may have offered change with good intentions to try to expand their diet, we may have created even less trust about change and increased worry that there will be a surprise on every plate, a surprise in every cup! This can just increase the visual vigilance or the detective-like analysis of food smells and flavors. This vigilance is their defense against change!

What is in a name?

These days there are lots of names and descriptors for these eaters. They have been called picky eaters, selective eaters, *highly* selective eaters, *extremely* picky eaters, behavioral eaters, food averse eaters, sensory eaters, avoidant eaters, restrictive eaters, chronic food refusers, food neophobic eaters, dysphagics, choosy of fussy eaters, problem feeders, pediatric feeding disorder, really, really choosy eaters! And the list goes on. Medical professionals supporting these children and their families have not been able to fully agree on a particular term yet. Therefore, many are used. I am always looking for the words not that *label* but ones that *describe* and give us an idea about how to help.

Think about the word *picky*. Does the word *picky* help us know how to help? Well, that depends. Is the child a little picky or a lot picky? Is the child two and possibly under the influence of toddler independence streak, or eight and picky about eating a worrisome few foods? *Picky* is a label commonly used in research, in parent magazines and at feeding clinics. And it is a common descriptor heard in conversations that parents of toddlers casually have together. But it means different things to different people. There are so many different definitions out there.

Is *picky* the toddler who is on a cereal jag and who has decided green, as in vegetables, is bad but then gradually does outgrow it? Or is *picky* the five-year-old who eats six containers of yogurt daily (must be pink and Mom must feed her). She drinks whole milk (from a certain cup) and apple juice (a particular brand). Is *picky* the four-year-old who screams, and cries real tears, if he is offered *anything* but the one familiar brand macaroni and cheese he knows? Is *picky* the eight-year-old who has seven very particular foods who cannot eat at the school cafeteria, restaurants or out with friends?

Picky, choosy or selective is what they *are*, but so are so many typically developing toddlers. There seems to be a continuum of *picky* from typically pickiness of toddlerhood to the REAL DAILY LIFE ALTERING **PICKY** of some of the children we know. So many parents will tell us, their child's eating is WELL BEYOND just *picky*. Some parents describe feeling insulted or frustrated when the term *picky* is used, as they describe feeling like their child's issues are minimized, and their efforts to help are misunderstood. The immenseness of their child's feeding challenges can feel dismissed.

 Picky, to me, implies choice and some of these kids just don't have any options. They aren't choosing to drive us crazy! They are struggling to feel safe with food. The pressure they feel is real. ~Lauri Ziemba

You will see the concept of continuum described throughout this book in a variety of different ways. A continuum is, according to the Oxford Dictionary[3] *a continuous sequence in which adjacent elements are **not perceptibly different** from each other, although the extremes are quite distinct.* So many of these terms and labels seem to be a continuum from milder to more complicated, from a developmental stage to a lifetime pattern, from an inconvenience to a serious worry. At what point does mild *picky* becomes seriously *picky*? For me, the term *picky* describes so many very different children and the term does not give me enough information to help. For example:

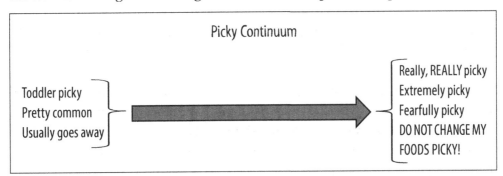

Picky Continuum

Toddler picky
Pretty common
Usually goes away

Really, REALLY picky
Extremely picky
Fearfully picky
DO NOT CHANGE MY FOODS PICKY!

There are lots of levels of *picky* along the way and we do not and cannot support them all in exactly the same way. The word *picky* does not inherently tell us how to help. There are common themes, which we will discuss, but it is my experience that some seriously *picky*, extremely *picky* children need extra special help.

A similar continuum of milder to complicated can be used to describe the variations of selective. Selective about a few foods? Or selective, really selective about many foods? Fussy eater is a term that has been used, but parents who know these eaters often laugh at that term. *Fussy? Choosy, Really?? If fussy was all it was, I would not be running to the doctor, I would not be worried. I would not be stressed at mealtimes! Our family would be able to eat out!* Parents of these eaters tell us *fussy* is NOT what *they* are talking about. Some parents of extremely *picky* eaters will tell us they do not even believe *fussy* is a whole continuum but refers only to the mild end of the continuum. And does the term *fussy* inform us how to help them? I do not think so. If picky, selective, fussy or choosy are not the perfect descriptors, what else is out there?

The term *sensory feeder* is often used and can fit (with qualifiers). However, it implies the main problem is a sensory problem, but that often does not describe the whole picture. *Sensory* is often part of the problem for these eaters, certain sensory properties, looks, smells, flavors or textures many define the sameness, but may not describe the contributing level of fear and worry about *change. Any* change. A child may prefer a smooth yogurt because it is easy to chew and swallow, but when that same child requires that the smooth yogurt be pink, (one brand AND FED TO HIM BY MOM) and absolutely falls apart with the introduction of a different flavor or different feeder, then we are looking at a bigger degree of challenge. This now goes beyond texture challenge. The parentheses can inform that level of complexity. It can help us understand that it is not just *sensory*. There is more. And I would consider that more to be the level of worry about **change**. By only supporting these children with sensory treatment, we can get stuck and they can get stuck.

Behavioral feeder may be accurate in that the child is not behaving in the way adults would prefer or expect, but many parents tell us the term makes them feel like their child is doing something wrong, being bad, or misbehaving. Could it be that the behaviors are your child's reaction to what you are asking of them? Becky Baily, PhD and author of Conscious Discipline tells us "misbehavior serves as a communication system. Adults must learn to read children's signs."[4] The food, the pace, the pressure? Could it be your child's way of communicating *wait, this is NOT working*? Maybe their behavior is a communication that *this is not a food I can try*. Period. By treating these children as purely behavior problems that need to be modified, we could bury the need to attend to the sensory challenges, what they are trying to say to us, and their level of worry about *change*.

And *problem feeders*? This whole eating experience is hard enough for the child, but to then also be labeled a *problem* when you are doing the best you can? We need to look at why are they refusing foods offered and not add the labels that could add blame? Is the problem that they do not know how to chew, or that they do not like the feel of the food, or that its new or it makes them feel bad? I just do not love any of these terms. And there are more. There are other terms parents find when wandering around the internet.

Food Neophobia

Some professionals have described these children as *food neophobic*. This is not an official diagnostic term but is descriptive. The term *food neophobia* was popularized by Leanne Birch[5] as she has researched the development of food preferences in children in the 1990's. This was described as a typical phase many toddlers enter where they are fearful of the presentation of new, novel foods. She characterizes this phase as *phob*ic (irrational fear) of new *(neo)* foods. Though she describes this stage in typically developing food preferences, most toddlers outgrow this phase with regular positive exposures to and interactions with new foods and maturation. Most toddlers move on and eventually eat many more new foods if we avoid creating a battleground. In her original writings and the writings of her team, she indicates that these children need multiple exposures to new foods (five to ten) to be comfortable enough to try them.[6] Others further compared and contrasted picky eaters and food neophobic eaters. They described food neophobic eaters as reluctant or unwilling to try new or novel foods and picky eaters were unwilling to try many familiar foods. Once the child had been exposed to the novel food, it was then no longer considered new and so then a subsequent rejection was considered picky.

The term food neophobia gets us thinking about food worry, fear, and novelty, but it does not yet capture the level of reluctance that parents describe with their children who cannot deviate from **their LIST**. The challenge for parents of children who have parentheses diets is that their children are often unable to eat, not just novel foods, but **any** foods **not** on their *List*. Their fear and worry about things different from their *List* is huge. Parents wonder, *why in the world will my child eat <u>this</u> particular brand or color of yogurt and not <u>that</u> one? And why so much reluctance, resistance, fear and worry?* The logic, their reasoning, may not make sense to others who care about them, but the logic is important, very important *to them*.

Many of the children we are talking about did demonstrate some type of *food neophobia* as toddlers but could never quite get past it. They then got stuck there with their parentheses. As we continue to look for the description that works for these children, we must start by believing each child. We can believe that even though we do not quite understand it, or have a label for it, their reaction is real, the worry is real and what we want to do is NOT practice more of that worry but find where IS comfortable and build from there. So, we keep looking for the term that helps better understand these children.

Sensory Processing Disorder

Some of these children do have a diagnosis of Sensory Processing Disorder (SPD). This is described as a neurological disorder in which the sensory information that the individual perceives results in abnormal responses (Star Institute).[7] It is strongly linked to many children with sensory related eating challenges. Many of our anxious eaters process the sensory information of eating in very unique ways. And, make no mistake about it, mealtimes ARE SENSORY! Their responses to the smell, sound, look, taste, and texture of mealtimes are abnormal responses that interfere with their ability to enjoy a variety of foods. But Sensory Processing Disorder does not always include food issues. We definitely know children who have SPD where food is not their challenge. And we know anxious eaters who do not seem to have generalized sensory processing challenges. This, again, may be part of the issue, but not all of it. Finding the right descriptor is complicated!

Autism Spectrum Disorder (ASD)

Many children diagnosed with autism spectrum disorders are described as picky eaters. Many children with autism diagnoses also have diagnoses of sensory processing disorder, anxiety disorder or may also be co-diagnosed with obsessive compulsive personality disorder. Many of our anxious eaters would never be described as on that spectrum. And some children officially diagnosed on the ASD spectrum do not have eating challenges. The prevalence of eating challenges in this group varies some in different studies, however, Zickgraf and Mayer reported their parent reports that 70% of their children diagnosed with ASD had difficulties with eating.[8] That means that 30% do not.

In order to receive a diagnosis of autism, children often have persistent challenges with socialization, communication and interaction.[9] They have restrictive and repetitive patterns of behavior, insistence on sameness and inflexible adherence to routines, difficulty with transitions and rigid thinking patterns. Children with ASD often have sensory processing challenges. And many of our anxious eaters like routine, sameness and have sensory processing challenges.

Think about mealtimes. They are times of socialization and communication, sensory richness and transition. Counselor and Feeding specialist, Jo Cormack writes "Many children with autism cling to routines with force - this can be especially true with food."[10] Mealtimes include multiple transitions: A transition to a meal. A transition from a full looking plate to one that has had parts eaten. Transitions from one texture as the food enters the mouth to changing textures as the food is chewed and readied for swallowing. Now think about children who have been diagnosed with ASD. These children struggle with communication and socialization and they often have sensory sensitivities and ritualistic behaviors. Many have difficulty with transitions. Mealtimes may cause a child with ASD to confront their largest social and sensory challenges. And, if mealtimes are a time of worry for them, they understandably may not want to transition *toward* the meal multiple times a day. They would rather transition *away* from it. So some of our anxious eaters have a diagnosis of autism spectrum disorder, but that diagnosis is not right for many of our anxious eaters.

Avoidant Restrictive Food Intake Disorder (ARFID)

In 2013 the inventory of psychiatric diagnoses, *Diagnostic and Statistical Manual of Mental Disorders*, Fifth Edition [11, 14] created a new eating disorder diagnosis called ARFID, or avoidant restrictive food intake disorder. This diagnosis was an effort to provide a name for an eating disorder that was not anorexia and not bulimia but that did effect diet and eating in a significant way. The diagnosis of ARFID is not restricted to one particular developmental period. It can be diagnosed throughout the life span.

ARFID describes an apparent lack of interest in eating foods often based on sensory characteristics of the food. Children may have one or more of the following: weight loss or faltering growth, or significant nutritional deficiency, dependency on supplements. An important component of the ARFID diagnosis is the marked interference with psychosocial functioning. The eating issues cannot be further explained by another diagnosis such as digestive issues or other medical issues. Characteristically, the diets of these individuals are narrow and the choice of foods often has a sensory component. A child may reject food based on how it looks, smells, tastes, feels or sounds. The interference with food interactions with others and the ability to participate in the social interactions with food is prominent.

This diagnosis *does* describe a number of the *very worried about change* eaters we know. Many parents have found this diagnosis online and had "Ahah" moments for their children who have narrow *List* diets with lots of mealtime struggle and diets that are often characterized by specific sensory properties: the look, the texture, the smell. These children and their families cannot begin to think about what it might be like for them to participate in a normal family meal together. The eating issues do interfere every day, every meal.

However, there are pros and cons about using ARFID as a diagnosis for these children. This is a mental health diagnosis and there is considerable discussion about whether these children should be treated in pediatric feeding clinics or eating disorder clinics and about the pros and cons of giving another big diagnosis or label. This is another label that may not be perfect but many families do describe relief that there might be a name for what is going on at their family meal and that other families may be struggling with similar issues.

Pediatric Feeding Disorder

Recently, a consensus paper was published declaring pediatric feeding disorder (PFD) a stand-alone diagnosis. This term, PFD, defined as impaired oral intake that is not age-appropriate, and is associated with medical, nutritional, feeding skill, and/or psychosocial dysfunction.[12] This effort, facilitated by Feeding Matters[13] works to enable practitioners and researchers to better characterize the needs of heterogeneous patient populations, facilitate inclusion of all relevant disciplines in treatment, and allow the health care team to use a common, precise terminology necessary to advance clinical practice and research. This diagnosis, if universally accepted, is intended to greatly help in diagnosing pediatric feeding issues. It does not yet more specifically sub-categorize different types of pediatric feeding issues. This diagnosis is just in its beginning stages of acceptance. The great news is that it is on the way. And yet, it is a general term that does not specifically describe the uniqueness of this group of worried eaters or how to help them.

Anxiety Disorder

Just as *picky* may well have a continuum from the mildest toddler form of picky to serious-and -worrisome-narrow-diet-picky, anxiousness can also have its own continuum from mild worry to anxiousness and all the way to a medically diagnosed generalized anxiety disorder. A Generalized Anxiety Disorder is defined as an "excessive anxiety and worry (apprehensive expectation) occurring more days than not for at least six months about a number of events or activities such as work or school.[9] Children who are fully diagnosed with a generalized anxiety disorder are usually being treated for it with medical and/or psychological therapies. The worry for some of the anxious eaters we describe sometimes reaches the level of anxiety disorder.

Yet we know many children (and adults) who do not have or need an official anxiety disorder diagnosis, who certainly live on the worried side of life. We hear, *it makes me worried* OR *it makes me anxious*. These are common colloquial phrases used every day throughout that continuum of worry intensity from the mildest worry temperament to the most complex diagnosable anxiety disorder. In between there are many degrees of intensity. Some children have anxiousness that shows itself predominantly around food and food choices. Other anxious eaters do have excessive worry that shows up both at mealtimes and during other parts of their life. Still others are fully diagnosed with an anxiety disorder and are being treated for it with medical and/or psychological therapies.

Anxiety temperaments and anxiety disorders tend to run in families. There is an increasing body of evidence that anxiety issues have a neurobiological basis. With or without an official anxiety diagnosis, many of our anxious eaters experience anxiousness or worry associated with eating and change surrounding mealtimes. No matter the label, the worry is there.

Worry wiring and worry temperament

Some children may just be born with a worry temperament. When taking histories from families of anxious eaters we regularly ask, *who else in the family struggles with these difficulties? Is anyone else anxious or worried, obsessive or compulsive, or have similar challenges with food?* The answer is so often yes! *Oh, yes, my husband or my cousin, my wife or the siblings, my uncle or my grandmother,* or multiple of these relatives. There is ever emerging research that confirms the neurobiological differences and genetic pre-dispositions that influence these challenging eating worries.[14,15,16] We will often tell parents to think of their child as having different "wiring." Some children might just be worry wired to perceive food, and life, differently.

> **Dear Parent,**
>
> Who else in your family has some of these issues?

Label?

Clearly there is not yet a label acceptable to all. I am not sure we NEED to new label these children, in order to move forward, in order to help them, especially in light of the multiple labels out there and the multiple different opinions on the labels. Different clinics, different professionals will provide a different label, if any at all.

Whether a child has one of the above labels, or another new one altogether, certain realities remain. It IS important that these children and families find their way to proper sensitive support that fully understands the individuality of these issues and the layers of worry these children experience. It IS important that parents find a way to understand their child's challenges and guide them toward more success. It IS important that the anger, pressure and frustration stop and we help them return to mealtime peace. It IS important that parents know there are other children out there who have issues like their child. It IS important that families find support in regaining some mealtime balance.

The fact that so many "names" are used underlies the complexity of the challenges for these children and families. As a feeding professional, I can say that none of these labels seems quite right to me because each of these children is so different in their response to food or their diet. It is not my intention in this book to find a new label or name. There are enough. It is only my intention to find descriptor words that provide us have common ground for understanding these children and how we can help them.

In my opinion, these worried eaters who maintain their worry well beyond toddler *picky* need extra help, therapy that takes into consideration the sensory challenges and the need for careful small changes so as not to push the directly into their worry. Diagnosis or no diagnosis. These strategies are described throughout.

Consider the descriptor "anxious"

I have been in search of descriptor words that describe the situation of the mealtime, the emotion of it, and give us a hint about how to help these children and families. For the purpose of this book I will describe these eaters as **anxious eaters** and will also use the word *worry*, often interchangeably. This is not meant in any way to label or diagnose an official anxiety disorder but more to refer to the **colloquial** terminology of the adjective *anxious, as in worried*, often *very worried* about change. And when children are described as worried, anxious about eating, parents worry and are anxious about feeding them, hence, **anxious eaters/anxious mealtimes**. I see eating challenges as a child issue **and** a parent issue since eating is a parent child partnership, a relationship. The challenges do not occur in isolation of each other. Here is my thinking. Here are some definitions of **anxious**.

1. Oxford Dictionary: Anxious (adj):
   "Feeling or showing *worry*, nervousness, or unease about something with an uncertain outcome. Causing or characterized by *worry or nervousness*."[3]

2. Merriam-Webster Dictionary: Anxious (adj):
   "Characterized by extreme uneasiness of mind or *brooding fear* about some contingency : WORRIED.[17]

3. Collins Dictionary: Anxious (adv):
   "If you are anxious, you *are nervous or worried* about something."[18]

4. The Free Dictionary: Anxious
   adj): "*Worried and tense* because of possible misfortune, danger, etc; uneasy," Or "raught with or causing anxiety; worrying; distressing: *an anxious time*".[19]

We can consider the term *anxious* here as it pairs colloquially with the words *worry* and *fear*. Most parents with extremely picky eaters will describe the significantly increased level of worry about mealtimes shown in their children. *Worry* with coming to the table. *Worry* with trying new foods. *Worry* with change, any change at all, about mealtimes. Selective, yes. Narrow diet, yes. But the factor that describes their eating AND gives us a hint about how to carefully and sensitively support them is, for us, *worry* or just plain fear. There are so many influences on eating for these children. There is pickiness, though extreme pickiness. There is a selective, narrow diet that is worrisome. There are behaviors that demonstrate refusal and sometime even es- cape. There are sensory preferences with color, texture, smell and taste and the visual appearance of the food. But, the term *anxious* helps us to also look at the *why*, the extreme worry or fear about change that influences so many children. By considering anxiousness and worry as the TOP-OF-THE-LIST issue for these particular children, we can carefully find ways help children feel calm, and tiptoe toward the *new*. We can support them as they move toward the changes they need and sensitively help them overcome fear of that change. Rather than demanding change, we can acknowledge that it's really hard for them to accept change. We can stop *pushing into their worry* and offer guided opportunities for worry reduction with foods.

Dear Parent,

What worries your child about food and mealtime?

When There is Fear and Worry

Imagine yourself as a worried eater. Imagine that every day four, five, six times a day you are offered unfamiliar food that makes you feel worried. My family loves to travel and we love to try new adventurous foods when we travel. However, I recently had an interesting experience that helped me understand worried eating in a new way.

We traveled to Hong Kong and tried so many new foods. I am less experienced with the cuisine of Hong Kong and almost every food, every smell, and every texture was new to me. New is often great for me, but the *new* smells and tastes there were unexpected. Sometimes they felt like taste or texture surprises. I was offered a round snowball-looking food with, what looked like a powdered sugar on the outside. It was an afternoon snack at a conference, so I assumed it was a sweet food. It turned out to be the texture somewhere between Playdough™ and Silly Putty™ and the surprise in the center was a kind of fermented bean curd, not sweet. It was a total sensory surprise, so much so that I accidentally dropped it. The next day the snowball-looking offer had a white coconut-like coating on the outside. I tried it, and this time already knew the texture would be different, so it was not as big of a surprise, but the inside was a surprising mango pudding. Tasty, but again, not what I had expected. This time, I was ready for fermented bean curd. I was on high alert. At least this time, I did not drop it!

Then the fish dishes! Oh my! I thought I was a fish person. I like many fishes, but apparently my experience is with fish, not as much with the richness of the seafood offered in Hong Kong. There were many slippery, rubbery, chewy, very different textures of fish parts. The unexpected textures got me! I would take a bite of my fish dinner and it would turn out to have a texture different from what I was expecting. It was hard to anticipate which new, slippery or rubbery texture I would find in my mouth. As a polite guest I would need to chew and swallow the slippery or rubbery fish. I realized that I became very cautious and actually worried. What would be next? I genuinely longed for some kind of familiar home food—something that would have predictable tastes and textures. Something that I didn't have to work so hard to taste and understand at each meal.

As a parent, you are entrusted with the responsibility of nourishing and nurturing your children. When your children do not want to eat or cannot eat, you, of course, worry. You worry about the overall nutrition, worry that the food you prepared will be rejected, worry that mealtime will end up as a battleground, worry that it will end in tears.

Imagine that your child is always in this state of worry when she comes to the table. When we are worried, our bodies may become tense, our appetite may decrease, our gut may be weird and it can be hard to find enjoyment in the meal. When children are anxious about eating, it can lead to anxious mealtimes for everyone in the whole family.

Common parent worries

Parents tell us that the following are some of their common concerns. Some families have all of these concerns and some have only some of these issues, but they all are real and they all impact the whole family mealtimes. Take a listen.

- *My child is a picky eater who only eat certain foods. I cannot find a way for her to eat or try new things. She seems so scared of new things!*

- *My child has a very narrow diet. The favored foods she likes are so limited that I worry she is not getting sufficient nutrition. Often whole food groups are ignored. I worry every day about her nutrition! Dietitians have told us she needs to eat a rainbow. Her current brown and beige diet is certainly not a rainbow. How can I **get** that rainbow in her?*

- *My child is unable to eat with our family. The stress, the sights and smells of the foods, the commotion of the mealtime environment, and the worry about having to try a new food makes it necessary for me to feed him separately. He cannot even tolerate being in the same room as the food!*

- *My child likes his food in only one texture and that **cannot** be changed. OR My child just wants smooth foods. OR My child only eats crunchy foods. OR The peanut butter sandwich MUST be toasted.*

- *My child has gotten stuck on food of a certain flavor and any attempt to change the flavor can lead to complete elimination of that food from his diet. I have to offer same brand of food all the time so as not to vary the flavor (or texture). He needs that predictability. And I hate it when a food brand changes its recipe or label or goes out of business and my child only ate the old recipe or trusted the old package! What other parents have to worry about THAT!? It feels crazy!*

- *I cannot change presentation, at all. Why does he need his juice in THAT red cup, or his peanut butter sandwich cut in triangles? Why will he only eat with ME around? That is a HUGE pressure on ME!*

- *We cannot change the brand. My child needs his nuggets from a certain fast food restaurant or his macaroni and cheese from a certain brand with certain shaped macaroni. It is exhausting!*

- *Oh dear, if those foods accidentally touch, he has a complete meltdown!*

- *We cannot change the mealtime environment. My child wants the presentation to be the same, the same feeder, same chair, same house, same look of the mealtime. I can only feed my child at home. We cannot go to friend's houses or to restaurants. It is a stress on the whole family. We used to like to eat out. This is so limiting! And imagine what this does to eating out at a restaurant? Impossible!*

- *My child's food choices are not logical. They do not make sense! Why would she like vanilla yogurt but not raspberry when they are BOTH smooth? Or why would she like only one brand of vanilla yogurt, but not another brand of vanilla yogurt? I cannot taste any difference! Aren't they really almost the same? Why would my child only eat toast but not an English muffin? Why only apple juice from the box, but not the same juice in a cup? It is completely impossible to predict when my child will like a food and when not. It defies my parent logic.*

- *There is a huge emotional impact on our whole family. I want my child to eat good foods and be well nourished. I want her to eat a variety! When this does not happen consistently (or at all) I am feeling like I am failing my child. I sometimes feel like I am failing as a parent. I lose my confidence! And the more I try, the more stressful meals become for all of us!*

- *My child's pediatrician does not understand! She sees my child as growing and says my child will outgrow this! He may have no medical concerns that she can "fix", but I am his parent and I have concerns that are not being heard. It is not helpful to be told, your child will outgrow this when my child is five and only eat six specific foods! He is NOT outgrowing it and I need help! I **get** that lots of toddlers do get picky and that they do outgrow this. I **get** that calming parents down by saying your child will outgrow this may be the right answer for many parents, but NOT FOR ME!*

- *Even my family and friends do not get it. My Mom talks about 'in her day children just ate what was in front of them!' {Oh, Mom, if it were that easy, my child would be eating lots of different foods}. Or I often hear, 'you know, if you did not just offer snack foods all day, your child would eat better'. {Dear friend, don't you think I have thought of that? Don't you think I have tried other foods? THIS is all my child will eat!}. I feel judged all the time! I end up avoiding family and friends.}*

- *I get told to just make him hungry. Believe me, I have tried that multiple times and if my child is not comfortable with the food offered, he just cannot eat it, even if he was hungry! I have tried waiting for him to be hungry and three days and lots of tears later he ate nothing! His worry about the new foods is so great, I think he could starve! It is isolating!*

- *No one at our house enjoys the meal. It is so hard to enjoy family meals when they become stressful for every person at the table. I am pushing, bribing, coercing, coddling, demanding, trying, trying, **TRYING** to get my child to eat more and different foods and he is pushing me farther and farther away. No one at the table is having a relaxed meal!*

- *My child eats all day. He hates the smells and experience of mealtime so much that I just put out a plate of the favorite foods, foods I KNOW he will eat, and let him eat when he wants to and when he can.*

- *My child has such a hard time transitioning to meals. The meals are just not fun for him and he would much rather do his thing at the computer or with his toys. I could **MAKE** him eat with us, but he becomes so upset, it is not worth it. I do not want to force him to the table if he is going to be miserable and make all of us miserable!*

Common child worries

We have described child worries about food. They are many and they are personal. The bottom line for most of these worried eaters is that they find little enjoyment in eating that does not involve their *List* foods.

- What if the food offered is not MY food?
- What if there is a surprise in it?
- What if the foods touch?
- What if I gag or throw up?
- What if the food smells bad, feels bad, looks wrong, tastes bad, or is too loud?
- What if my sandwich has crust?
- What if I am hungry and I cannot eat what is on my plate?
- What if my cracker is broken?
- What if I expected a red apple and they gave me a green one with specks on it?
- What if my milk is in the wrong cup?
- What if I HAVE to try something?
- What if I have to touch it?
- What if I make my parents mad?
- What if….
- What if….

Dear Parent,
    Fill it in.
    What if_____?
    What if_____?
    What if_____?
    What if_____?
    What if_____?

Parents want to get to "normal." It is exhausting and can sometimes feel like a kind of meal-time prison when your kiddo is so selective. Your choices are so limited. Some days, it can feel like shackles robbing your family of freedom and joy. Every decision you make must consider possible food interactions. For example, you cannot go to a museum all day because their cafeteria has peanut butter and jelly sandwiches only with strawberry jam, and my child only likes grape! Other parents do not need to deal with this! ~Lauri Ziemba

There is lots going on at these worried mealtimes for anxious eaters and their families and so many things to consider. First and foremost, we have to help each family find their own **mealtime peace**. We have to support the feeding relationship between parents and their children and bring that back in balance, bringing back family mealtimes and pleasant comfortable, less pressured, meals for all. From that starting point of mealtime peace we will need to find a way for children of the parentheses diet to learn about and become comfortable with change since, as we have described, change is so hard for so many of them. We can sensitively teach them **change happens** and it will be okay. And then, and only then, can we embark on the journey of teaching **new food trying skills**. We will discuss many different strategies for new food trying since each child will need his support in his own way. We will discuss the importance of teaching new food trying away from that peaceful family meal...to keep that family meal peaceful. Once children have skill and confidence in their new food trying we will support bringing those skills back to the table. And lastly, you will notice throughout the book that we will think about all the ways to tiptoe toward change and offer little tiny steps that help children and families succeed without pushing directly into their worry. Change will happen **at the child's pace** and at the family's pace. Now first, let us consider what mealtimes are all about so we can look for what mealtime peace might look like.

The Journey

Mealtime peace
Change happens
New food trying strategies
Always at your child's pace

What is a Mealtime?

"I am the boss of my eating."
Anonymous, age six

Mealtime for many families who have an anxious eater is out of balance and probably has evolved into something other than the mealtime of your dreams. To re-find mealtime balance, we must first look at what we mean by *mealtime. Mealtime* means different things to different families[20].

Why do we eat? We eat for calories, health and enjoyment. Yes, but we also create meals as time to be with family and friends, to socialize, to communicate, and to celebrate togetherness with others. Don't we catch up with a friend over coffee and a bagel, where the food is secondary to the conversation? Don't we have anniversary dinners where the purpose is a romantic evening rather than all about the food? We may eat to try new foods and new mealtime situations. Sometimes we just eat from habit or because we MUST.

Anxious eaters often eat because they *have* to, not because they *want* to come to the table. Food can be such a worry that they dread transitions toward every mealtime. Enjoyment is *not* what they are experiencing. Many parents of anxious eaters describe the *why* of mealtime as a time to *get in* a certain number of calories or certain amount of food.

Where do we eat? Healthy eaters have flexibility. We eat at home, at the family table, in front of the TV, at restaurants, at Grandma and Grandpa's house, in the car, at the park, at school, and at playgroups, at work, at parties. We eat in lots of places. We have choices!

Anxious eaters often eat in one familiar place. New places often increase their worry so much that parents find themselves offering food in the same place and quit eating in other places altogether. Restaurants and even Grandma's house can become impossible.

When do we eat? We usually eat on some type of meal and snack routine. We allow ourselves the privilege of being hungry at a meal, eating when hungry and stopping when we are full. We usually have some variation on breakfast, lunch and dinner and maybe a couple snacks. We know toddlers seem to grow best when they are offered this type of mealtime routine.

Many anxious eaters have their eating volumes closely directed by their worried parents and do not get to decide when to finish a meal. Some meals can take an hour or two to "finish" only to turn around and declare it time for the next meal. Entire days can be spent in feeding an anxious eater. Some families have given up on having family "meals" altogether since no two people in the family eat the same foods. Some children have such negative reactions to food that their *List* foods are put out on plates around the house so the child can just snack whenever he is willing and able to eat just to have calories available to them. Though this provides the opportunity for child-directed calories and reducing mealtime stress, it unfortunately removes hunger as an influencing support at all. The *when* can become all confused.

With whom do we eat? We eat alone and with others. We eat in big groups and in small ones. Sometimes we eat with the whole family, sometimes a sibling snack, sometimes with Grandma and Grandpa, with friends, and co-workers, or classmates. The social context of eating is a plus for many eaters, but often, anxious eaters are only comfortable eating with one person as their feeder, or companion. When an anxious eater is only comfortable eating with one parent, it puts a tremendous amount of pressure on that parent meal after meal, day after day.

What do we eat? We eat different foods, a variety of foods. Dietitians encourage us to eat a rainbow. Sometimes it is a home cooked meal, and other times it is eating on the run. Sometimes it is food picked from a garden and other times it is a quicker processed meal or fast food. Our anxious eaters often eat from their *List*, only *their* foods, and encouragement to try anything else has become pressure.

And about nourishment

Mealtime can also be thought of as a time of nourishment. Yes, food is caloric nourishment. But can we find a way to *nourish*, not just your child's body but also nourish their being, who they are? Can we find a way for our children to feel celebrated beyond the calories? When children have become discouraged about mealtimes and feel like they are not pleasing parents, maybe disappointing parents, they are not feeling the celebration, but may be feeling "not good enough," not emotionally nourished?

Division of Responsibility

Ellyn Satter has described a division of responsibility in feeding.[21,22] She describes the different roles parents and children have in the feeding relationship. She tells us it is the parent's job to provide the toddler with the *what* of eating (the menu), the *where* of eating (the lap, the highchair, the family table, the snack table? Somewhere, but not wandering). It is also the parent's responsibility to determine the *when* of eating. As a dietitian, she encourages us to offer meals and snacks with breaks in between to allow for the privilege of being hungry at a meal, hence the *when*. She tells us, though, that it is the child's responsibility to decide whether they are going to eat the foods offered, and *how much*. Satter has helped us better understand the dynamics of mealtimes and the importance of allowing the child to make her own decisions about the food offered and the how much. She has reminded us that children's meal sizes and caloric intake can vary from meal to meal and day to day, but that most of the time they grow appropriately with that variation. The important element here is that THEY decide volumes. They know what foods they like and can eat. She encourages us to reintroduce foods that have been rejected in the past. She encourages us to offer family style meals so children can help serve themselves since they know their own appetite and for us parents not to get in the middle of their "how much." But, how do we manage when they just won't eat?

> Dear Parent,
>   Can you describe the why, when, where, what and with whom of your child's mealtime?

Offer or demand?

Let us look at the importance of *offering* food (*not demanding*) and allowing the child to *give permission* if she wants it and not give permission if she doesn't. We grownups offer and the child controls the pace, the pace of accepting the food we offer on a spoon, or the pace of their independent eating. The pace is influenced by the acquisition of new foods, and more maturing eating skills and independence.

When we believe it is the parent job to provide the food and the child's job to decide how much to eat, essentially the adult **offers** the food and the child can take it or leave it. **Most** children will eat when hungry and eat enough. To help us look at the evolution of mealtime pressure as we consider the words *offer* and *demand*.

> **Offer:** *To present for acceptance or rejection.*[23]

Basic to this definition is the option of accepting *or* rejecting. An offer is a choice. When grownups offer food to a child, if it is really an offer, children can accept or reject that food. (That does not mean they can reject the food and demand a whole new version of the menu, but they can eat it, or not. It is *offered*.)

Demand: *To call for or <u>require</u>, to ask with proper authority.*[23]

When we demand, the division of responsibility is off balance. The word *demand*, in and of itself, connotes pressure. When we are deciding what our child is to eat or how much, we step into the child's side of the division of responsibility equation[21]. As a general concept if we grownups are making demands about food, we are externally motivating the food decision making and not allowing the child to develop her own internal motivation to eat enough. We are confusing the mealtime responsibilities.

> **Dear Parent,**
>
> Are you offering or demanding?

Positive tilt

We discuss the positive and negative tilt of mealtimes in the Get Permission Approach to Pediatric Feeding Challenges[24]. This tilt of mealtimes matters. When we offer a breast or bottle, or food from a spoon if a baby wants that food, she leans forward toward it and toward the feeder. She leans toward the food in a *positive tilt* that says, *I want it. Yes!* She is motivated to explore that food. She indicates she wants it by opening her mouth, or reaching for the food or utensil, or maybe feeding herself. The tilt is positive, toward each other, with child and feeder meeting at the middle, either **physically or emotionally.** There is a coming together of the parent and child toward each other.

A child can also let us know she needs a pause in a meal by turning away, not opening her mouth, or distracting herself with the spoon, chasing a piece of cereal around the tray or leaning over to feed the dog. These can be examples of a normal pacing of the meal and, when ready and, if still hungry, she will again engage with the food and have a positive tilt. Gradually she will be full, stop eating, will no longer reach for the food, and the meal will end. These are natural parts of the mealtime communication but not a negative tilt.

The tilt is very significant in early feeding where the parent and baby are building a feeding relationship based on trust and sensitivity. However, the philosophical underpinnings of this concept continue to apply with older children as we feed responsively during each developmental stage.

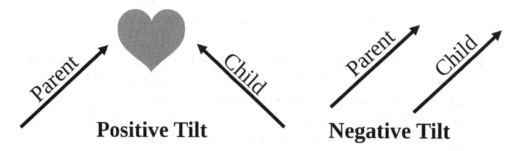

Positive Tilt   **Negative Tilt**

Negative tilt

However, sometimes the tilt of mealtime actually becomes **negative**. A negative tilt should not be a natural part of *any* mealtime communication. We see this negative tilt when we make and offer and the child is **adamant** in pushing the food or us away, turning away from the meal, and trying to leave the high chair or table or finding some way to protect herself from their perceived pressure of the food demand. The interaction is a negative one when the child feels pressure and more of a battleground scene ensues. Negative tilts do not help her like new foods. They do not help *anyone* enjoy the meal. Would you like a food you were forced to eat? What children do in response to that kind of pressure is RESIST! And, when we are trying to help them like new foods, resistance is absolutely what we do not want. So, how can we create more positive tilts, eliminate resistance and find enjoyment? If we have negative tilts and adamant responses of worry, we need to **change** something in our offer.

> Dear Parent,
>
> Is there a negative tilt going on at your mealtimes?

   The children we are helping here are, by definition, worried or anxious about trying new foods. Consider whether we want to offer or demand that they eat certain foods in a certain way. We know from more and more research that children tend to eat better when multiple people around the child are eating and offering food around them.[6] We know that an encouraging approach rather than in an authoritarian approach inspires more eating. We know when we follow children's cues in eating and are responsive to their needs, eating goes better.[25,26,27] You can find scholarly research in journals, as well as opinion papers, current parenting magazines, blogs and news stories. It is in the news! Many families have gotten discouraged that their attempts or their therapist attempts to get their child to eat more have ended in a struggle. They describe what feels like a battle of demands and resistance. We want to find ways to offer and get rid of the demand approach.

Enjoyment, Confidence, Internal Motivation

In the Get Permission courses, we are also looking for enjoyment, confidence and internal motivation. First, enjoyment is all about the sensory aspects of the food. Sensory **enjoyment**. Does it look good, smell good, sound good, feel good, taste good? Secondly, we look next for **confidence**. Through the lens of the Get Permission Approach, confidence is developed as the child has positive experiences in her motor interactions with food? Can children skillfully and confidently manage the motor skills of eating? And then thirdly, we are looking for **internal motivation**. Is the child internally motivated to eat enough to grow well? Internally motivated (and healthy, skilled) eaters take in what they need and grow accordingly.

It is important that children listen to their own bodies, eat until full and be allowed to stop the meal when they have had enough. By listening to their own bodies, they learn to be internally motivated eaters. We want children to grow up internally motivated to eat well and to eat enough. We want them to understand and respond to their own hunger. When we make the demands, require eating certain foods and certain amounts against the child's wishes, the motivation is clearly not internal and the division of responsibility is unbalanced. Even the wording *get my child to eat more* indicates a lack of balance in the mealtime where the whole responsibility of eating ends up on the parent shoulders, not the child's. The motivation becomes external and that is not where we want to end up. Our goal should be internal motivation and enjoyment, not external motivation and struggle. Internal motivation and enjoyment are sustainable. Any parent of an anxious eater will tell you that external motivation and struggle are NOT.

> **Enjoyment**
> **Confidence**
> **Internal Motivation**

When we pressure children to eat more or differently, we tell them not to listen to their bodies and to eat for the external reasons that WE want them to, **because we**

said so. The relationship can get off balance. When we want them to eat more they push back from our external pressure. They resist. The conversations of mealtime can get stuck in the reverberating cycle of *try this* or *eat another bite*. Forget about manners, celebration, and enjoyment, because the goal often becomes how to *get in* food. The foods offered become limited and, forget about exploration, *just eat*! It gets confusing when they clearly are not eating enough or cannot eat enough.

I have worked with children who are anxious eaters for most of my career, with children who have a multitude of medical, sensory and emotional challenges relating to eating. This group of children, the children of the parentheses diet, are especially challenging. Their parents repeatedly tell us their child would rather fight than eat a new food, would rather sit at the table until bedtime in order to avoid new foods. Parents often shyly admit, *I waited out three days offering my child the good and healthy food I made and not the List foods, and my child cried, and cried, and ate NONE of it. His Grandma said 'just make him hungry', and I tried, but IT DID NOT WORK*. Because the balance is off at many levels, we want you to partner with medical support for your child. This is where you need the **support and guidance of a medical and nutritional team that knows YOUR child** to help you understand the nature of your child's eating and where nutritional or medical support may be necessary.

Toddler Independence

To complicate all of this, babies become two years old developmentally. Toddlers are notorious for their need for independence. They get good at *NO* and that is their toddler job, figuring out who they are, figuring out and challenging the limits. And, of course, their *No's* show up at mealtimes! And some toddlers have a bigger *NO* than others! It can be confusing when they tell us *NO* around food. Is it because they do not want it today, or they are just not hungry right now? Or they are just practicing NO, or they are getting sick, or they do not feel well, or they genuinely do not like the flavor or texture? Or they are worried about it? Are they sensory sensitive? Or the planets are poorly aligned!? Or all of the above? It is hard to know. But we do know if they tell us NO and we repeatedly push into their **NO**, it can lead to worry and more **No**. This can be so confusing to parents.

> Dear Parent,
> Are you stepping into your child's job at mealtime? How did you get there?

Response to pressure.

Why is it that many parents say "the harder I try the less my child eats new?" That could well be the case. We know from lots of research that pressuring a child to eat, or authoritarian practice geared at making them eat a new food (because we are bigger and because we can) do not actually help.[6] Could it be that the methods we grownups use to help children try new foods do not work with these children and can actually push them away from food? Could it be we need new methods? Could it be that pressuring does not work and can make worried eaters eat less?

You tell us if you just take away the pressure your child will not eat. You tell us that you have tried that and he sat there, or only ate his food. You tell us you are afraid not to pressure because what if your child loses weight. All of those are very good concerns. We ask you to consider your child's eating issues in the big picture perspective of his medical, growth and nutritional needs. There are many very usable ideas in this book but they do not take the place of sound medical evaluation and care. They are meant to compliment sound medical decision about your child's health. Throughout this book we will discuss ways to work back toward child directed eating, food enjoyment and reducing the pressure and finding more balance. Let us look at pressure. Read on.

What is There to be Worried About?

"Food fears are loud. It would be like eating in an earthquake!"
Lauri Ziemba

Children do not start out as worried eaters. But past medical experiences, sensitivities, and other worrisome experiences can make mealtimes a place of discomfort for them. Parents mean the best in wanting the best for their children. You want to offer healthy food and see your children eat well. But when children start experiencing worry, parents begin to worry. Worrisome experiences lead to worrisome mealtimes.

How do worried eaters get there? Where did the worry come from? Maybe your baby had medical problems, pain and/or discomfort in early infancy and learned that mealtime is **not** an enjoyable experience. As she got older she began to worry about what if I feel badly again when they feed me, and the cycle of worry develops. Maybe she got there from a typical toddler phase of worry, independence and a hefty practicing of "no" that got worse and did not go away. Maybe she got to worry from communication mismatches. Maybe worry is linked to her temperament. Maybe it is in her "wiring." Maybe she is extra sensitive about "sensory" and meals **are** all about sensory experiences! Maybe she was made to eat when she just did not feel well. Maybe she has learned to worry. The challenge for these anxious eaters is that their worry has led them to be particularly worried and rigid about CHANGE. Helping them with change in tiny careful ways will be the focus of this book.

Worry defined!

Worry is defined as *to feel or cause to feel anxious or troubled about **actual or potential** problems.* (Oxford Dictionary[3]) OR *to think about problems or unpleasant things that might happen in a way that makes you frightened and unhappy.* (Cambridge Dictionary)[30] Synonyms: anxiety, disturbance, uneasiness, unease, disquiet, nervousness, stressfulness, tension, strain, agitation. These are words many parents use in describing their mealtimes and their child's reaction to new foods. Children worry and parents worry and in the partnership of feeding and eating, worry influences the pace of skill development and growth.

- Actual problems. Some worry comes from **actual** problems with eating such as systems problems, skill problems, structural problems, sensory problems, choking, severe allergic reactions to foods. For example, a four-year-old girl who had a severe choking incident and then quit eating solids completely. From her perspective, there was an actual very frightening experience that scared her, and her remedy was to protect herself by stopping choke-able solids. Or the child who tries that new offered food and then has an anaphylactic reaction, a scary trip to the hospital and terrified parents. Or, what about the child who has extreme sensory sensitivity and experiences the sensory aspects of food differently. The smells trigger their PROTECT ME response; the texture feels wrong and the taste is experienced as unpleasant. Or for parents the actual problems can be watching their child's weight go down, or their gagging, vomiting, their inability to eat enough food to grow, the medical challenges, hospitalizations, the number of hours in the day required for feeding, feeding enough.

- Fear of potential problems. Sometimes the worry comes from fear of potential real or imagined problems. As parents, we worry about potential problems, and so do children. We all worry based on our experiences. For example, if the child has had a choking incident, we (and they) worry it will happen again. If the child has had a bad food reaction, we (and they) worry it will happen again. If their child's growth chart begins to dip down we worry they are not eating or a eating a properly balance diet; we worry we cannot find or afford help. And children worry that mealtimes will be stressful because they cannot eat what is offered, how it is offered, that they do not have the energy to eat that much, that they do not like the feel, the look or the presentation of the food. So, the mealtime worry is complicated by thinking about potential problems that "might happen and make us frightened or unhappy." Let us look at what there might be to be worried about.

Winston is a two-year-old who was cautious about change. He liked breast feeding. Parents described him as a sensitive baby. When offered baby food at six months, he pushed away. The more his parents tried to get him to take foods at seven, eight, nine, ten, eleven and twelve months, the more he pushed back, started to gag and now vomits with the presentation of solid foods. Now mealtimes are a big struggle for Winston and his parents.

It is hard to say if Winston was just on his own slower schedule for learning to enjoy foods, or if he had a physical or sensory reason to be more cautious. He continued his caution, learned more caution, and continued to practice *no*. Now he and his parents are in a cycle of worry that has turned into a **battle-ground of stress** for all. Parents want and need help in figuring out what to do next.

Jerry is a bright twenty-eight-month-old who has a severe allergy disorder. He drinks a special baby formula for babies with allergies. The first five foods his mother introduced to him landed him in the hospital with life threatening reactions. The next three foods his mother introduced also caused him to have severe allergic reactions, vomiting and retching. Jerry's mother discovered the best place for him to try new foods was the parking lot of the local children's hospital, right near the emergency room! Jerry quickly figured out that this "new food stuff" is bad for me! Jerry continued to worry when he was faced with new foods. His mother finally discovered that he could eat two different kinds of baby food: mango blend and baby food applesauce. He lived on these two foods and that special formula. It is no wonder that at twenty-eight-months of age, Jerry only wants one variety of pouch food made with mango and applesauce and rice cereal. He eats at least six of these a day. He knows the color of the pouch and knows it is safe. He runs from any offer of a new food. His worry decreases when he knows exactly what he will be eating.

Jerry learned to be afraid of food. His actual **severe allergic anaphylactic reactions** taught him to worry about food. His fear has contributed to his rigid self-protection from new foods. His family is now stuck offering the same foods in the same way, and still do not understand the full extent of his allergies because he vehemently will not try *new*! He protected himself from change and potential problems he wanted to avoid. He is an anxious eater, and his worry came from **fear**.

Penny happily ate a variety of baby foods when she was an infant. But, by the time she was 24 months old, she quit talking and she began eliminating many of the puree and finger foods she had enjoyed when she was younger. Penny restricted her food intake to a small number of specific foods prepared in specific ways. Her communication skills were delayed. She started demonstrating rituals and repetition in her play. At four, she eats seven *foods*! She is very **afraid** of new foods and cannot tolerate any mealtime change. Actual or fear of potential problems worry?

Penny ended up with a **diagnosis** of autism spectrum disorder (ASD). Characteristic of that disorder is a need for routine and ritual and enhanced sensory sensitivity. We know there is a neurobiological basis for the ASD diagnosis. Her mealtime worry dominated her approach to new foods. Why worry? It could have been her wiring paired with her experiences.

Quincy was born in China and lived in an orphanage until he was adopted at about a year of age. When his new adoptive parents offered him foods from a spoon or finger foods, he screamed, cried and pushed them away just at the sight of them! Clearly, his reaction was out of balance. Had he had some type of negative experience with foods that were not presented in the bottle? What happened? His new parents would never know, but they were left trying to help him deal with his fear response to new foods.

Quincy had some type of **negative experience** in the orphanage before his adoptive parents even met him. The experiences were apparently negative enough that introduction to food caused a significant fear response. He clearly had some type of trauma around food (actual worry). His food refusals may well protect him from re-living whatever negative experiences he endured as an infant. He has clearly learned to worry. (Fear of potential problems worry).

Marcus is a three-year-old. He breast-fed well. As a matter of fact, he has never stopped breast feeding. He *could not tolerate change* in his feeding routine. From the beginning he gagged or vomited with the presentation of any baby foods or finger foods. His reaction was clear and STRONG. He could NOT manage the change from breast feeding to other types of eating no matter what his mother tried! No one other than his mother could feed him. He has grown into an absolutely delightful, bright three-year old who eats yogurt and one specific kind of apple juice, other than breast feeding. He has no specific diagnosis, but he is anxious and has lots of worry about every day experiences in his life. He worries about new people, new feeders, new foods. He clearly has sensory processing sensitivity and is worried in other areas of his life. Mom also describes herself as anxious. That is a tough combination. Add worry to sensory sensitivity and it is a big challenge for Marcus and his parents. Maybe it started as fear or discomfort with the sensation of the purees but has turned into **fear with anything new**.

Marcus did **not like change from the beginning**. He sought out routine and sameness from the start. He presents, at three, as an anxious, worried child, who lives in a family where anxiousness is part of the family wiring. Could it be that he is wired to be worried?

Lana was not a good breast feeder and ended up on a bottle. She was an okay, but not great, eater and at nine months was hospitalized with a respiratory virus and quit eating. She needed a feeding tube. She had poor tolerance for volume and formula and ended up "practicing" the routine of being fed and throwing up for two years. She learned eating was absolutely no fun, and actually downright sickening. When she was older and healthier she was pressured to eat in her home and therapy sessions by well-meaning grownups who just wanted to help her learn to eat with her mouth. She hated all food presentations. She protected herself from all new food presentations.

> Lana learned not to like food. She was worried about any food presentation. She had to **feel well and trust** her grownups and learn to take on the skills of eating carefully before her tube could be removed. She managed her worry about food by refusing and worrying about *new*.

Jim is eight. He does well in school. He has no diagnosis. No allergies or medical issues, no diagnosis of autism spectrum disorder, no diagnoses of anxiety disorder, and no specific sensory processing disorder. But he is an anxious eater. He has eight foods he is comfortable eating. His mother describes herself as *a bit obsessive and* describes Grandma as having an anxiety disorder. Two cousins have diagnoses on the autism spectrum. Jim's worry seems to be focused on food though he is also described as somewhat obsessive in play and a bit of a "clean freak." The food fears are real, and they are debilitating for him.

> Jim comes from a family with histories of obsessiveness, anxiety and autism spectrum disorder. Could it be that *worried* is the temperament Jim inherited, that he is wired for worry?

Jaime is an eight-year-old child with a diagnosis of a **sensory processing disorder**. His therapists call him a "sensory avoider." He does not like to touch wet things, cannot walk barefoot on the grass. He hates the tags on his clothing and requires extra soft T-shirts. He likes his food to be pureed and will eat many different foods if they are pureed and offered in the same bowl. He is very observant about visual changes in his food and can tell a texture change from across the room!

> Jaime is highly sensitive about sensations in general. Mealtimes include so many sensations and his sensitivities play havoc with his mealtime choices and his willingness to try new mealtime textures. He has become very narrow is his diet, favoring specific foods of specific textures and specific looks. He wants the foods he *knows*.

At four years of age Elijah had a bad choking incident on a hot dog. It terrified him, his parents, and there was a 911 call and trip to the hospital. After that he refused any solid foods. He was only willing to drink his nutrition.

> Elijah was afraid. Multiple medical tests showed no structural reason for his change in food choices. He wanted foods he KNEW would be safe and not cause another choking episode.

Melissa's Mom came to her first feeding therapy session and summed it up. "I just think Melissa is afraid of food!"

> We need to believe parents AND children! A more in-depth history may give us clues why Melissa is afraid of food. Her team needs to understand how she feels physically, what kind of experiences she has had around food, what systems work and want don't, but her starting point during that process is that mealtimes are fearful times.

Worry starts

When little eaters worry about mealtimes, they worry that they are not ready, that the food will send them back to the hospital, that it may not be safe, that it doesn't feel right, that it may cause them to choke, that it may make them feel bad, that they will not be able to chew or swallow it, that the mouthful is too big, that it doesn't look right, that it is too cold, that it is too hot, that it is not the right person feeding them, that it is new, different, that it will be pressure. The actual-problem-worry can easily lead into fear that problem will occur again. So, children can end up in Protect-Themselves-Mode of refusal and rejections as they worry about potential problems. It can reduce any confidence in trying new foods. Their initial caution can turn to worry and then lead to more worry. They bring their past experiences and worry to the table and the mealtime becomes crowded with their worry and the subsequent parent worry. Their worry is actual, real to them and they anticipate potential worry around many corners.

> Dear Parent,
> What might your child be worried about at your family mealtimes?

Why children might worry about eating

Eating is complicated. There are so many reason children might not eat or want to eat. As a feeding therapist it is often quite amazing to me how well things work for most children most of the time. When the eating apparatus and systems above go wrong and the child does not have an eating system that allows good eating, enough eating, confident eating and enjoyable eating, those issues **must** be addressed. Children need to feel well and capable to eat and eat enough. Your feeding team will help to identify some of these layers of eating challenge and find the treatment and support that can help you and your child navigate successful and enjoyable mealtimes and figure out influences on his current mealtime challenges. Let us look at some common challenges.

Medical challenges: To successfully and comfortably eat and feel appetite and motivation to eat, your heart and lungs need to give good support. You need endurance to make it through a meal and need to breath comfortably. When children have to choose between eating and breathing, they choose breathing! You need a well-functioning gastrointestinal system to move food through its entire digestive and metabolic processes. Your brain needs to help and control the whole process. Allergies and intolerances of foods certainly can affect how a child feels about foods. When children have poorly functioning systems, or when their health is compromised, it is hard to prioritized good eating, efficient eating, and eating enough.

Physical challenges: Eating is a very muscle connected activity. You have muscles to support your posture which supports your internal organs. You need muscles to feed yourself and muscles to chew and swallow. When children have challenges influencing their muscles these activities can become inefficient and even unsafe. If the physical systems of eating do not work well, or consistently it is hard to trust your body's ability to eat.

Sensory processing challenges: Children can have sensory imbalances in any of the senses. Poor vision or hearing can complicate their interaction with the world. If children are not able to see others eat or see the food coming, they miss a lot of cues about food and mealtimes. They may have heightened sensitivity to sounds including the sounds of chewing and food preparation. They may have enhanced sensory sensitivities that cause them to overreact to the sensations of mealtimes. They may have very heightened responses to particular smells, touch and texture, flavors and taste. They may respond to every smell as a danger alert! Or they may have dampened response to the sensations of eating causing them to have challenges finding and organizing the food in their mouth or enjoying the touches of food. And the sensory challenges go on and on…

These sensory challenges can influence their demand for a very narrow diet of predictable foods where the smell, texture and flavor and sound are very predictable. Lucy Skye, a Trainer Consultant with the national Autistic Society in June 2018, wrote a paper on "Autism and Controlled Eating: Making Sense of Food and Feeding."[29] Ms. Skye describes her own sensory challenges with eating. She describes how she controls the (food) variables for herself to control the unexpected, the worry. She says "I don't want to eat, not because I am scared of the food, but because I am scared of processing every single pre, during and post-eating sensation and thought spiral. It's exhausting and takes any enjoyment out of the act of eating." She helps us understand that when sensory is the challenge, it is exhausting and difficult for those of us who are not sensory worried eaters to understand.

Past Experiences

Children bring their past experiences with them to the mealtime, as do parents. They bring their memories of that choking incident or the time they had a severe allergic reaction. They bring memories of chronic vomiting and gagging or pain associated with eating. They bring memories of how this food or that smell, or that texture made them feel. And they bring memories, their mealtime experiences and our pressure. They bring their worry and we bring our worry.

When we worry about our children, their growth, their diet, their eating, we want to help, encourage, entice them to eat more. Our past experiences lead us to pressure. And, too often a child's response to our pressure is resistance and a mis-match of communication has begun.

In general, children want to eat. But negative experiences can teach children NOT to want to eat. They can learn not to want to be around food or come to the table. If they eat and feel pain or discomfort, they learn not to want to eat. If they eat and have a severe allergic reaction they learn not to want to eat. If they eat and feel uncomfortable sensations, texture or flavors, they can learn not to want to eat. If they come to the family meal and there is pressure to eat, pressure to try just one more bite, pressure to clean their plate or try a scary food, they learn not to want to come to the table. If they try a food and it has a new flavor or texture snuck in, they can learn not to want to eat, AND not to trust their grownups. We know children bring their memories of those negative experiences to the table and these memories impact their perceptions of food and mealtimes.

Mismatch of Communication?

In a mismatch of communication, children tell us NO for whatever reasons they need to and, because we care, we sometimes try to override their NO. We aim for YES and our anxious eaters may insist on NO. This can lead to a mismatch of communication where we try harder for YES with coercion, bribes, coddling, force, anger and they get stronger in their NO with anger, tears, or even gagging and vomiting. The battleground is established. Their mealtime worries turn into mealtime worries for all!

> Dear Parents,
> Might there be a relationship between your child's worry and his parentheses diet?

Worry is a two-way street

Parents and children both bring their past experiences and expectations to each mealtime. No way around it! It just comes to the table with us. Just as feeding your child is a relationship, a partnership, so is worry. Worry can come from the child, but it can also come from the grownups. And sometimes their worry leads to our worry which leads to their worry! The worry relationship can be quite daunting. They worry about the food or the presentation and we worry about growth and balance diet. We push, bribe, coerce, force, the child to eat more. We become pressure makers! Many children become food resisters! Our pressure increases as does their resistance. Katja Rowell and Jennifer McGlothlin describe this "worry cycle" so well in their book, Helping Your Child with Extreme Picky Eating: A Step by Step Guide for Overcoming Selective Eating, Food Aversion and Feeding Disorders.[30] Pressure, worry, and resistance is a tough cycle to get caught up in!

Worry temperament and wiring

Some children seem to be wired to have a worry temperament. They are just plain worriers and have been from the beginning. They may experience seemingly the same challenges others may experience, but where others get over it, and move on, the worriers may well stay worried and get more and more worried.

Research supports these wiring tendencies for our worried eaters. There are demonstrated links between both moderate and severe selective eaters and significantly elevated symptoms of depression, social anxiety and generalized anxiety.[31,32,33] There is an increasing body of evidence about the neurobiological basis of both anxiety related issues and autism.[14,34] Our research community is continuing to delve deeper into these relationships. There is research that is linking anxiety, sensory sensitivity.[35,36,37] They seem to be very related.

Worry impacts the body

We all have experienced the intricate ways our guts and our emotions are connected. We feel "butterflies in our stomach" when anticipating an exciting event. We feel "sick to our stomach" when we see terrible news on the television. Some of us respond to stress with eating lots more. Some of us respond with eating way less. Some of us "just cannot eat today" when we are seriously worried. Some of us get diarrhea when stressed and others get seriously constipated. We now know there are significant mind and gut connections and relationships.[38] Research is most recently describing this as a bidirectional.[39] The information can go in both directions, brain to gut an gut to brain. It relates the cognitive and emotional centers of the brain with the gut. The brain seems to be able to influence the gut and the gut seems to be able to influence the brain.

Chronic worry and stress have their own impact on how the body functions and are well defined.[40] When we perceive a significant threat, it is natural to try to protect ourselves with a fight-flight reaction. It includes an increased heart rate, increased blood flow and changes in gastrointestinal motility. During that reaction our bodies release neurotransmitters and stress hormones that prepare us to flee. Digestion slows down as the body priorities *escape*. When the body is chronically stressed, it releases the stress hormone corticotrophin releasing factor (CRF). This hormone acts within the brain to suppress appetite, increase anxiety and improve selective attention to fine tune the body's stress response. We know this can influence gut function by causing inhibition of stomach emptying and stimulation of colon function. Your digestive tract is not meant to be chronically stressed. Children who are constantly stressed by their mealtimes can have gut and brain reactions that negatively impact appetite, and mealtime enjoyment.

Trauma around feeding

In some cases, worry comes from negative experiences that could be considered trauma. Trauma can result from an event or series of events that are experienced by the person as physically harmful, or emotionally threatening that can have adverse effects on their mental, physical, social or emotional well-being. It can be the result of a variety of experiences and is being studied more and more extensively in relation to pediatric feeding.[41,42] Trauma can be defined as "the result of exposure to inescapably stressful events that overwhelms a person's coping mechanism."[43] Children can experience trauma influencing feeding from multiple medical procedures and from life threatening medical procedures.[44] It can occur for children or parents as a result of frightening situations such as a traumatic choking episode, from traumatic medical procedures or events, or even from chronic negative forceful eating interactions that were emotionally stressful. It is important to remember that trauma is individual specific and what is no big deal to one child may have traumatic effects on another.

Past experiences of trauma may significantly impact a child's growth and development. Specifically, past trauma may change a child's ability to self-regulate, make sense of sensations, emotions, and develop motor skills and social skills.[45] We know that feeding is a complicated activity that requires children to actively utilize all of these developing skills. Research is describing how early experiences and environmental influences can leave a lasting signature on the genetic predisposition of emerging brains It describes how toxic stress can literally adversely affect the developing brain.[41]

Children who have experienced chronic stress or discomfort may attempt to protect themselves in ways that seem irrational, are not understandable, to an outside observer not familiar with the child's past. Past trauma has a real effect on children and has the potential to make mealtimes more worrisome. Chatoor and others are describing post traumatic feeding or eating disorder as behaviors exhibited when an infant relates a painful or frightening experiences with eating.[45,46]

Trauma also has the ability to significantly influence parents. We have a growing body of knowledge that looks at post-traumatic stress in parents whose children have had significant early medical challenges and feeding challenges.[41] Sometimes significantly stressful experiences families have endured continue to influence the ways they interact with their children. Parents who have experienced trauma might have more worry or hypervigilance than we or they would expect. It could be harder for parents who have experienced trauma in relation to their child's health to be fully in the present feeding moment responding to their child's cues.

But there is also a growing discussion about the effects of traumatic interactions as they relate to feeding and emotions. As you read this book, you will realize that I do not believe children should be force fed, or traumatized, EVER, as a result of therapies to better help them eat. Katja Rowll, MD, tells us "Parents so often share that what they were told to do went against their instincts and felt wrong. It is unconscionable that desperate parents are unknowingly engaging in (force feeding or trauma inducing) therapies that may do more harm than good. These therapies are failing children and families, not the other way around. As one mother warned, Bad therapy is worse than no therapy."[47] Practitioners and parents need to work together to help children struggling to eat in ways that do not further contribute to their trauma. Both need to proceed with full understanding that past trauma affects both children and their parents and help parents find the support they and their children need to heal.

> Dear Parent,
> Can you have a conversation with your health care professional if the feel of therapy is going against your instinct or causes traumatic responses in your child?

The Many Faces of Pressure

"Food is pressure!"
Brady, eight-year-old worried eater

Eight-year-old Brady has always had a traumatic relationship with food. He assumes food trying will be challenging. It is intimidating for him and only on a rare occasion is he pleasantly surprised by new foods. Brady helped inspire the writing of this book. After he learned to try new foods in a comfortable way, he wanted to teach kids about new food trying so he made some YouTube videos with his sister. The link is in the acknowledgement section of this book. When asked if he wanted to share anything with parents and professionals in this book, he gave the above quote, unprompted. Anxious eaters know!

Your child does not eat for reasons that are personal and specific to him. You worry when your child is not eating enough or receiving adequate variation in his diet. Sometimes you might have even tried what later seemed like counter-productive strategies to get your children to eat. While well-meaning, these strategies can feel like pressure to your child. Our children respond to demands, pressure and authoritarian feeding strategies with push back, resistance, refusals and reduced interest in the meals. So, the pressure continues. What a cycle!

Pressure all around

When we grownups get worried about our child's diet, we try to find ways to *get them* to eat more, to be healthy. (The phrase *"get them to eat"* is, by definition, pressure!) We can feel pressure knowing that this current *List* diet is not a healthy diet and believe it is our job *get better food in him.* The reality is that we can offer a great diet but finding ways for your child to WANT the food is the challenge! We may pressure because we feel shame and judgement from relatives and friends who scold about the narrow or "junk" diet. We may feel pressure because our idea of good healthy eating is organic, fresh and home grown and our child's diet is processed! We may feel pressure from pediatricians or grandmothers who say *just let them get hungry and they will eat* knowing we have tried that and our child did not eat when we "just let them get hungry."

We may pressure because we know that healthy food will help our child have more energy, have more focus, or help overcome other health or medical challenges they may be facing. Yes, we need to nourish children, but HOW to get them to enjoy that food is a challenge!

Your child's feeding therapists may also feel pressure to help you and your child experience progress, make change. Much of our parental and therapeutic support can be interpreted as pressure from your child's point of view. We all need to find ways to offer support and find ways that do not feel like pressure to your child. It is a balancing act! We pressure in ways that are obvious and ways that are not.

Obvious pressure

Here are some common mealtime situations that will sound too familiar to many. You may even be doing or have said all of these things. Know it was because you wanted to help. You tried to make things better. If these techniques were working well, you might not even be reading this book. And know we can discover a different way of supporting your anxious eater tomorrow.

1. We tell children to eat their food, clean their plate, while they are refusing.

   > It is not our grownup job to tell children they must eat. They are supposed to be in charge of how much they eat, not us! And if they are refusing do we understand why?

2. We shame them by saying, *see your brother is eating it.*

3. We threaten the loss of favorite toys or privileges or punish.

   > Threats and shaming do not help and can only make your child feel like he is disappointing you. It erodes self-confidence when children are asked to do something they cannot (due to skill or worry). Punishment is just plain sad when your child does not have the trust, skill or confidence to try that new food.

4. We tell them to *eat four bites and then you can have that.... Or finish your meal then you can have your electronics."*

> Requiring a child to eat before they can have treats can teach them dependence on grown up prompts. They then may need their grownups to cue each bite and reinforce each bite. Children learn to eat for parents, for the treats, and not for internal motivation.

5. *If you don't eat this, then you will go to bed hungry.*

> The child role of deciding how much to eat has been taken over by the parent. And, why is the child not eating the food offered? Do we understand? Does the child feel well? Does the child like that food? Is that a familiar food or new food? Is there worry?

6. We get angry, at our wits end and demand *JUST EAT IT!!!*

7. Parent leaves the table crying.

8. *Just touch these three foods then you can have your pretzels,* while the child is crying.

9. Mealtimes are described in battleground terms.

> Crying and anger do not help children learn to enjoy food or want to come to the family table meal after meal. Battlegrounds are pressure for all. If parents WIN and the child does eat that food, was that really a WIN in the long run? It was not self-motivated eating.

> Dear Parent,
>
> By describing these pressure situations, my goal is to create awareness. It is absolutely NOT my intention to create more pressure on YOU. There is already enough pressure to go around. Many parents who have read this book tell us how badly they feel that they have done or are creating many or all of these situations. This is not blame. Put that guilt aside. I believe these situations come from caring and

concern for your child. These were yesterday. This is today. Throughout this book I hope we can help you find gentler, more effect ways to help your child (and you) get to enjoyment at his mealtimes.

A hug,
Marsha

Less obvious pressure (It comes in many disguises!)

Sometimes our pressure is much less obvious and we might not have looked at pressure in these ways.

1. We *feed children* to get them to eat the whole meal, even though they can feed themselves.

> Children should be allowed to feed themselves when they have those skills. They know their pace, they know what they like and what tastes or feels good. They know when they are full. When we decide the amount and determine to feed them the whole amount, we have taken over their job of deciding how much to eat and when to end them meal. They are eating to please US or because we essentially made them eat it all.

2. We say nicely "C'mon, you can do it," and wait (hover) until they try the food.

> We imagine if we are nice about it, it is not pressure. But, for some children it still is pressure. When we provide a food and bribe, coerce and cajole them (and hover over them) until they try it, it is pressure.

3. We sneak a new food in the mix.

> Many parents have had the experience of sneaking in new foods, food groups and calories only to be quickly found out and rejected. We want children to trust their grownups, so sensory surprises can erode trust.

4. We fill the child's plate with a mountain of food to eat or try.

> That mountain of food on the plate can look so daunting, overwhelming. It can feel like pressure as the child imagines they are to eat the whole thing!

5. Dad said "try it" and Mom says "do not worry about it."

> When parents disagree if front of children, there is pressure to take sides. It adds to the overall emotion of the mealtime.

6. Parents gently but persistently coerce their child to eat, only to have him not eat. Parental disappointment is common and not always easy to hide.

> Our praise and our disappointment can both be interpreted as pressure for children. They feel pressure to get our praise and they feel pressure not to disappoint us.

7. Parent or therapist says "Just lick this food."

> Is what we asked even possible? Maybe he cannot even stand the smell, let alone the texture and flavor of the food on his tongue. It can feel like pressure when he just cannot do what we asked.

8. Parent or therapist says "Just put this food on your plate."

> As a feeding therapist, I need to put in my two cents worth here. Children who are really worried about trying new foods do need to learn safe and comfortable ways to try new foods. Smelling, touching, kissing or licking can well be a systematic way to check food out. It is my experience that we can offer these as "new food trying strategies" *without demanding* and while going at the child's pace, thereby eliminating the pressure for extremely worried/anxious eaters. New food trying strategies can be learned at the child's pace away from the table and gradually used at mealtimes as the child is comfortable. But if the grownups demand three licks of the new food before the familiar food, or make the crying child kiss an unwanted food, it is absolutely pressure.

9. "Let's make a chart so you can try it ten times every meal."

> For some children that chart is fun and a celebration, but for others it can feel like ten bites of pressure. We want children to eat because they want it, not for an external motivator. For a child who has begun to try new foods and feel less pressure, we have used charts as a focus of celebration (Check it out later in the book).

Pressure can be everywhere

Once you have made the commitment to reduce the pressure, you will look around and may notice that pressure can be everywhere. It can be at grandparent's home, with the baby sitter, at school and even in therapy clinics. Think about it.

> Dear Parents,
>   Are there some obvious and not so obvious ways you or other love ones are pressuring your child?

Therapy can be pressure

Your child may experience pressure at feeding therapy and this is a conversation to have with your team. Therapists can also be part of the pressure problem. Just like you, therapists want to help and provide lots of ideas on how to feed worried eaters. We have our favorite strategies for helping anxious eaters try new foods. We often include a sequence, a set of recommendations, a protocol of how parents are to present foods. We mean well and want to help but our therapy can be unintentional pressure from your child's perspective. The activity that was playful and fun to one child may feel like big pressure to another. Keep those conversations open with your team to try to create the best learning environment for your child.

Robbie's story

I recall a darling five-year old who drove with his mom to our clinic, three hours from his home. The pressure on the mother was great. She would do <u>anything</u> to help her child, and there was no local support. Her child ate seven or eight specific foods in specific ways. She was worried about a balanced diet. She was worried about what to send him to school for lunches as he was just about to start Kindergarten. There was pressure on Robbie as he had a parentheses diet and did not want foods that were different. His loving parents wanted him to try new foods. He wanted to please them but couldn't handle the big *asks*.

And there was pressure on me, as his feeding therapist. This family did, after all, drive three hours to get to the clinic and would need to drive three hours back after our consultation. I wanted the family to feel that their trip was worthwhile, and that they better understood their anxious eater after attending the session. The sessions with him were extended in length because of the distance the family had traveled. Robbie, Mom, teacher and I explored foods together as we got to know each other. I made absolutely sure that he enjoyed himself and was a part of every activity we tried. We had multiple food exposures and sensory rehearsals as we discussed these ideas. Mom and I practiced them with Robbie. Robbie discovered that he liked crumbs so we made crumbs of his familiar cheese flavored fish crackers. In the course of playing with the fish cracker crumbs, Robbie found that he was interested also in the crumbs of pretzel fish crackers, then crumbs of crispy rice cereal, "O" cereal, and two other cereals. He learned to drink his favorite pouch fruit puree in a cup with a straw as a precursor to smoothie drinking. We were all excited. We began to see change already!

The next week, the family made the trek to the clinic again and Robbie, again, had a good time, tried new things and parents went home with more ideas. But he was much more nervous to try his new foods at home even though Mom had been central to all the activities we had done in clinic. But by week three, Mom reported that Robbie was not comfortable trying these new foods at home <u>at all</u>! AND he came to the clinic that week having had an entire three-hour car ride to think about all the things that we might do in our therapy consultation, all the things he could worry about. He was a bright guy and had figured out that new food trying was what was happening, and though we had had fun with no tears, no meltdowns, and lots of celebration, he was determined to have NOTHING to do with therapy that day. Despite the fact that we tried our best to make it fun and not pressure, to encourage and not provide judgments, or any criticism, HE felt the pressure because he had figured us out. Here is the challenge. We absolutely MUST respond to his pullback. We must listen. But he had already made progress, we already found some strategies that worked, so the challenge was finding balance again.

It is imperative that he feel we are listening, but also that we find ways to continue to help him have the confidence to make changes to his environment. We decided that he could be helped best in a more distant face to face computer session where we gave him and his parents new food trying ideas by video screen while at home. This was the distance he needed. He and his mom prepared a variety of foods that we predetermined prior to the conference call. (And she had other options available in the cupboard or fridge as ideas came up in our explorations). He had weekly support sessions that we divided into parent update chat without his listening ears, and then we explored foods together and then he went off to play while parents and therapists summarized together and made plans for the next week. Robbie established those foods he had tried in the first two sessions, learned to eat them in different ways, learned about crumbs, dips and foods touching. We made plans for the next week of practice at home and he and parents made videos of his food interactions during the week. Robbie needed to be in the safety of his own home to feel comfortable enough to explore new foods.

Children tell us. We must LISTEN

Some children seem to have the same positive first few sessions that Robbie had and they return and have a good time learning in the playful environment of therapy. However, if parents say, *my child did not want to come to therapy today*, or that *he was crying in the parking lot*, it is NOT okay. Therapy has become too much pressure. None of us want this to build up into a BIG WORRY. Something MUST change. We all need to fine tune our *asks* the best we can and try to avoid pressure…and then we adjust whenever we need to. We believe each child. Only your child knows how he is feeling about trying new foods today. By responding to the worry, he will learn to trust that we are trying not to push him **into his worry**. By giving rehearsals, he will know what is coming and not stress.

Pressure happens

Robbie was an important teacher in helping us look at pressure. Our entire goal in clinic is to minimize the pressure. We thought we had! Robbie let us know, *no way, I still imagine pressure. I need extra help.* The most important thing is that we be responsive to HIS cues, that we listen to what HE is saying to us in words or actions. AND, we must adjust, change our asks, change the environment, and dilute the pressure. Can you create a mealtime pressure free zone?

> Dear Parents,
> Are there obvious or not so obvious ways your child's feeding team members are pressuring your child?

Parents feel the pressure

Robbie's therapy needed to be changed to work for him and work to reduce <u>his</u> worry. But parents also tell us feel pressure in scheduling any therapy appointment. One Mom tells us of the pressure of therapy on their household. Imagine. She describes that it takes forty minutes to drive to a therapy clinic or hospital. Then time is needed to find a parking spot and walk with a toddler to the waiting room. Then there is the check in and the wait. Then parents describe the chit chat (actually it is the *how are things going at home* chat), and then the actual "therapy time" and then pack up, walk back to the parking garage, and drive back home. This could easily be a four-hour chunk of time or more. Half of a day. Though the parent may be motivated to bring the child for treatment, therapists need to understand how this actually fits into their day. In order to get to therapy on time, a meal might need to be eliminated or shortened. Siblings may need to be farmed out to sitters. The parent may have the expectation that the child will make up those calories in therapy and maybe that does not happen. The child is then too tired when she gets home to eat her afternoon snack, so in order to attend a therapy session which is supposed to help, the day's meals and intake are disrupted. Of course, I am not saying therapist does not help or is not warranted, but therapists should understand what the parent does to get there and the pressures on parents just to participate. Imagine it you are the parent and part of this interaction is that you are sent to the waiting room because your child is "not compliant," or if your child ends up in tears!

Re-calibrate the mealtime

Research tells us that when our parental worry turns into *pressure to eat* tactics it can lead to even more food avoidance.[25,48,49,50] In other words, our pressure can cause them not to eat more as we intend and hope, but to actually eat less.

We ask for a family to make a commitment for change. What needs to happen at YOUR mealtime to re-calibrate the mealtime, to get rid of the pressure altogether? Can reduced pressure become a new way of life not reduced pressure one day and increased pressure the next? Can the whole family get on board with reduce pressure? That will involve changes in conversations, body language and expectation. How can your child re-learn to trust that mealtimes will be a comfortable and that from now on?

But for you to feel good about reducing the pressure, you may need help in understanding your child's eating and in learning what specifically it will take for you to see progress. It is hard to eliminate the pressure that you thought would help, without an alternative way to help. You need new ideas, new strategies, and you must be able to see progress. This book offers those strategies.

Dear Parent,

What needs to happen at YOUR mealtime to re-calibrate the mealtime, to get rid of the pressure altogether, to make it a NO PRESSURE ZONE?

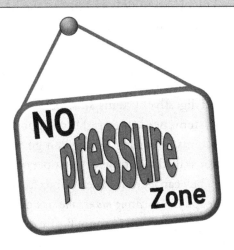

The Now, Then and Yet of Mealtimes

"Children and parents bring their past mealtime memories to the table."
Suzanne Evans Morris

Eating is complicated and involves multiple systems in the body. It involves internal and external muscles for sucking, swallowing and chewing and moving food through the body for proper digestion. It involves muscles to help bring food to the mouth and muscles for postural support. It involves all the main senses of smell, touch and taste, sight and sound. It involves breathing systems and cardiac systems. It involves the brain and emotional and digestive systems. It involves having all the anatomy and physiology work. Lots of systems need to go right to support eating.

When any of these systems go wrong, eating can go wrong. Children who do not feel well, or who are not skilled at eating for multiple reasons, can *learn to be very cautious* about mealtimes. They can learn that new foods cause anaphylactic reactions and stressful trips to the hospital. Or *eating makes me sick* or causes pain. Or children learn *I cannot breathe and eat.* Children who cannot figure out how to chew, can worry about big, or maybe even small, pieces of food in their mouths. Or children can learn that food just feels wrong in their mouth. Children can then learn that mealtime feels like BIG PRESSURE when their grownups feed them, want them to eat more, want them to eat less, or want them to eat differently.

The NOW of eating

As we are trying to understand each child's eating issues, we need to look at the **NOW** of eating. What are mealtimes like for your child right now? What is working **NOW** and what is not? Here are some of the things therapists will want to know when working with you to understand the layers of influence on your child's **NOW** of eating.

The *Now* of Eating- The Current Mealtime Situation

What is the current diet?	What are the foods on your child's *List*?	Your thoughts? What is working and what is not?
What is your current mealtime routine?	When does your child eat? Where are meals held? Is there a family mealtime?	
What is the current level of independence?	Does your child feed himself part or all of the meal, or does your child want to be fed? If you feed your child, does he look at the spoon, or help you with the utensils?	
Who does your child eat with?	Who feeds your child? Is anyone else present and eating?	

Where does your child sit turn eating and is his posture supported?	Do feet touch the floor? Is the table a good height?	
What is the current level of mealtime worry?	What worries your child at mealtimes?	
Does your child experience pressure to eat?	Is your child asked to eat, try, taste new foods that worry him? Does he feel pressure to finish his food, clean his plate, eat a certain amount before he can leave the table?	
Does your child feel well?	Constipated, allergies, vomiting, gagging, other health problems? Your child's medical team will ask many questions in this area to be sure your child is feeling well enough for good eating and good growth. Together you will make a list of further questions to explore with medical professionals.	

Does your child trust his grownups?	Is he calm at the table? Is he worried that you might sneak a new food in his foods, offer a sensory (texture or flavor) surprise?	
Does he know how to try new foods?	Is he being asked to try new foods in a way that works for him?	
Does he have positive mealtime modeling?	Does your child get to see others eating enjoying foods, and eating food beyond his List?	
Does your child have opportunities to interact positively with foods without pressure or expectation?	Does your child get to help prepare foods, or be around you as you prepare food?	
Does your child have the mouth skills to chew and swallow food?	Is chewing and swallowing easy or challenging for your child? (Your child's feeding therapist can look at this with you).	

Does your child have the motor skills to feed himself or be an active participant in the meals?	Can your child use utensils independently or help you to feed him? Do the utensils fit? Does he let you know when he is hungry or when he wants more?	
Does your child enjoy the sensations of eating?	Does your child enjoy the smells, textures and feels, tastes and sounds of the food?	
How is the mealtime working for you?	How do **you** feel about the mealtime? Is it stressful? Enjoyable? Are other family members enjoying the mealtime?	

Think about these aspects of the **NOW** of your family mealtime as a starting point for looking in depth about what is happening. Your feeding team will also want to look with you the past experiences that got you both to the **NOW**. What has happened in the past that might influence how your child feels about food and mealtimes today? What caused your child to not want to eat? Where are the layers of worry? We call this the **THEN**. The **THEN** is what past experiences and memories your child (and you) bring to the mealtime which influences your expectation and enjoyment of the meal. The **THEN** helps you understand how your child got to this place with all this worry, this **NOW** of eating.

What food and mealtime experiences has your child had?	Did early feeding go well? Were these experiences positive or negative?	Your thoughts? What worked and did not work?
What eating challenges has your child had?	Muscle challenges, sensory challenges? Scary experiences?	
What medical/ health challenges have interfered with feeling good about eating?	Tummy problems, teeth problems, ear and throat problems? Breathing problems? Children bring those memories to the meal!	
Has there been pressure?	From where, what kind? Obvious, not so obvious?	
Has there been nutritional supplementation?	Special formulas? Tube feedings?	
What have been the influence on appetite?	Medications? Constipation Is there a mealtime routine at your house that allows for hunger at meals?	

The *Yet* of Mealtime

Once you and your feeding team understand the **NOW** and **THEN** of mealtime, you will begin to piece together the puzzle of what is going on, where it might have come from, and you can start to understand how to piece together help. You can begin to look forward. I will call this the **YET** of mealtime. The **YET** is what is to come, the **hope** of change in the future.

Instead of thinking about how your child does not drink from a straw, how about, *he has not YET learned to drink from a straw?* This reminds you that hope is around the corner. **YET** is possible. Instead of thinking that your child only eats crunchy foods, how about that he is not **YET** comfortable with wet foods? **Yet** reminds us of hope. Understanding that the top challenge is medical allows us to find medical treatment. Understanding that the problem is sensory allows us to thoughtfully support sensory. Understanding that top the problem is worry allows us to reduce our pressure and their need for worry. Understanding that change is really hard allows us to offer change much more carefully. Understanding prepares us for **YET,** for hope. Carol Dweck has made a TedTalk™ entitled "The Power of YET." [1,2] I encourage you to check it out. It is a great one that will give you hope.

Maximize the Meal

To help your child be as successful as possible during eating you will want to use the information gained in your child's evaluation, the NOW, THEN and YET to maximize his meal. Eating may be hard enough all by itself, so we need to be sure to set you and your child up for success.

Feel well

When talking with your child's pediatrician or other professionals on the feeding team, you will want to be sure your child feels well. Are there specific medical challenges in the THEN and NOW of eating that will decrease your child's health and appetite for eating? When we do not feel well, we do not want to eat. Our appetite can be negatively influenced. Appetite helps in new food trying! It is important to work with specialists for systems affecting your child's health and well-being to optimize how your child feels. Eating is complicated and has lots of layers so if you have a concern about your child's health ask it! Your pediatrician is a good place to start in asking those questions.

I would like to especially call out the gastrointestinal systems. They can influence appetite, and how well the food is being digested and utilized and moved through the body. Many children have or have had GI pain and discomfort from gastroesophageal reflux, allergies, and imbalances of gut bacteria. Allergies can negatively influence appetite and interest in foods. Chronic constipation happens. This gets its own mention because it is so common with anxious eaters. Bowel health can be negatively influenced by chronic stress. And when children are constipated, they may want to eat less. Work with your child's pediatrician or dietitian to help your child have regular bowel movements. You will be glad you did.

Postural support

All the muscle systems affect the efficiency of eating from overall posture, to muscles for self-feeding, chewing and swallowing to internal muscles of breathing and digestion. In the NOW of eating you and your team will look at your child's posture during eating. What kind of a chair is used? Does the chair support his trunk in a nice upright position? Are feet resting solidly on the floor or a support? Is an added foot rest needed? Is the chair at a good height at the table for self-feeding? Posture is important from infant feeding in arms where all the support is external to highchairs, booster seats, and family dining chairs where increasing amounts of internal postural control is needed.

One area that is often overlooked is foot support. We move children from our arms to a high chair as they learn to sit and be upright. The challenges increase as children are brought to the family table. The chairs are big and the children are small. Extra cushions and booster seats certainly help bring the child up to the table, but often feet are the challenge.

There are short children-sized tables and chairs where bottoms fit nicely on chairs and feet fit nicely on the floor. But as we bring children up to the table where we want them to experience all the great learning and interaction of the family meal at the height where they can feed themselves, we lose the feet. They can dangle. Work with your child's team to see if the chair and table situation at your house supports your child's overall posture and especially look at the feet. If your child's therapy team comes to your house, have them take a peek and brainstorm with you about how you might better support his posture. OR if you go to a clinic, take a picture or video of your child eating at your family table to review with your team. Especially look at your child's posture, including feet. Your child may need a foot rest added. (Those phone books you never use could be covered and stacked to be used as a foot rest.) Many families especially like some of the chairs on the market today that are adjustable so they can grow with your child to be at the right height for self-feeding while also having a foot rest that can be adjusted as your child grows and those legs get longer! It is easier for all muscles in the body to function best when your child is sitting with bottom, back and feet supported well.

Environmental support

We want the environment of eating to attract your child to the table and support his focus and attention into the meal. Take a moment to look around and listen to your meal. Is it quiet? Is it loud and enthusiastic? Music, no music? We encourage meals to be conversational and enjoyable so your child can focus on the meal. Some environments can be very distracting for our anxious eaters, who already are not even sure they want to be around the new foods. If the TV is on nearby, it could be quite a distraction. (You may have determined that the TV distraction helps. We can talk about that later). But for many children it takes attention away from the meal and you as a feeder. Consider it carefully.

School cafeterias can be one of the most challenging environments. Lots of children, lots of enthusiastic conversations, lots of smells, the clanking of utensils, opening and closing of lunch boxes, crumpling of bags, and the inevitable dropping of things can make it quite a noisy place. Some anxious eaters are more comfortable eating at a table with fewer children or in an alternative situation so as to minimize the distractions and mealtime noise as they are gaining expanded confidence in their eating. Work with your child's school to best meet your child's needs. (Check out the Anxious Eaters at School Chapter).

School Cafeteria

My son often doesn't eat anything at school because he "ran out of time." They get 15 minutes, at most, to eat and if he wants to get in line for food there is much less time available! If he gets distracted at all, his lunchbox comes home full. He does not drink water. He only takes apple juice or chocolate milk to drink, but he can't have those in the classroom. So, if he does not drink them at lunch, he often hasn't had anything to drink all day either.

I went to the school to have lunch with him a couple of times just to try to understand the situation. I didn't like it either! The lighting, tremendous noise, smells, kids not doing what they're supposed to... and knowing we only had a few minutes was all very stressful, even for me! No wonder he often does not eat his lunch!

Parents might consider going to their child's school to experience their child's cafeteria mealtime. I found that it helped me understand a bit more of what my son was experiencing and how to work with the school to help him. ~Lauri Ziemba

Transition support

Transitions matter at mealtimes. Consider this. So many children we are talking about are already not enjoying some parts of mealtime. The smells, the sounds and the expectations can be overwhelming. New food trying can be overwhelming. It is, therefore, understandable that going **to the meal** may well NOT be their favorite activity. Now imagine your child is doing something he enjoys, playing on the screen time, playing with favorite cars or action figures, coloring, and NOW you want him to be interrupted, to leave THAT favored activity, and go to the meal. The transition can be tough.

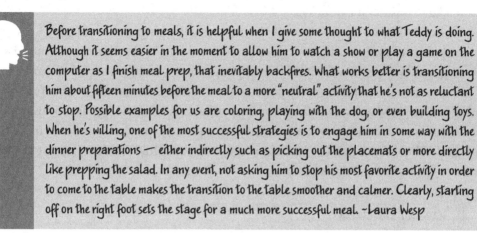

Before transitioning to meals, it is helpful when I give some thought to what Teddy is doing. Although it seems easier in the moment to allow him to watch a show or play a game on the computer as I finish meal prep, that inevitably backfires. What works better is transitioning him about fifteen minutes before the meal to a more "neutral" activity that he's not as reluctant to stop. Possible examples for us are coloring, playing with the dog, or even building toys. When he's willing, one of the most successful strategies is to engage him in some way with the dinner preparations — either indirectly such as picking out the placemats or more directly like prepping the salad. In any event, not asking him to stop his most favorite activity in order to come to the table makes the transition to the table smoother and calmer. Clearly, starting off on the right foot sets the stage for a much more successful meal. ~Laura Wesp

These step downs are a great idea. They could be going from one preferred activity to a less preferred activity as Laura describes. Your child may also need a **sensory step down** on the way to the table.

Sensory support

Mealtimes are sensory. We will describe all the specific sensory aspects of food including the look, sound, smell, texture, and taste later in the book in great detail as we try to find ways to not overwhelm children with our food offers. We will describe ways to rehearse those sensory aspects of the foods ahead of the meal.

However, there are other components to well-functioning sensory systems. Many of the children we are discussing have diagnosed (or un-diagnosed) Sensory Processing Disorders, problems with sensory integration. You and they may need some extra sensory support in the transition to the meal. Some children who are more excitable in their senses may need some *sensory calming* before the meal. Some may need some sensory *waking up* if they process sensory information on the calmer side of the sensory continuum. Some sensory therapists recommend preparing your child with some massage prior to the meal, or some deep pressure as you march with them to the meal with your hands on their shoulders giving some focused downward pressure to let them know YOU ARE HERE and together we are going to the meal in a focused and calm way. Other children clearly need to know the mealtime routine. First, we wash our hands, then we set the table, then we eat. Knowing what is next helps many children.

Other children are given the recommendation of wearing a weighted vest or sensory pressure shirt to the meal and during the meal to see if it helps them focus. Your child's sensory therapist will make those recommendations as she or he gets to know your child. You can observe and see if those recommendations help.

Utensil support

Shoes need to fit feet. Spoons and forks also need to fit hands. If your small child is learning about and becoming proficient with utensils, take care that they are toddler or child-sized and fit his hands. When spoons are too big, it is harder to be coordinated with them and if we are trying to maximize the meal, can the utensils fit his little hands? We also increase success, for example, with new spoon users if we give them food to use in practice that sticks well to the spoon when it is dipped in the bowl. Yogurts, oatmeal, refried beans and puddings are the kind of food choices that can stick to the spoon so it is less likely to all fall off between the bowl and the mouth! Dips and dippers are a great utensil practice as the dipper becomes a utensil. (Check out Dips and Dipper Chapter).

To optimize beginning spoon skills, you will want the bowl to stay steady and not move around the table. When the bowl moves your child has the spoon AND the food AND the bowl to worry about. Consider the non-skid mats that have bowls and divided plates built in to minimize the skid. Children and parents love them!

Mouth support

To maximize the meal, mouths need support. Your child's feeding therapist will help you look carefully at your child's chewing and swallowing skills and provide support as needed. Many anxious eaters need improved oral skills, either due to lack of experience or due to coordination challenges. If your child eats one yogurt brand only (and nothing else), he is probably very inexperienced with chew-able foods. HOWEVER, within the category of new food trying, he may be able to learn more about new food trying with other yogurts and purees before having to learn a new food (CHANGE!) AND new chewing skills. To chew, the texture needs to be quite different, so it becomes TWO changes, texture change AND food change. Some children do better with one change at a time.

Nutritional support

Nutrition is a concern when children have parentheses diets. You will need to work with your pediatrician or dietitian to look at the Big Picture of your child's growth and diet and determine priorities. Change is hard, so these recommendations need to be made carefully considering nutritional needs, as well as growth and your child's level of worry. There will be more about his later.

Emotional support

And to maximize mealtime support for your child, it may help to reintroduce yourself to him as his food helper, the person who will help him and guide him, not the enforcer of scary big new food trying rules. Throughout this book we will explore together some ways to help him be successful in new food interactions one tiny step at a time.

The Stories

When I first started learning about feeding children as an occupational therapist there was very little information out there. Back then we did not learn about feeding at our university programs and the books, chapters and research were not yet out there as they are today! I was working at a day care for fragile babies and due to their medical complications and neurological challenges most needed to be fed at mealtimes. As a young therapist, I wanted to be of help. So, I jumped in and offered to feed babies every lunchtime. The staff were still learning about feeding these children so I learned from each parent about what worked for them at home. My goal in feeding each baby was to nourish them and…not to do harm. These babies had complicated challenges! I learned from carefully offering foods and carefully watching their reactions. I adjusted, as needed. I learned from their parents, and I learned from them. Decades later, we have more books, more courses, more research, but I still believe we have much to learn from parents and children.

I would like to share stories that have been most influential as I have gathered ideas on how to help children eat. There is one from my own life, one each from two adults who could articulately describe their own eating worries, one from a parent of triplets, all of whom had eating challenges, and one from an eight-year old, Brady, the boy who is the inspiration for this book, the handsome boy on the cover.

Grasshopper Story

Of all things, grasshoppers helped me imagine being a worried eater! Here is the story. When my sons were ten and thirteen we traveled to Oaxaca, Mexico to study Spanish for a month in an immersion program. We lived and ate with a local family. We were served absolutely delicious food for the entire month and on our last day, our hostess went to the mercado and brought home a *surprise*. "What is it?" we asked in our newly emerging Spanish. Her response was "chapulinas." We had to look up the word in our Spanish dictionary as she could not translate it into English. It was *grasshoppers*. Yes, really, *grasshoppers*.

We wanted to be polite. We wanted to appreciate our surprise, but *grasshoppers*??! Really?! My children looked at me as if to say, *Mom, YOU are going FIRST*, so I started checking them out. First off, they were dead. That seemed like a good start as I had read that in some parts of the world people eat *live* bugs. Next, they obviously smelled like garlic and I like garlic. However, the very large bowl of grasshoppers was all *parts*, head *parts*, body *parts*, leg *parts*, antenna *parts*…parts! Now I began to seriously get worried. I asked our hostess, "how do we eat them?" She demonstrated as she piled some guacamole on a flour tortilla and then put on a handful of them, yes, a handful of *parts*, folded the tortilla and ate the delicacy! All eyes were on me. It was my turn to eat grasshoppers.

I took a tortilla, which I like, and put on LOTS of guacamole, which I also like. Then I bravely felt one little *"part"* with my fingertips, put it on the pile of guacamole, folded it and ate it. My mouth felt a tiny little crunch, but I expected a crunch because it had crunched between my fingers. Everyone giggled. I was proud I did not embarrass myself by gagging. But, the *trying* was not over. This was not a little snack for the *gringo family*, it was LUNCH. So, by my fourth one, I still had a lot of guacamole, but I could put on a whole cluster of *parts*. They did not *taste* particularly bad or good as my generous mounds of guacamole dominated the flavor but they were noticeably *crunchy* in the center of the mouthful. We all lived through this experience with lots of laughter and photos.

I realized later that I had just experienced being a worried eater and I naturally did the things we do to help our worried eater friends. First, I *looked* at the new food, and asked about it. I *smelled* it and could relate to a smell that I already liked (garlic). I *watched* someone else eating it. I *felt* it with my fingers while preparing it. I got to try it at *my own pace* with lots of guacamole and tortilla initially to camouflage the worrisome taste and texture. I added a little more of the worrisome food at my pace and I fed it *to myself*. It was clear to me that if someone else had put a pile of grasshoppers on a spoon and tried to FEED ME, I would have gagged or vomited and it would have been an overall very bad experience. Because I was able to go at my own pace, I ended up having a good time (even though grasshoppers may never end up on my favorite food list!).

I learned, first hand, we need to respect the *worry* when children are anxious about trying new foods. We need to help them learn something about the new food ahead of time through watching us and through all their senses and *absolutely* let them go at their pace. New food offering may well be easier if parents of worried consider every new food they offer their child to be a *grasshopper*. Throughout this book I will use this powerful grasshopper story as a reference in our strategies for support of children worried about trying new foods. Check out the YouTube video or the Grasshopper story and share it![51]

Kind Dad's story

Years ago, we had a support group for parents of children who had both a diagnosis on the autism spectrum *and* feeding challenges. New parents shared their story and worries and veteran parents shared their experiences and insight. A new Dad came to the group and had realized as his child was just diagnosed with Asperger's Syndrome, that he probably had the diagnosis himself. This was eye opening for him that his child had this diagnosis and that the criterion for the diagnosis in the literature provided by the psychologist described him as well as describing his child. And this was not surprising to him as he had always described himself as "quirky" and shared that he, too, had and has many, many eating challenges. He told us he still does not like to eat, but knows he has to eat to stay alive and has found ways to eat that work for him.

He described growing up with his own very serious eating challenges and at that time there was not help for his parents to guide them or him. He liked only a few foods. The foods were of a certain color and texture and familiarity. His well-meaning parents wanted him to eat more and different foods, a balanced diet! He remembered that when he was about twelve, his parents would make him sit at the table *until he finished dinner.* The challenge for him was that they were not offering him *food.* To him, he was offered random stuff that was not *food.* It was not on his *List.* Of course, he could NOT, did NOT eat it. So, he would sit at the table *"until he finished,"* and in the end, he did NOT eat it. By ten in the evening everyone was sufficiently frustrated that he would go to bed without having eaten the food. He told us what he learned was that 1.) He hated mealtimes; 2.) He was more powerful than his parents and that they could not make him do *anything* and that 3.) He HATED his parents.

His parents, who probably just wanted him to eat a balanced diet, tried. They believed that if they pressured him into eating new foods, they could get to a balanced diet. But, they unintentionally pushed him away and caused even more problems. From this man's perspective looking back on being twelve, *no one understood.* When remembering the foods his parents would want him to eat from his current grown up perspective, he gave this analogy. Imagine someone offering YOU a glass of kerosene and a piece of carpet and told you it was lunch. YOU would know it absolutely was not lunch. YOU would know that was not food and was NOT going in YOUR mouth. He said, for him, everything offered that was not *his* food, he KNEW was not food and, of course, he would not eat it. Imagine?!

He told the group that, as an adult, he still hates food, but has learned to live with his very quirky eating. He *knows* he must eat to survive. His wife knows just how he likes food presented and served so he knows there will be no food challenges at home, unless she inadvertently mismatches the bread shape when putting together a sandwich. They have learned to navigate the world of eating with others. At buffets he always eats at home first so if there is nothing that appeals to him, at least he has eaten. On the off chance there is some food he knows, it is an extra. Dinner invitations are hard because he knows they will have to sit down at a table and be served a particular (not familiar) meal. They have learned to suggest, *let's just go out to eat* (at one of three restaurants he likes in our town). Of course, he orders the same foods at the restaurant every time they go and hates it when the restaurant change the menu! And, he still prefers to take those offending salad parts away from touching his lettuce. He puts them on the side of his plate and *prefers* that his wife removes them, but, if she can't, he can now tolerate the lettuce, even with those offending parts on the side of his plate! And he was so proud. He had just learned to eat pizza! He had realized that eating pizza was a *social thing* that he should work on and work on it he did. It took him a while. Now he likes pizza. Of course, he likes cheese pizza from one particular local restaurant!

This concerned Dad looked at the group so seriously and said, *If I can share one thing with you all who have picky eaters, please... do not teach them to hate you! Pressuring them will not help. Try another way.* Goodness, there was not a dry eye in the group. He shared from his heart.

From Kind Dad I learned, we must find a way to help our anxious eaters with love and understanding and without the pressure. We must prioritize the relationship between a child and his parents. This is hard work and anxious children need a guide, a partner, not a PRESSURER. And, as a feeding therapist, I want to NEVER make recommendations that draw a wedge between a parent and a child! We must honor that relationship. And I learned we need prioritize goals that help each child learn the lifelong skills of eating with others. They will need to learn how to say "no thank you" and survive eating out.

Marta's story

Marta, a co-worker, described herself as a very picky eater enjoying only a handful of foods, mostly in the brown, beige and potato *food groups*. She wanted to find new foods that she could like to expand her short list of favored foods, as she had recently married and was very aware of the narrowness, the *extreme* narrowness of her diet. She wanted to eat out more with her husband. But, she was discouraged. When asked about her usual strategy for trying new foods, she relayed this story:

> Marta: *I put the new food on a fork. I plug my nose with one hand and with the other I quickly grab the glass of water and wash it down.* While describing this technique, her face was scrunched up and miserable as she demonstrated choking down the food!
>
> Me: *And how is that technique working for you?*
>
> Marta: *Terribly, I HATE trying new foods and I am not finding any new ones I like!*

Is that a surprise? Can you imagine? If that was the technique you needed to use to try new foods, you probably would not find new enjoyable foods either! Instead of finding new foods she liked, she was overwhelming herself each time she tried a new food. No wonder she hated trying new foods. For starters, she needed to hear the Grasshopper Story!

Then, we discussed a possible new food trying strategy that may make it easier for her. Could she pick a food that she wanted to try? Could she start *small* taking a tiny bite of the food? OR Could she *pair the new* food with a food she likes already to dilute the taste, smell and texture of the new food?

The first food Marta wanted to try was salmon as her new husband *really liked* salmon and it was a frequent choice. Here was the new strategy we imagined for her. She could be around the salmon when her husband prepared it and sit with him as he was eating his (a kind of rehearsal). She liked bread, so I suggested she make a tiny sandwich (quarter or nickel size) with two small pieces of bread surrounding the tiniest morsel (pea size) of salmon. (The flavor and texture of the salmon would be diluted). She could *try* that. How tiny would the salmon piece need to be and how big would the bread pieces need to be so she did not feel the need to chug a drink of water as it landed on her tongue? When if she found that the first tiny sandwich was OKAY, she could try more and more salmon with bread and gradually make a tiny open-faced sandwich bite? The bread could be decreased as she was ready. She could increase the amount of new food at HER pace. She learned to like salmon, and seven new foods in that first two-week period after our cheerleading support! I could not help but think, if a bright and thoughtful adult thought THAT was trying, my goodness, we have work to do in teaching about new food trying! And we need to **Re-Define Try It**! *Just try it*, for anxious eaters can be way too scary.

Instead of thinking of *try it* as that mound of a new food or a mound of grasshoppers on a spoon, let us think of *try it* as a series of little food explorations that help the worried child get more comfortable all along the way. We want to start way back at safe and comfortable. We, then, want to tip toe toward the worry without pushing them into a *too scary* place.

Kind Triplet Mom

I knew a family who had triplets. All three of them had feeding tubes. You can imagine that all you do all day long when you have triplet babies is feed them! I tried to sensitively share ideas for feeding them. Lots of ideas. Looking back, I functioned on a philosophy that boiled down to "offer as many ideas as possible and some will fit!" I thought I was being helpful. I thought I was offering choices. But this incredibly kind mother was able to tell me the ideas were too many. It was hard to even have any idea about where to start. I had made an assumption that an overwhelmed mom could get from all these ideas to success, that she could just adapt them as needed. I did not take into careful enough consideration the three babies, the all-day feedings, the grief, worry, and details of their daily life. I learned from this Kind Triplet Mom that we need to partner carefully with our ideas and that each family will need to let us know what they can do, what they think might work for them, and where THEY want to start. It is our job to help them be successful, not to add to the stress of feeding challenges.

Brady's story

Brady was eight when I met him. He has had lots of challenges trying new foods. But, he loved videos and wanted to use the knowledge and skills he learned about trying new foods to make a video to help other kids. When we asked him, *"Is there anything you would like to share with parents of other kids who are worried about trying new foods?"* He said, *"Yes. When your kids do not want to rush in to try new foods, it is okay...Give them time...Help them."* Check out and share Brady's You Tube link.[52]

Brady reminded us that this is a slow process. We must be patient, give children time to go at their own pace and, most importantly, help them. After meeting hundreds and hundreds of these worried the specifics of new food trying so they have ideas and confidence to figure out how to even go about to try a new food.

Circle of Sensitivity

These stories have provided the foundation for the support of anxious eaters and their families that you will see described throughout this book. The grasshopper story is the foundation that helped me imagine being in the child's shoes, being an anxious eater. Marta's story inspired us to reconsider what we mean by "Try It." Kind Dad inspired us to love and celebrate our children and that they are doing the best they can. He told us pressure does not help and most importantly to support and nurture the special relationship between children and their parents. Kind Triplet Mom taught us that parents are in the middle of these complicated stories and they need to be the ones to have success. *They* are at mealtimes a number of times per day. *They* are the ones doing the hard work and *they* need to be celebrated. And Brady. Eight-year-old, Brady has told us that this is a slow process and anxious eaters need time. He tells us, "give them time, help them."

Throughout this book you will find little stories and examples from parents who live this journey. They too are helping us continue to grow and expand our understanding of what children and families are going through and how best to help them.

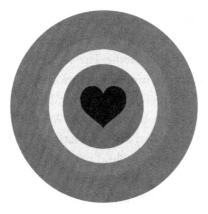

This Circle of Sensitivity is a visual starting place of caring that you will see adapted throughout this book. It helps us visualize the child's many layers of protection and worry that surround joyful eating. The heart at the center of this diagram is your child and her enjoyment of eating. The heart can be the confident trying of new foods. It can be enjoyable mealtime interactions. The heart represents the goal of happy mealtimes. We want to find a way to help our worried eaters get from their starting point *here,* to their new comfortable place with eating, new foods, and new mealtime enjoyment, *there,* in tiny, achievable, successful steps that do not create more worry along the way.

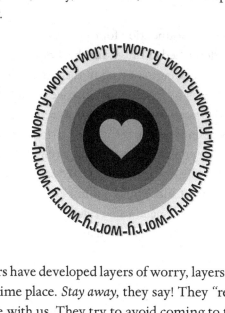

But anxious eaters have developed layers of worry, layers of protection, surrounding that happy mealtime place. *Stay away,* they say! They "refuse" the food we offer. They try to negotiate with us. They try to avoid coming to the table. They tell us *no thanks.* They tell us, *No, really, NO THANKS!* They push the food away, or even gag or vomit. As we bombard them with our loving pressure to eat new foods, we can unintentionally **push into their outer worry layers** fortifying their worry rather than reducing it. When we say *have another bite, finish this, just try it,* or *eat it,* children worry more, protect more, resist more, build more layers of protection increasing their mealtime stress and the stress of those around them. Some even describe these layers of protection as behavior problems. I don't. What if we think of their responses as protection from worry rather than a problematic behavior? Jennifer McGloughlin, CCC-SLP, co-author of <u>Helping Your Child with Extreme Picky Eating</u> [32] tells us "a child with problematic behavior is communicating that there is a problem. It's our job to listen and pay close attention to determine what the problem is and help the child solve that problem—then they can focus on developing skills."[53] Are we listening?

> Dear Parent,
>
> Has your child exhibited any problematic "behaviors" at mealtime? Can you imagine what your child might have been communicating?

When we see resistance as layers of worry instead of behavior problems, we can carefully tiptoe toward their worry place, their vulnerability, one layer at a time so each child can be comfortable and successful at each layer before moving closer to their worry. We can offer, listen and respond with empathy as we try to help them find that center heart of food enjoyment. By tiptoeing, we are guiding them and making this journey WITH them sensitively watching their response. We will call this the **Circle of Sensitivity Hug**. It is the visual that defines our embrace of the child as we lovingly guide him. As we gradually reduce those layers of worry in tiny asks to help them get to happier eating at the center heart. Can we help it feel like a **hug rather than a push**? Can we reduce their need for protection and help them get to *enjoyment*? Can we be their loving, understanding food guide?

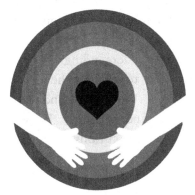

Circle of Sensitivity Hug

We can encircle the child with love, teach them and *guide* them into mealtime enjoyment. We start with the child's comfortable place, comfortable list foods. You will see many different food interactions in this book described through these circles of sensitivity. Each strategy will be described as offers that help you help your child break through layers of worry one layer and little tiny steps at a time.

Grade the *Asks*

If we want a child to respond differently to foods, WE MUST CHANGE SOMETHING. We are giving our children experiences to see what foods, what exposures, what interactions inspire them to be curious about a new food. We want to engage children when we can and when they can to talk about new food trying. I might say things like, *I would like to help you try new foods when you are ready. Sometimes it takes a while for tongues (mouths?) to find new foods to like. We can try some foods together. I can help you.* (Remember our Circle of Sensitivity Hug!) TOGETHER you will get there!

It is my experience that children are more confident at new food trying when they are partners in the decision making and when they know we are helping them, guiding them, offering or asking not demanding. We want to find ways to sensitively help them *want* the foods we offer, to lean *into* the meal with a positive tilt. We will offer, but they can tell us *yes* or *no*. We want to find ways that our food invitation is careful so our anxious eaters can find enjoyment. We want to make the food invitation comfortable enough that they are curious about it and *want* to interact with it!

Grade the *ask*

The *ask* is what we, as grownups who care for these children, do. Can we grade our *ask?* By this we mean, can we carefully ask your child to try a new food in a way that does not push into his worry? An *ask* is just that, an offer and not a demand. *Asks* have many layers of influence. We can carefully grade our *ask* in its safety, developmental appropriateness, sensory challenge, motor readiness, emotional worry, and independence opportunity. Let's consider our *asks*.

> **Safety *Ask*:** Are we asking the child to try a food that is safe for him? If he is scared that he will choke or cough and aspirate and increase fear, he will probably want to resist. If the safety *ask* is too great, the right response from the child is to protect himself from the food offered.

We can grade our safety *ask* by being careful to give a food or liquid that will be safe. Maybe a child who aspirates and has an unsafe swallow needs his liquids thickened to improve the likelihood of a safe swallow or the drink may need to be offered in a different way. Your child's feeding therapist will let you know when and how to gradually change the thickness as your child demonstrates skill and confidence with a maturing swallow. Or maybe your child has trouble organizing food in his mouth for chewing. We might give him smaller meltable or tiny crumbs of a solid rather than big pieces of hard-to-chew cookie or provide a type of food net that does not allow pieces to scatter. We generally start small. We want our *ask* to be safe. It is distressing for children to trust their grownups, only to find themselves with food offers that are very scary, or even life threatening. They want to trust us and we need to be trustworthy and grade our safety *ask*.

> **Developmental *Ask*:** Is the food we are asking them to try developmentally appropriate? If the developmental *ask* is too great, the child will fail and increase the worry.

We can grade developmental *asks*. There is a continuum of developmental steps to being an independent eater. Babies suck breast or bottle then are introduced carefully to solids. Some get to solids through purees and others through tiny soft and safe tastes. They are fed and then learn to feed themselves. Developmentally we do not ask babies to eat solids before they can suck and swallow efficiently. We do not make children feed themselves when they do not have head control. Development follows sequences, tiny steps of progress, each step building on the previous step, the previous skill and the previous experiences. Our developmental *ask* needs to match their skills in this sequence.

> **Sensory *Ask*:** Are the sensations of the food the best sensory *ask*? Is the change between comfortable, favored food smell, texture, sound and appearance too different and too big of an *ask*? Can we grade the *ask* into smaller achievable, less scary little steps? Have we combined too many new sensory variables into one *ask*? Do we need to separate out the sensory variables such as flavor from texture, look from taste?

We can grade the sensory *ask*. We can very carefully look at each child's sensory preferences and start with their *here*. If your child likes only the thin smoothness of baby food pureed apricots, it will be a huge sensory leap to offer Irish cooked oatmeal. Both are purees, but the *ask* is BIG. If your child only likes a particular vanilla smoothie, a green smoothie may be too big of an *ask*. If he is worried big food smells, offering aromatic salmon or Brussel sprouts may be a big *ask*.

> **Motor *Ask***: Does the child have the chewing and swallowing skills needed to eat this new food? Will the child be successful with motor coordination of chewing and swallowing this food without getting scared? Is the motor *ask* appropriate to the skills the child demonstrates?

We can grade our motor *ask*. Sucking, swallowing and chewing are motor skills. These are coordinated activities that the mouth does. We need to ask children to interact with food that requires a motor response that is *possible* for them. If they have experience, skill and confidence only with purees, they will not yet be ready to chew a piece of steak or piece of dried apricot. That is too big of a motor *ask*.

> **Emotional *Ask*:** Children bring their past worried food experiences to the table with them. Anxious eaters can be emotional about eating and their parents can emotional about mealtimes. Trying new foods can be hard for everyone. Is the *ask* starting at a place where the child is comfortable and tiptoeing toward the new flavor, texture, smell, and trying of the new food? Does the emotional *ask* allow the child to be comfortable along the way?

We can grade our emotional *ask*. Children who have been worried about eating can be emotional or fearful about mealtimes. Are we asking our worried new *food try-ers* to just try a mouthful of shrimp? This may well push right into their worry and be too big of an emotional *ask*. If he has choked on a piece of pizza, asking him to eat a big mouthful may push too close to the worry memory.

> **Independence *Ask*:** Remember the grasshoppers? I would have vomited or, at a minimum, gagged if someone else had plopped a spoonful of grasshoppers on my tongue. Each child should be allowed to participate in the process of bringing food to their own mouth. Are we allowing the child to pace the trying by allowing them to actively help in the approach to their mouth? Is our independence *ask* appropriate for success and reducing, not contributing to their stress?

We can grade our independence *ask*. If we ask a baby to completely feed themselves before they are ready, they would starve. We offer a period of co-feeding where we do it together with supervision and tiny successful opportunities. Babies are given the safety net of breast feeding or bottle feeding while they develop the skills to eat foods and feed themselves. On the flip side, if we insist that we do the feeding when they are perfectly capable of feeding themselves, it can be a poorly grading independence *ask* as we are interfering with their ability to be independent.

> Dear Parent,
>
> Are you grading your asks? Is what you are offering possible?
> Or might it be too big of an ask?

Systematic de-sensitization vs flooding

To find more information about helping anxious eaters and our *asks,* we have looked in nutrition literature, sensory literature, behavioral literature, therapy literature. Lots of different professions describe the challenge of supporting children who are picky, really anxious, worried eaters. Each profession has added knowledge and strategies of support for these children and families. We have developmental strategies, sensory strategies, diet strategies, coordination strategies, relationship strategies, behavioral strategies and medication strategies. All have a place. However, I have found a great deal of help from the psychological literature as I read about phobias and fears. Phobias can be defined as irrational fears. Don't some of the fears of anxious eaters appear to us as irrational, not logical to us? This has made sense as I think of many of these eaters as, first and foremost, being worried and fearful.

Psychologist Kay Toomey, PhD has described the relationship between systematic de-sensitization and little steps of progress with feeding with her SOS Sequential Oral Sensory Approach to Pediatric Eating.[54] **Systematic de-sensitization** is a type of classical conditioning that helps us carefully and systematically replace a person's phobia, or fear response, with a new response. In the simplest of terms, it creates a hierarchy of situations (tiny little steps along a continuum) that trigger a fearful response starting with the most comfortable starting place (the *here*) and working toward the most fearful, most worried response, the *there*.

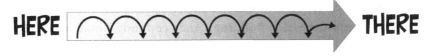

(Little tiny achievable steps in progress)

The steps from the starting place to the new place are tiny. This is described in our continuum of *here to there.* We start by giving the child the slightest challenge toward worry, finding a relaxed comfortable reaction, and then trying a small next challenge again and again until the child has reached the goal place without the fear (or phobia).

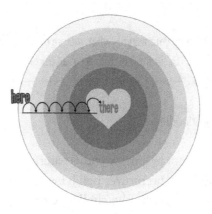

The secret to systematic de-sensitization is to use a continuum of tiny options to help find a comfortable place at each challenge along the way before going to the next step and to help them get comfortable *there* before progressing forward. Going directly to the worry would be called **flooding,** or an overstimulation of the *ask*. We help a child get from here to there systematically, carefully without flooding them with worry about the *there*.

Remember how I was worried about trying the grasshoppers? It is a prime example of systematic de-sensitization 101. It worked. I created little tiny steps toward my worry. I put the tiniest piece of grasshopper on the tortilla with lots of guacamole. I tried that. I survived. It was okay. I got comfortable there so I added more grasshoppers next. I ate it, survived and got comfortable so I added more grasshopper, and less guacamole the next two times. Each time I ate it, survived and got comfortable. By the fourth trial, I put a small handful of grasshoppers on the tortilla and guacamole and ate it. Tiny step by tiny step, I made the challenge harder, kept moving toward my worry, but went at the PACE I COULD HANDLE. No steps pushed me right into my worry. I got comfortable at every step along the way before I made the decision to challenge myself more. Now, if someone had placed a whole mouthful of grasshoppers on my tongue it would have been **flooding**…and I certainly would have vomited!

Some medical professionals have used an elevator analogy in thinking about various approaches to feeding therapy, tube transitions and anxious eaters. It goes like this. If you want to get to the top of a very tall building, do you want to take the elevator to the top, or stop on every floor? The implication could be, do you want to use a faster more direct "behavioral" approach, or a slower sensory or child directed, responsive approach? This so clearly depends on each child, and I will add, his worry and skills. Going directly to the top in a fast elevator may make sense if you have no fear of heights, but if you are afraid of heights, it may be better to stop at comfortable heights on your way to the top. The same can be said for children with worry about feeding. We could go right to the top-**making** them try new foods-but we would risk flooding some with worry like Marta did to herself in her new food trying method. But, as Marta found out, it was hard to find trust, enjoyment or confidence in new food trying when she continued to put too much in her mouth without any new food trying help. She just plain was not finding new foods to enjoy in her method. Instead of *here to there*, taking the elevator went directly to *there,* and in Marta's case, the worry. Perhaps the approach described in this book is a stop-on-every-floor-approach, systematically de-sensitizing your child's worry each floor along the way, so that he can confidently get to the top. There are lots of methods to help children progress in feeding, and this systematic way is just one of them. Can't we find a way to blend approaches in careful and sensitive ways?

Now let's think about a child example. You could take the elevator to the top and MAKE him eat it and may end up with tears, anger and even gagging or vomiting. If your child wants to try a hamburger, but is worried about eating it, you might start by letting him get used to seeing other people eating hamburgers. Then can he sit closer to that person eating a hamburger? (And get comfortable). Then can he hand that person a hamburger? (And get comfortable). Can he smell that hamburger? (And get comfortable). Rub his finger on the burger and put that flavor to his lips, then on his tongue? (And get comfortable). Lick that hamburger quickly, then multiple times? (And get comfortable). Then can he take the tiniest piece of a hamburger and put it between two pieces of a familiar bread and eat it? The taste, smell and texture are diluted in between the bread. (And get comfortable). If that goes well, can he take tastes with gradually bigger pieces of hamburger and less bread? (And get comfortable). Then taste it with only one piece of bread with the hamburger taste on top? (And get comfortable). And finally, can he comfortably eat separate tiny pieces, then bigger pieces of hamburger? The *get comfortable* part is most important in this de-sensitized tiny step approach.

The concept of systematic de-sensitization is to create tiny steps of offers and the watch the child's response. We want each child to **be fully comfortable at each challenge** offer before making the challenge greater. If he likes that offer, we can inch a bit toward the worry, toward the *there* of hamburger eating. If he doesn't, we can stay at that same level or back up. The sequence is written in questions so we can be careful to move closer to the worry ONLY if the child is ready. This is not written as **THE hamburger trying sequence**. This example is only one option but there could be many other variations on hamburger sequences **depending on each child's responses.**

Here is another example. Say we want to help your child like a fortified powdered chocolate breakfast drink. If we offer it him full strength in milk, it may be too great of a push into his worry. It could be flooding. In a systematic de-sensitization continuum sequence, we can offer the taste change in tiny ways. We could add one half teaspoon of the very chocolate drink into your child's whole milk. Your child can add help add a little amount with a spoon or dropper and stir. He tries it. If that change is okay, together, we can add a teaspoon of that flavor change and see how that goes. We can help him stir more and more until he is fully comfortable with the new rich chocolate flavor. Along the way if the flavor change is too great, we can back up a bit and add less chocolate or back up with a bit more milk to return back to a lesser concentrated version of the flavor. We can stay at that level of concentration, that comfortable place, until he is really comfortable, and then together tiptoe toward more concentration of the chocolate. Your child will let you know his readiness for more and give you feedback along the way.

Another way to systematically change the flavor might be to add an ice cube of the frozen chocolate drink to the familiar milk. As the ice cube melts, he gets a tiny taste of the new flavor mixture. The flavor gradually gets *bigger*, more concentrated. You and your child can add two ice cubes of the chocolate drink then three, then four and eventually got to the fully concentrated fortified breakfast drink. The important part is to only go as fast as he is ready and adjust as needed. You are systematically helping your child become less sensitive to the new challenge in little achievable steps rather than in a big worried way.

Foods can be presented in tiny steps of change along each continuum of sensory variables of the look, smell, touch, flavor, taste and eating skill needed as previously described. The sensory variables can be distant, farther from the worry, or up-close sensations, that get closer to the worry. The important part is a tiptoed approach, little steps with comfort at each step before increasing the challenge. This systematic de-sensitization is the foundation of the continuum concept which we will use throughout this book. We will use principles of continuum and systematic de-sensitization as we *Re-Define* what me mean by *Try It* in a later chapter.

Dear Parent,
Can you think of a time when your child had a flooding experience with food?
Can you think of a way you might be able to offer a new experience with
that food in a systematic de-sensitization continuum sequence?

The Art of Active Encouragement

"Celebrate and encourage the effort and the
experience, but not just the outcome."
Jennifer Berry

We need to find ways to take the pressure out of our asks. But how? Most people naturally enjoy eating. The taste and flavor of food is pleasurable. When we are hungry we eat, we eat foods we love, and we eat more. The food tastes and feels good, fills our tummies. when are enjoying food, we are motivated to eat more. We often return to favorite recipes and favorite restaurants for food we enjoy. The sensory properties of the food help us find those foods we love! We want to help children find enjoyment AND internal motivation to eat more.

But for our anxious eaters, enjoyment is not as easy to find at mealtimes unless they are eating their same old *List* foods. Eating, especially the "trying new food" part, is not as motivating and can feel like pressure. The sensory properties of the food are **not** enjoyable for them. The smell, taste, texture of the new foods is **not** what anxious eaters appreciate. These are often the parts of eating that leads anxious eaters to push away from the table. It is no wonder parents and therapists have tried so many different ways to reward or praise the child for eating because so many of these **children do not naturally enjoy the foods or the trying of new foods**. They have had difficulty enjoying new tastes and flavors and have gotten stuck with predictable *List* foods. Mealtimes do not feel like celebrations.

As loving grownups. we have succumbed to using external motivators to help our children gain some motivation—any motivation to eat, since their internal motivation is not there in ways we can predict. We praise them to see if THAT helps. We say, *good eating, good boy, nice eating your green beans! Wahoo, you ate some bacon! Yay, here is a sticker or treat*! We say it nicely and without anger, so doesn't that help?! Well, our praise can be pressure too.

We want our words to help. We mean well. We are trying, often desperately, to find ways to *get them to eat more* and *differently*. But, we do need to remember that the starting point for coming to the meal is different for anxious eaters. For food celebrators, the starting point is enthusiasm and for anxious eaters, the starting point can be just plain worry.

We can all agree that we want children to make food choices based on their own internal cues and physiological needs. We do not want them to eat because someone else TOLD them to or because of external motivators and treats and toys. But what do we do when the internal cues and physiological signals have become confused or are just not there? What do we do when children do not naturally respond to their own hunger cues or look to foods as satisfying? What do we do when the sensory food properties WE enjoy so much are not there? Or worse that they are a repellent to the meal? What do we do when anxious eaters do not want or cannot possibly try the foods we offer? What do we do when natural curiosity and sensory reinforcement for eating is not there? Here is where the whole *praise thing* gets complicated. We have to find a balance between external and internal motivation, pushing and supporting, by actively encouraging and celebrating with love and not pressure. Let us look at how **praise** and **encouragement** can influence mealtimes and where loving grownups can find the balance of support.

What is praise?

Praise (v) *To express warm approval or admiration of, compliment, applaud.*[3]
Praise (v) *To express strong approval or admiration*[60]

Wait, I thought praise was good!? What does praise look like? *Great job. I am so proud of you. Good boy, you ate your peas! I like how you ate your broccoli. I like how Daddy is eating his corn.* These statements are all warm approval or admiration, compliments. We are trying to be positive, but at closer glance, we might unintentionally be pressuring or judging. *Good job* can be interpreted as *bad job* on those days our *ask* is too great, or when it is just not a new-food-trying-kind-of-day. *I am proud of you* may work at this moment, but what about those days or times the child cannot possibly try *that* offered food? Does this mean *I am NOT proud of you* on those days? Does this mean *you are disappointing me today?*

What about when we tell a sibling, *great job eating YOUR vegetables?* Though meant as a positive statement and a hopeful way to role model that you celebrate vegetable eating, what it can also be saying to your anxious eater is, *I celebrate your brother as he tries vegetables,* and *do not celebrate you because you don't.* You may feel like being judged, you are less good, you are a disappointment. Of course, we never meant *any of that* in our praise efforts, but too many of our anxious eaters unfortunately get the impression that they *are less, inadequate, wrong.* If praise, by definition, suggests *approval,* worried eaters can feel that they are disappointing us meal after meal and constantly being judged. Praise can focus on the *right or wrongness* of the eating, the *goodness or badness,* the *pride or disappointment,* the *perfection* rather than the process. When children eat for praise, they are eating to please YOU and not to satisfy their physiological needs or enjoyment value. The motivation becomes external, even though we were aiming for internal!

Praise can be pressure

Lots of experts are weighing in on the influence of pressure on eating. Yes, praise **can** be interpreted as pressure. We want children to grow up internally motivated to eat, and when praise is heaped on the meal, we could be pressuring a child in a way that could stunt their own internal motivation. By praising too much or being critical of the child eating, we mess with that mealtime balance and responsibility. Children may begin to ignore their own internal cues and volume satiety.

Ellyn Satter tells us "pressure can be hard to detect: Ask yourself why you are doing something with feeding. Is it to get your child to eat more, less or different food than he does on his own? If so, it is pressure."[22] Speech pathologist Heidi Liefer Moreland, writes about the "pressure of praise."[56] Jo Cormack in her Emotionally Aware Eating blog tells us "Do not praise or criticize your child for what they eat."[57] So, if praise is not good or creates too much pressure, then what are we to do? We want to help! Let us look at encouragement.

What is encouragement?

> Encouragement (v): *To give support, confidence of hope.*[55] *To inspire with courage, spirit or hope. To attempt to persuade.*[17] *To suggest that someone does something that you believe would be good. OR To provide conditions that help something happen.*[55]

Praise tells children what we like about them or their behavior such as *you are such a good girl to eat that* OR *I like how you ate your cheese.* It can become a reward system and we can be training them to be approval seekers eating for our approval rather than for their own enjoyment. By contrast, encouragement supports the effort. (*You tried the carrot by licking it*). Encouragement offers an internal framework to look at your child's own choice or actions by commenting on them. (*You picked the short straw. You tasted that with your finger. How was that carrot?*) Encouragement offers observation about what your child is doing. (*You smelled it then touched it to your lips. What was that like?*) Encouragement acknowledges the effort or bravery. *You did some serious food trying today! You must be proud of yourself.* The goal is to promote self-esteem and confidence so each child spends less time asking the world for evaluation of their eating and learns to make her own assessment of his own efforts. Encouragement can help your child build her own internal motivation to eat and taste new foods.

Another way to see the difference between praise and encouragement is that encouragement needs to support the **journey** of new food trying, whereas praise waits for end result to be *perfect*. When we say *eat this* and then you will get the reward (toy or our praise):

1. The child is eating on demand (Oh no, where is the offer?),
2. The child is not eating because *they* want it (Oh dear, external motivation, not internal), and
3. The *ask* may be much too big of an *ask* (The child will fail and worry about being a disappointment).

Even though we gave the reward by saying, *Good job*, it still was eating for the treat and approval and not eating for the enjoyment.

When we teach the skills of new food trying, and offer new foods without a demand, we give the child confidence in new food trying and do not judge their efforts. Trying is not one event, pass or fail. It is a continuum of encouraging little steps. These are the little steps to **YET**. We celebrate where they are in the new-food-trying journey. The child then has choices that work for him. He is encouraged to try new foods as he learns that even saying *no thank you* is a kind of early trying, a multiple food exposure, a rehearsal. (*You said no thank you to bananas, this time. Your tongue might not be ready to tasting that YET. You must be proud that you were so polite.*) This time he may pass it on to someone else, and next time, he may smell or explore the texture! He will know trying can happen *at his pace*. Our encouragement is for him to do what he can today, in this environment with the foods offered. And we celebrate his efforts, not the amount eaten. *You passed the bread bowl to your sister.* OR *What did your tongue think about that bacon taste?* OR *Did you like the smell of the biscuit? Did it remind you of a food you like?*

Part of our taking the judgment and shaming out of our comments is taking the judgement and shaming out of our beliefs. We need to find ways to celebrate tiny steps along the continuum of little steps of progress so we can be encouraging rather than setting our expectations of 7 bites of Brussel sprouts, a huge *ask* for many. Too big of an expectation can lead them to failure and lead us to actual disappointment.

As loving parents and grownups we want to give support, and we want to build confidence and hope. If we are encouraging in order to **get** children to try new food, to **make** the try a new food, we are still tilting the balance toward pressure. We do not want our encouragement to become pressure too. We want to offer the encouraging conditions that ALLOW success, that allow the child to be brave enough to participate and allow choice but again we must be careful that we do not use these strategies to add pressure toward our desired goal.

Encouragement in new food trying

One goal throughout this book is to help parents help their very worried eaters learn the steps and gain the confidence to try new foods. By teaching your child the skills and a sequence of new food trying, we give them options and offers. When we give them a sequence of steps in trying methods, we are encouraging them to try the foods in the way they can, in the steps they can. We will be **re-defining try** it so children can get as close to trying as they are comfortable in their own time.

When we say *you decided to lick that food today*, we are neutrally commenting on the choice the child made without judging it. When we tell the child to pick which straw they want to use, we did give a choice, but inherent in the wording was *you will pick a straw* and **you will drink this**. A demand. Be careful. We must be careful that we are giving the option of *No Thank You* when we give choices. The difference is the child's perception of our *ask*. However, we do give choices in novel and encouraging ways all the time. Offering different interesting straws provides and invitation into the activity so the child can try them when ready and curious, when he wants to, feels different for the child. Having the child know that he CAN choose one straw, or if he decides *today is not the day I want to drink that drink,* he will KNOW that that choice is also okay. This is why we call this the Art of Encouragement, because our encouragement reflects our attitudes and responsiveness to the child's reaction.

What is active encouragement?

Active encouragement is a sensitive and responsive way to encourage children to learn something new. In this case, we are encouraging children to try more foods, using new food trying skill training, encouraging words, choices and novelty when making the offer. It respects the wishes, preferences and sensory sensitivities of the child. The child can choose to participate --- or not. Active encouragement invites a child to eat more. But**, it is *an ask* with a choice.** Remember the difference between an *offer or ask* and a *demand*? The difference is that the child is offered, and can say *no. No* is completely accepted. *Not today, not at this time, I am not ready.* When we are actively encouraging, the child knows we are their partner. We are supporting their process. We are trying to create a safe environment for them to succeed and be celebrated for attempts, whatever they are, for their bravery. These are the foundational principles of active encouragement:

Active Encouragement Principles

1. The child **knows** we **know** new food trying is hard and that we will help them learn how. We will be their guide, their food partner, their teacher, their support.
2. The child knows we will make **offers**, provide opportunities, but that **he** gets to decide when he is ready. We must accept that when he is ready he will let us know by trying, in the trying way that he can.
3. The **choices** we offer are our best thoughts on what would be good next foods that could be comfortably tried (See Sensory Rehearsals and Food is Sensory sections), but that we are prepared to adjust the *ask* right then and there. We are prepared that the child may or may not try that food.
4. We offer choices so **the child** can be the one making his own decisions about the trying.
5. We let the child know that it is okay to try the food, and okay if he is unable to try it today. We remind him he will know when his mouth is ready to taste it or fingers are ready to touch it.
6. Our choices are meant to give the child the power of the decision make internally motivated decisions, but also to add some novelty and interest to tip the offer toward more interesting and toward possible. We are following part two of the definition of encouragement, that is, *to provide conditions that help something happen.* We are providing the conditions that may help the new food trying to happen, to be more comfortable

---

Choices

Let's look more at choices. Choices give the child some power and child power is good when the history has been all about grownup power. Choices are good when the child is learning that he will no longer be pressured and no longer have no choice. It helps him *get* that he is an active participant in this meal. We are giving him power, but not asking him to take over the process. Grownups still choose the menu and the place. Grownups still decide on the choices offered, graded choices, graded *asks*. The rule is to offer a choice that is appropriate for the child, but choices that you, as a grownup, can live with. For example, do not offer potato chips or broccoli if you are going to be upset that they choose potato chips! By the same token, try to make choices your child can live with also. Do not offer an entire plate of octopus or an entire plate of cooked kale when both are extremely *big asks*!

Novelty

In addition to choices, we also use *novelty* as a way to inspire interest and to dilute the worry. Novelty spices up our *asks*. It works really well for many children. And, some children see right through it and perceive it as pressure. We do not want pressure. This is not a demand. If they are feeling pressure, we need to recalibrate our offer and work on our art of encouragement. Novelty is an invitation to participate more, to eat more bites, to practice with this new food more to establish it as a familiar food. It is an art. Novelty may be about interesting utensils, special spoons, tongs, chopsticks, straws, bowls, napkins or interesting presentations. (See Thoughts About Novelty Chapter). Novelty can create the interest that draws the child toward the mealtime. Novelty can be an anxiety diluter to bridge the gap between newness and confidence. We certainly do not want children to require novelty at every meal in order to eat, but the novelty can be a bridge to a new food or mealtime presentations.

Active Encouragement

- Adult provides consistent emotional support, circle of sensitivity hugs, preserving the parent-child relationship.
- Teach skills for new food trying.
- Make it interesting (novel).
- Choose encouragement over praise.
- Give choices so the motivation is internal.
- Accept the child for wherever they are along the new food trying continuum.

Dear Parents,

Can you think of encouraging ways to support your child?

Consider Evan

Evan was described as an anxious eater. He had spent time learning ways to try new foods but was still cautious. He did, however, seem very comfortable with guiding the pace of therapy sessions, happily participating when he could and saying no when he needed to. He knew that when he said no, the adults in his world would change the *ask* and that all along the way, he was celebrated. And, therapy was enjoyable and fun.

Therapist: *Evan, would you like to try this pepperoni?* (An offer)

Evan: *No.* (A decision)

Therapist: *Okay, shall we count how many we have?* (He is great at counting. Counting was a way to see if he could get comfortable touching them and being around the smell, taste from a distance, and feel. The counting question was open ended and could have meant we touch them, or he touches them…less pressure)

Evan: *Yes!*

Therapist: *Hmmm, shall we count them into this bowl or this bowl?*

Evan: *THIS bowl!!*

Therapist: *Who is going to put them in the bowl?*

Evan: *Me!*

Therapist: *Do you want to count them with Mom or with Miss Karen?*

Evan: MOM! (Evan picked up, placed **and counted 37 pieces of pepperoni**. Miss Karen noticed he enjoyed the activity. He did not require coercion, bribery or pushing to participate. He was having fun. The conversation throughout the counting revolved around how many pepperonis there might be with everyone guessing. Everyone was having fun!)

Therapist: *Mom, can you smell a pepperoni?* (This is a sensory rehearsal, more on this later. Mom brings a pepperoni to her nose to smell it and likes it!)

Therapist: *It is my turn to smell a pepperoni.* (Miss Karen modeled the smelling of the pepperoni, liking the pepperoni SHE smelled)!

Therapist: *Wait, wait! Whose turn is it to try the pepperoni?*

Evan: *My turn, my turn!* (He smells his and seems to enjoy it!)

Therapist: *Hmmm, what do you think about the smell of pepperonis?*

Evan: *Good.*

Therapist: *I can have a finger taste.* (Miss Karen demonstrates rubbing her finger on the pepperoni and then bringing it to her lips, then rubbing her lips).

Evan He rubbed his already pepperoni flavored fingers on a pepperoni and brought his finger right to his tongue. (Hmmm, he is liking this!!)

Therapist: *I can lick my pepperoni. Mom, can you lick your pepperoni piece?* (Miss Karen demonstrates. Evan brings a pepperoni to his own tongue and licks it in an enthusiastic noisy lick.)

Therapist and Mom start eating pepperonis.

Therapist: *Do your teeth know how to take a teeny tiny mouse bite?* (Therapist and Mom demonstrate.)

Evan took the tiniest bite, then more, then bigger. He finished that first entire piece of pepperoni and started on his second one announcing he LIKED pepperoni!

Now, let's look at this. He was given choices all along the way. There was no judgment whether he tried the food or not. The *ask* was graded- reflecting that he said *no* he did not want **to try** the pepperoni in his mouth at first. Rather than stopping the activity there, we broke down trying into the tinier steps and went through the new food trying steps together. There were choices and rehearsals; he was in charge of the pace and he was internally motivated to make the decisions along the way. HE decided to taste and chew pepperonis when end as HE was ready. He was encouraged to try the new food. He found enjoyment in the food. (Just like with the grasshopper story, had we said you need to eat a whole mouthful of these, the response and enthusiasm would have been MUCH DIFFERENT. We would have lost his trust as we pushed him hard into his worry).

And this whole story could have gone differently. We could have asked Evan *would you like to try this pepperoni?* He could have said *NO* and could have been much more worried about it with wide eyes, trying to leave the situation, moving farther from the pepperoni and withdrawing hands. At that point we would realize this is not the day or time for this activity, therefore we need to adjust our *ask* to end the activity on a positive note.

Now there are choices as we watch his reaction. There are always choices and our adjusted asks depend on the watching each child's reaction.

Option #1

Therapist: *Thanks for telling me. Should we put the pepperoni away then?*

Evan: *Yes.*

Therapist: *Okay, can you help me put the pepperoni away?*

Evan: Reaches for the package of pepperoni.

Therapist: *Can you put it over here on the counter? Thanks, we are all done with that.*

Option #2

Therapist: *Not today? Okay, Evan maybe we should put the pepperoni away then? Do you want to put it away or shall I do it?*

Evan: *You!*

Therapist: *Okay, I will put it away, will you help me? I will touch it, and you can help me put it in the bowl.* (and the therapist guides *his hand* to guide *her hand* as SHE picks up and puts away the pepperoni). His hand is on HER forearm as she picks up the package and puts it away. His hand is not on the pepperoni as per his request, but we ended the activity on a positive note.

The Exit

We do not want to inadvertently teach children that you just say NO to everything that relates to mealtime. We do want to help them trust food and trying. If we offer and the child always says NO then perhaps our *asks* are too big and our hover is too "hovery!" ☺ So, let's look at our *ask*. But also, let's look at the power structure. Let's look at how we exit from an *ask* while still respecting the child's need to control their own mealtime.

Here is an example. If we are teaching new food trying and your child is happily learning he can smell a food, touch it, and then carefully bring it toward their mouth with finger flavor tastes, lip flavor tastes, texture tastes, we are watching for their limits, the edges of their worry. We are teaching the *trying skill* and encouraging it, but sensitively understanding when your child indicates his limit has been reached. So, if we said, *hmmm could you smell this? What is it like? Is it a good smell?* (And the child smells it). Then we might say, *I wonder if you could you check it out and touch it? Or bring it to your lips to kiss it?* If your child says "no," we do not end there. Instead we say, *that is okay, can you just hand it to Dad?* We back down the continuum and end the *ask* at a more comfortable place. This provides two experiences. 1.) It is okay, we only try as far as YOU can go and 2.) We still are the askers and your child does not learn to say *no* and everything stops. There will be one more, (lesser worrisome) ask. "Can you just hand it to Dad?"

Or, if we asked if a child wanted to try licking it, and he says *no thanks*, we can say, *it is okay, but can you just kiss it good bye?* What makes this work is that you already KNOW that kissing that food has been fine. We do not ask an *ask* that will be too hard for him. We end on an easier *ask* so your child *gets* the sequence. If they did not want to lick it we can also say, *it's okay, but can you just put it in the bowl."* These are examples of adjusting our *ask*, but the grownup is the one to end the *ask*. (Check out the chapter, Adjust! Adjust! Adjust!)

How can you say *have another bite* without saying *have another bite*?

You know how we just want them to try more of the new taste? To practice it? We do not say *have another bite*, because that is jumping directly into the child's role, but we do some artful active encouraging when he shows an interest and willingness to participate and does not become too worried. Active encouragement is about choices and novelty opportunities that we would also give to non-anxious eaters. They can ALWAYS say *no* when they are not ready.

Do you want this drink or this drink? (You make the decision of what choices will be offered. This can be a familiar drink or a new one, one they usually drink, or the new one *you* are drinking. You are giving them the chance to choose the new one, or not).

Do you want your drink in a blue cup or a red cup? (You have made the choice of the drink. This might be offered when a child has tasted, and liked, a new drink, such as a smoothie. You know your child likes it and you are providing a structure to have more. If you child says *yes*, great. If he says *no*, that is okay too, maybe it was too big an *ask* today.)

Do you want a big taste or a little taste? Wait, wait, do you want two tastes or four or eight? (We have a little friend who loved the number eight. He always chose eight. He got the chance to try new foods eight times and quickly moved toward establishing more foods on his *List*. He made the choice. If he had said NO, we may well have made too big of an *ask*. If he said NO, we might say, *that is okay, can you just give some to Dad?*)

Do you want to take a noisy bite or a quiet bite? (You picked the food, hopefully a graded sensory choice, and you offered it. You probably gave a rehearsal and asked the parent to try first, or you demonstrated the biting.) You may have commented, *there are teeth marks in mine, are there teeth marks in yours?*

Can I help you serve yourself some of this food? Would you like it on your plate or on the nearby plate? (No? *Then can you just give some to Mom on her plate?*)

Do you want your drink out of this straw or this straw? OR, I am having a bouquet of straws, would you like a bouquet of straws? A bouquet of straws is three or four or five straws in one cup. The next questions might be, *I am going to choose (to drink with) this straw. Which one will you choose? Now which one? Now which one?* The choice of which straw encourages another sip and another sip, but it was made as an offer and not a demand. If your child acts worried, you back off and let him know it is okay if they need to be done. These requests allow you to ask, but to be sensitive to your child's response. He gets experiences where, though there was an offer you did not demand and you did respect his choice. (If your child says NO, you can tell him, *it is okay, but can you give these straws to your brother?*

Dear Parent,

How can you say *have another bite* without saying *have another bite*?

Big Picture

"Celebrate the small victories and keep peace at the table."
Lauri Ziemba

Let us look at the BIG Picture as we move forward together to figure this out. This book has just started and there may already be lots to think about and lots to worry about. You are reading this book because of your concern about an anxious eater. You are not alone. This is a problem that many families are dealing with and there *is* help. Lauri has described the Big Picture. It is small victories and peace at the table.

One of my biggest concerns as I meet families is that by the time I meet them many are already frustrated with mealtime battle grounds, sometimes at wits end! First of all, I believe and *know* this is hard and you have done the best you can. And your child has done the best he can. From my years of experience, I do believe that it would actually be simpler on anxious eaters if they could just eat the food you are offering... but they don't. It is clearly harder to say *no* under the spotlight of loving grownup pressure. Just eating what you offer would reduce the stress of the meal... but they CANNOT. Maybe their appetite cues are confused from their GI and stress experiences? Maybe their worry is just too big at the moment? Their reasons for not eating offered foods are personal, quirky, or maybe even completely illogical from your perspective, but they are real! Children tell us they *don't want* to be like this! We must believe them.

So, from this page on, can we think about *this*? We are their helpers and guides. We are giving those Circle of Sensitivity hugs! Can we work together to reduce, and actually eliminate, the pressure and learn more ways, different ways to guide them? Can you create that no pressure zone? As we have said, these really worried, anxious eaters are not the picky toddlers that outgrow a "stage." They are different. Their level of worry is exponentially different. They are likely "wired differently" from birth or from experience. They have parentheses diets. They build qualifiers around their food to protect themselves and so they can predict the food being offered. They are avoiding sensory surprises. Change is very, very hard for them and helping them with CHANGE will be or starting focus. That will be the starting place. From this starting place we want to help you take care of you so you can take care of your child.

Take a deep breath

Mealtimes have been stressful for everyone. Having an anxious eater is a challenge and it can get so out of balance. Take a moment to close your eyes and breathe. Find that calm place within you and just pause. Think about how the mealtime challenges have affected everyone in your family. Can you commit to making some changes? It won't be fixed all at once. It will be slow. But commit to change, even a little tiny change, a little tiny step forward.

Put yourself in his shoes

In my career, whenever I am stuck on how to help a child and a family, I try to put myself in their shoes. I ask, "What might it be like for this family, for this child?" Can you think about all the things your child needs to worry about? Maybe past experiences? Maybe the sensory sensitivities? Maybe the overwhelming environment of the mealtime? Maybe something new lurking around every corner? Maybe a desire to please you but the inability to do so? Maybe, Maybe? I think it helps to think about standing in their shoes or think about sitting at their place at the mealtime.

> Dear Parent,
>
> Put yourself in your child's shoes.

> Dear Medical Professional,
>
> Put yourself in the parent's shoes.

Celebrate your child

We want children to feel celebrated for who they are. Set aside the anxious mealtimes for now. Who is your child besides all this food stress? What does he like to do? What does he love? What is he good at? Many parents tell us they spend all day trying to *get their child to try new foods*. That is no fun, for you or your child. If parents are spending all day pressuring, their child may feel that he is always disappointing his grownups if food trying is hard and he needs to reject each offer. Children may get the idea that they are not good enough. You can change that. Celebrate the great things your child does. Is he good at counting or computers, karate or trains? Does he know about dinosaurs? Is he sweet with his younger sibling or good at letters and reading, music or dance? Is he a helper in the kitchen making food to take to Grandma, (even if he cannot **yet** eat or try it)? Find ways to celebrate your child today, and every day!

Dear Parent,

How can you celebrate your child each day and focus on what your child is great at?

The principles of this approach can be described in this hierarchy. Each of these topics will be described in further detail in subsequent chapters but here is the overview so you see where we are going.

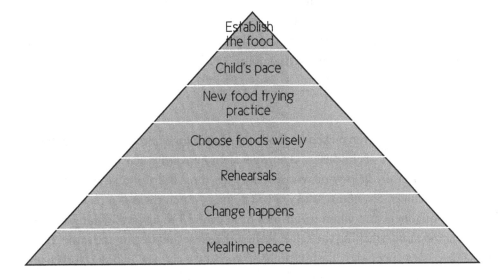

Mealtime peace

Let's face it. **Mealtime peace MUST be the starting point in your journey**. Most families seeking support for their anxious eaters are coming from a starting place of worry. You have worried you cannot make change in your food offerings because your child has just plain become too upset with change. It is stressful for ALL! Can we re-calibrate the stress? Can we find that place where mealtimes are not stressful, where the emotion, worry and pressure are reduced? You and your child may need to find that less pressured, less worried, more positive and supported peaceful mealtime as a foundation for mealtime learning. We want you and your child to want to come to the table, to want to be together around food, and support that feeding relationship in positive and comfortable ways.

Children learn so much from positive mealtimes. They learn how others eat and what others eat. They see grownups using utensils, trying new foods, enjoying their meals and having conversations. Can you find a way to take away the "take another bite" conversations and bring back family conversations? Can you create a mealtime routine that works for your family so your anxious eater knows what to expect? A positive mealtime starts with *mealtime peace* and elimination of pressure. It is eating and talking and socialization and togetherness and enjoyment.

Think about what it would it take to find mealtime peace at your house? What would mealtime peace look like? Can you start the new journey there? If the family could once again find an enjoyable, pleasant family meal, would it be worth it? If you can find mealtime peace as a starting point and then consider tiny steps of changes to guide your child into new directions carefully and without so much stress, it could be worth it! Mealtime peace is the starting point, AND the along-the-way point.

Change happens

You knew before you even picked up this book that change needed to happen. It needs to happen in support of children and families struggling with anxious mealtimes. We will need to carefully help your worried eater get more comfortable with *change can happen at mealtimes, Sweetheart, and you will be fine."* When there is a parentheses diet and many qualifiers and when mealtimes have evolved to always looking the same, sounding the same, smelling the same, feeling the same and tasting the same, EVERY change becomes a neon sign, flashing light of worrisome change! In order to even imagine this anxious eater managing any change in foods, we will need to start with **farther away change**, change in the environment. With the safety of the familiar and favored parentheses diet foods, can we make changes around the edges? Can table clothes, cups, plates, feeders change and can your child first become comfortable with that change? In my experience, when children become more comfortable with *change happens* around the edges, the closer, more sensitive food changes become easier to manage.

Rehearsals

When children are anxious, they worry about what is next. They can find ways to worry about every aspect of the meal. What will be served? What IS that smell? Who will feed me? Will there be a sensory surprise? We want to give children a heads up about what to expect at mealtimes and as they interact with foods. We will be calling these *rehearsals* throughout the book.

If children are only around *their favored* foods, they only know *their favored* foods. They need rehearsals around other foods in order to know they exist. They need to see *you* eating them and smell them, touch them and get comfortable with them. Can you provide multiple food exposures naturally within the day? Can your child be included in food preparation, and in mealtime preparation, in serving foods, passing foods, and being around other people who eat foods other than the few they eat. These interactions can be enjoyable, playful, pleasant. They do not need to be stressed or forced. They can be offered opportunities, not demanded opportunities. Anxious eaters often need *multiple positive exp*osures to foods before they feel familiar enough to even try them!

Rehearsals give children previews of foods so they can decide what foods they think are worth trying. Rehearsals are why we encourage mealtime modeling, family meals, and serving foods family serving style. So many anxious eaters **eat** only their *List* foods and to find peace your children may only ever **see** his *List* foods? It is hard to know what new food you might want to try if your world never provides an exposure to new foods. Can your child be at the family meal? Can they watch you eating foods not on their *List*? Can they see you eating your foods? Can they help in food preparation?

Later, we will describe two levels of rehearsals. The first is the mealtime modeling level where we provide multiple food exposure rehearsals to family meals and others eating and preparing foods not **YET** on their *List*. The second level of rehearsals is to provide sensory rehearsals *with foods* that give your child distant sensory and up-close sensory experiences with the foods. We can carefully help them see, smell, hear and touch new foods, from a distance at first as a rehearsal for bringing foods closer to their mouths. Then they can taste and touch the foods from lips toward tongue and mouth and get comfortable carefully and in a tiptoe approach.

Choose foods wisely

Choosing new trying foods can be an art. Of course, in the course of the day and the mealtime, children will be exposed to many family foods. And each child is free to try any of these new foods where and when they are comfortable. No pressure, no push. But for the children that need extra help in figuring out **how** to try new foods and what foods might feel safe enough to try, we can pick the new food opportunities wisely.

We want to be careful that we are grading our *ask*. Be careful that we are offering new foods to try, to rehearse, that are the right safety, developmental, sensory, motor, independence and emotional *ask*. We want to be sure we are calibrating the sensory variables so that, for very worried eaters, we offer only one change of sensation at a time. We can make our sensory food interactions easier to harder so let's pick easier. We will consider flavor before taste. Perhaps dry before wet or wet before dry. Perhaps predictable before unpredictable. We will discuss the sensory properties of foods in depth.

We also want to be careful that the food chosen at home or in therapy settings are worth the effort. Are these foods worth the effort that your child and you will go through in the sensory rehearsal? Are they foods you eat at home and can practice at home? Do they fit your beliefs about food you offer your family?

New food trying practice

This is the part of this book that is different from most and is presented in detail. It is my belief from years of experience that our most anxious eaters actually need to learn *how* to interact with the sensory properties of food that seem inherently scary for them. They need to learn *how* to go about trying a new food to give them confidence in mealtime change. As we saw from the Marta story, we all think of trying as something different. Some trying methods work and other just do not. Her method was clearly NOT working for her. Remember we cannot keep doing things in the same way and then expect different results. Let's help our worried eaters get different results by Re-Defining TRY IT. More on this later.

There are certainly children out there who, if left to their own devices, will find new foods they like just by watching others. We know from a wide body of research that children do try more foods when others around them are eating those foods.[58,59] We know they try more new foods when multiple people are trying them and they also try them when their peers are eating them. We encourage all of this eating together! It is important, but also, my experience says we need to teach ways to approach new foods so our worried eaters have the skills and confidence to break down new food trying into tinier less worrisome steps so they succeed in their efforts and actually find new foods.

New food trying can happen naturally as children see what we are doing and decide to try new foods. It can happen when we give children opportunities to be around new foods, to be exposed to others eating, preparing and interaction with foods. Children get these experiences by participating in family mealtimes and family food interactions. And, some children will need to have specific new food trying learning opportunities. We will encourage those opportunities to be away from the table, away from that family meal, that mealtime peace. Once the child has learned those trying methods away from the table, he can bring those confident strategies and those new foods to the table, so as to maintain that environment of mealtime peace.

Establish the foods

Each new food your child tries and enjoys will need to become an *established food*, one that can become a part of the mealtime routine. This will allow your child to practice that food and also to recognize it, want it, like it and choose it. We cannot just assume that because your child tried a new food today that it is automatically a favored food or one that will end up on the *List*. Yes, for some children it will work that way. The day my son, at five, decided he liked cucumbers, he ate an entire cucumber and ate them enthusiastically from that day on. However, many of our worried eaters need to have a number of tiny positive experiences with a new food to establish it. We cannot pressure with *"you tried it yesterday and liked it, why aren't you eating it today?"* They may not even be able to tell you why! Remember it is *their* body. They know when it feels good and when they feel brave enough to try more. It may make no logical sense to us, but it is their personal logic, not ours.

To *establish* new foods, these foods need to show up in your regular family meal food rotation. When your child first likes a new food, she will probably want it in that presentation, that texture again until she fully trusts that food. Many children will not allow change with it initially. Others allow change. Listen to them, watch their responses and be patient. But, keep offering that food regularly until it is established.

Sometime families celebrate a new food try with their child before it was fully established, and then forgot about it. This might happen if they tried a new food at Grandma's' or at school or therapy. If the food is not offered in the family food rotation for several months the child can forget about it and need to re-learn that food. If there is a positive response to that food in other places, families and therapists will need to make a conscious effort to transition that food home and offer it there.

Enjoy

And very importantly in the Big Picture, we are looking for what foods your child LOVES! Offer many different foods, offer what you are having as a family, and offer foods in restaurants and other places where your family eats. Just eat a variety of foods around your child, give them exposure to many foods and give them the new food trying skills and confidence and they will let you know what foods they are adding to the *List.* Here is a Circle of Sensitivity that will describe some levels of support.

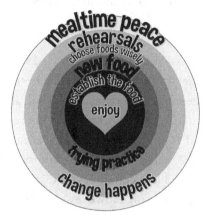

Circle of Sensitivity
Foundations

This may be the most obvious and yet the most important point I can make to another parent. Don't forget that your child's relationship with food is just one small part of his spirit and personality. Make time every day to enjoy your child, and to the extent possible, to enjoy helping him along his journey — no matter how that looks. For my son, feeding is literally a matter of life or death and he is reliant on a feeding tube to provide nearly half of his calories. It's a struggle to keep mealtimes and calories in their proper perspective. Even if your child never tries another new food or never gets off her tube or never eats mixed textures, it is okay! Enjoy the now! Maintain your focus on enjoying your wonderful child who is a delight in many other ways. The struggle and frustration are real but remember that they are not the only thing in his life. Remind yourself that working toward future progress shouldn't rob you of today's joy. ~Laura Wesp

Re-Define Progress

"Think about your daily routine with your child and identify one
thing that, if improved, would greatly improve your day."
Shannon Goldwater

In the Big Picture of this book you will notice that parents are central to every part
of it! You are the ones who are feeding your child multiple times a day. You are the
ones trying to find help, change and success. Many of you have told us you are stuck.
Change tends to be slow with anxious eaters and that it can be discouraging. This
book offers strategies for helping you find a starting place of mealtime peace and help
your worried eater regain trust and find ways to find lifelong strategies for food and
mealtime interactions. We will look at **Re-Defining TRY IT** later for more success in
new food interactions. But we also will need to **Re-Define Progress** so both you and
your child can turn your **YET** into progress, hope, and change.

To re-define progress, we need to consider re-defining the goals. Of course, we
will have big goals, but what about the littler ones? As Shannon Goldwater told us
in her introduction letter at the beginning of the book, when therapists initially
asked her what she wanted to work on most, she would immediately say to get her
triplet children off their tubes. (For most anxious eaters, the big goal is probably not
tube-related but may well be adding a large number of new foods to the *List* diet). She
tells us, perhaps a better question would have been: *I'd like you to think about your daily
routine with your child and identify one thing that, if improved, would greatly improve your
day?"* If your goal is for your child to eat the same foods as your family, and he is currently drinking one smoothie or one kind of fruit pouch or only brown and crunchy
foods, that goal is FAR away. Can there be goals that can improve your day, small
goals, little steps that tiptoe in the right direction but also allow you to see progress
and enjoy your NOW along the way? The **NOW** of mealtimes could end up being
disappointing every day and every meal because you and your child have not **YET**
met that big goal, whatever it might be for your family. Maybe we need to look tiny?

Too many parents describe their frustration with therapy that *we have been working on the same thing for two years!* OR *He has added NO NEW FOODS to his diet in eight
months.* When you see no progress, it is hard to go back to therapy. It is hard to pay

for therapy. It is hard to get enthusiastic about suggestions. It is hard to believe in **YET**. Anxious eaters do tend to make changes slowly, but we all need to be better at breaking down our asks into tiny achievable goals that allow you and your child to see that you are going in the right direction. You need to find those reasons to celebrate!

Systematic de-sensitization

In re-defining TRY IT and re-defining progress, we will look to those sound principles of systematic de-sensitization to help us find little steps for success for you, too. Comfortable, peace, is the starting place for *here*! The distance between *here* and *there* may be great, but the distance between the little steps is small and achievable. If we define little steps of progress in ways that are too big and you and your child are NOT successful, then we need more steps, plain and simple.

The **here** might be the *List* and the **there** might be the family diet but, as you well know, there are many steps in between. If you are holding out for that family homemade, organic, fresh diet for your **there**, and your child is only eating three processed foods and two drinks, you are going to need to re-define progress in tiny little elements of the continuum to find a pathway for change. This goal might be too big if an *ask* and hard to see ANY progress. You may see no progress for quite a while.

But let's look at this request in a variety of little steps. There could be many ways to approach this goal in little steps, depending on your child's skill and response to each step. (Check out the many stretches described later in the book). But let us look at some possible littler steps. Can you see how you may be able to re-define progress by seeing real progress in littler steps along the way, in a continuum, each step not perceptibly different from the last, until you get to **there**?

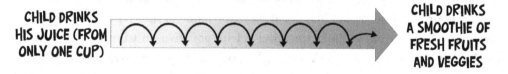

CHILD DRINKS HIS JUICE (FROM ONLY ONE CUP)

CHILD DRINKS A SMOOTHIE OF FRESH FRUITS AND VEGGIES

Little steps could be:

- Your child drinks his juice from another cup
- Your child drinks his juice from another cup with a lid
- Your child drinks his juice from another cup with a lid with a new juice ice cube in the cup

- Your child drinks his juice from a lidded cup with a nectar ice cube in the cup
- Your child drinks his juice from lidded cup with three ice cubes of nectar in the cup
- Your child drinks his nectar juice
- Your child drinks his nectar juice with stirred in puree fruit (1/2 ounce)
- Your child drinks his juice with two ounces fruit puree added
- Your child drinks his juice with half pureed, fruit half juice in the cup
- Your child drinks his juice with 3/4 pureed fruit, 1/4 juice in the cup
- Your child drinks pureed fruit from his cup
- Your child drinks pureed fruit made in the blender
- Your child drinks pureed fruit of different proportions as a smoothie
- Your child drinks a fresh fruit/veggie smoothie ordered out at a smoothie restaurant

There are many different ways to tip toe toward a smoothie from a juice. (See Smoothie Stretch chapter later). This is one set of tiny steps. Some possibilities will need more steps, and others can leap past several steps. But what all of the ways have in common is that the steps are tiny, and can you see how you could be encouraged seeing that steady sustainable progress? At the end of the day, that would be a win, right? That your child could drinks a smoothie at a restaurant. But, along the ways he and you can experience progress and more little wins.

Additional little *here to there* steps could be:

- Your child sits at the family meal and eats his own food while you eat yours. No one says "have a bite" of this or that.
- Your child sits at the family meal and helps pass the family foods.
- Your child sits at the family food and is comfortable with a little of that family food in a little bowl near, but separate from, his plate.
- Your child helps put a garnish food on everyone else's plate at the beginning of the meal.
- Your child allows a garnish food on his own plate with no requirement to eat it, while eating his own food.
- Your child allows some family food on his plate while eating his own foods.
- Your child learns to try the new food on his plate. (This one can have a number of extra tiny steps).

The little steps described here, again may require more steps along the way for some children and fewer for others. The whole trying sequence at the end can add many more steps. The thing about the steps described, is that each could be the little steps of improvement that Shannon Goldwater described as greatly improving your day. That is re-defined progress.

The **here** is that starting point or the **now** of your meal and the **there** is your goal. But what if your **there** is to have your child eat twenty new foods, but he cannot even comfortably come to the table? What if your child is so worried about trying new foods that he cannot even touch them? What if your child cannot even manage to eat one of his *List* crackers if it is broken? There are lots of little steps to work on along the way that still hope for a big long-term goal of lots of new foods, but that can allow for success while NOT deliberately pushing into worry.

The *here* could be that your child likes four foods and the **there** can be that you would love for her to enjoy eating twenty-five new foods. The **here** could be that he is very worried about trying new foods and the **there** could be that he knows how to confidently try new foods in little steps he can manage. The **here** could be that he always must have his juice in the green cup and the **there** might be that he can enjoy drinking his juice out of any cup. The **here** can be that she is only comfortable with baby food apricots. The **there** might be to help her enjoy apricots mixed with some baby food pears, or baby apricots offered off a different spoon. While you and your child are tip toeing toward progress, your anxious eater who does not like CHANGE, is comfortably experiencing change. We will discuss *change happens* in a later chapter in more depth.

The anxious eaters we are supporting have demonstrated that change is hard for them. If it were easy and the usual techniques for *getting* a child to try a new food worked, you probably would not even be reading this book! We want to remove the struggle. By starting where the child is comfortable and tiptoeing through a continuous sequence of tiny steps in which this step is not perceptibly different from the next step we greatly reduce the worry and increase the child's chances of active participation, worry reduction and enjoyment!

In the circle of sensitivity, the layers of worry complicate the journey toward new food trying and enjoyment. We start with where children are comfortable in the outer layer and tiptoe toward the **center heart of** enjoyable mealtimes and new food trying.

What are parents being asked to do?

Parents tell us they are told follow recommendations they do not believe in or cannot possibly implement!

~ To require their child to eat three tastes of a new food before getting to eat their familiar brown and crunchy foods and that this demand is met with tears and crying and mealtime disruption.
~ To just make him do that, be strong, be neutral faced and he will get over it.
~ That you are told you are not trying hard enough.
~ That you are supposed to keep data and write down every bite your child takes.

I understand how you might feel overwhelmed, blame and pressure! Where is the mealtime enjoyment? Where is the mealtime peace? There must be a solution that helps parents and children enjoy the process and find those little improvements that improve your time together with your child. Recommendations MUST match your child's needs **and** your family needs.

Goals can be *your child's* goals made smaller, or *your* goals. The goals do not always have to be how many bites, or new foods. There are lots of less stressful little steps along the way. Consider some of these samples.

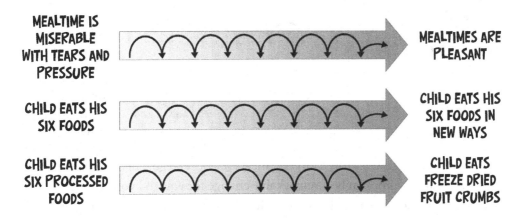

MEALTIME IS MISERABLE WITH TEARS AND PRESSURE → MEALTIMES ARE PLEASANT

CHILD EATS HIS SIX FOODS → CHILD EATS HIS SIX FOODS IN NEW WAYS

CHILD EATS HIS SIX PROCESSED FOODS → CHILD EATS FREEZE DRIED FRUIT CRUMBS

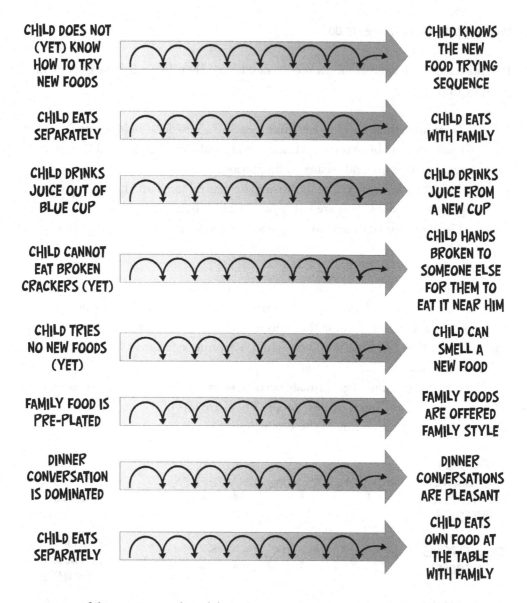

CHILD DOES NOT (YET) KNOW HOW TO TRY NEW FOODS → CHILD KNOWS THE NEW FOOD TRYING SEQUENCE

CHILD EATS SEPARATELY → CHILD EATS WITH FAMILY

CHILD DRINKS JUICE OUT OF BLUE CUP → CHILD DRINKS JUICE FROM A NEW CUP

CHILD CANNOT EAT BROKEN CRACKERS (YET) → CHILD HANDS BROKEN TO SOMEONE ELSE FOR THEM TO EAT IT NEAR HIM

CHILD TRIES NO NEW FOODS (YET) → CHILD CAN SMELL A NEW FOOD

FAMILY FOOD IS PRE-PLATED → FAMILY FOODS ARE OFFERED FAMILY STYLE

DINNER CONVERSATION IS DOMINATED → DINNER CONVERSATIONS ARE PLEASANT

CHILD EATS SEPARATELY → CHILD EATS OWN FOOD AT THE TABLE WITH FAMILY

None of the continuum listed directly meets the big end goal of adding new foods to the diet, but each one can be a remarkable change for you and your child. You can see that your child is learning, gaining confidence and moving in the right direction. You have re-defined progress! We know this can be an exhausting road, that it is so easy to get overwhelmed. We know that it is hard when yet another person has an enthusiastic idea that requires **your** time, **your** energy, **your** money and **your** patience, all of which may be in short demand. By finding tiny steps of achievable progress, essentially, re-defining progress, throughout this book we will help you and your team think in smaller steps so you do see the path and you do see the progress.

> Dear Parent,
> Can you identify one thing that, if improved, would greatly improve your day?
> Could that be your starting point?

Re-Defining Progress

It has become clear that we, as parents, may need to expand our definition and readjust our expectations of progress. A broader, healthier view frees us to see and celebrate the small successes along our path.

Marsha gave me a new list of possible successes to consider. She helped me re-define progress in a qualitative versus quantifiable way and in doing so, she revolutionized how I was thinking about our journey. Rather than focusing on weight (or "bites") alone as I had been, Marsha highlighted these other important milestones: happily joining the family at the meal-times, confidence in new food trying, enjoyment of food flavor and texture exploration; safe, confident eating and drinking skills; participation in family food preparation and internal motivation to eat enough. I found ways to see progress in this expanded definition of success.

Now when other parents reach out to me in frustration or agony over their own feeding struggles, I refer to this list and share it. Momma after Momma finds glimmers of hope and discovers new ways to see the progress her child is making. "Well, yes, he loves pizza now!" or "She'll eat waffles," or "We ate out Friday as a family." Or even "He tried green beans!"

As we expand our definition of progress, so too must we re-evaluate our expectations. In his new book *Atomic Habits*, James Clear[61] astutely states, "We often dismiss small changes because they don't seem to matter very much in the moment." He goes on to explain the exponential effects of making small, consistent changes over time. I'm convinced this is the approach we need to take with feeding our children. We need to focus more on the opportunities we are presenting each and every meal and less on the outcome. I am convinced that you will see progress over time, but it may be so tiny and imperceptible that you may not notice it yourself. The change may be so subtle that you miss it entirely. For this reason, it's extremely helpful to have a therapist or friend remind you of how far your child has come. Or you may simply want to make some videos or take some notes for yourself to keep track of where you started.

Once I'd fully embraced the slow, but steady, approach to progress my overall happiness as a mom improved. I was freed to enjoy all the many aspects of parenting again. We can be so hyper-focused on calories and meals that we lose sight of our ultimate goal: enjoying our kids in the present moment and guiding them to become happy, well-adjusted adults. I carry a notebook to all of Teddy's appointments where I write down notes and also keep track of noteworthy changes at home. On the inside cover in big, double-underlined, pink letters, I wrote this quote: "You will NEVER regret making a choice to focus on HELPING THEM ENJOY THE PROCESS, and not just reach the goal." Originally written on Kristen Kill's blog, *Hope with Feathers*[66], this quote had nothing to do with feeding in its original context, but became my defining mantra. What good would it do to be weaned from a tube, but not to enjoy food or thrive on a varied diet? Or to resent eating or rely primarily on external rewards or cues?

Here's just one final word about this journey. As a recovering perfectionist, I'm always relearning how many factors are 100% completely, out of my control. Progress with feeding is slow, and it is also non-linear. You are guaranteed to witness your child making steps forward only to be followed by days of regression. Many, many external factors influence your child's meals with stressors such as travel, a new school year, illnesses, allergies, and even developmental milestones. The list could go on and on. Rather than face discouragement, accept that each day will not necessarily be better than the last, but that does not mean that you are spiraling backward. Keep going, Momma! Your efforts will accumulate — maybe one lick, smell or taste at a time. ~Laura Wesp

Mealtime Peace

*"Food is often hard work for children. Helping
your child rest from food is your work."*
Heidi Moreland

In order to survive mealtimes with your anxious eaters, you have found what works and may offer the same foods, with the same brands, with the same presentation, same cups and utensils, in the same room, at the same table, with the same TV or screen on and with the same feeder. Some would describe you as *enabling* your child to continue in his worried patterns of eating. However, the reality is that we parents do what works and try to find ways to reduce our child's overall mealtime stress. We do what it takes to survive. This is completely understandable. By using screens and toys or distractions at the table, I really believe you have been are *enabling mealtime p*eace. It is your starting point. It is your peaceful place. It may be the way you have survived your mealtimes. However, most parents cannot imagine their mealtimes looking like THIS in five years! How did we get here and how do we move forward to our **YET** from here? You need sensitive support in helping your child tiptoe toward healthier eating habits with less worry.

As we consider the layers of worry and the tiny steps of progress toward enjoyment, our home base starting point will be to find *mealtime peace*. It will be your outer layer in the circle of sensitivity, the layer where trust starts, the layer that invites your child back to the table in a peaceful step by step way.

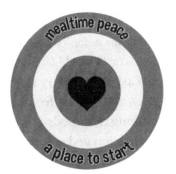

Circle of Sensitivity
Mealtime Peace

NOW is out of balance, no peace

Unfortunately, many families who have very anxious eaters have felt that mealtimes have become completely out of balance at their home and in their child's therapies. Eating has become the parent responsibility. That responsibility has become a huge burden. Parents who are worried about their child's growth, their nutritional variation, and their child's eating volume have stepped in to help and are right smack in the middle of the child's responsibility. The parent has come to be in charge of exactly how much the child is to eat, and how. The parent has been in charge of *getting the food in* (or trying to). Therapies have defined the way parents are to provide the food and what experiences the child is to have at each meal. Rather than a trusting partnership with parents, the meal has become a battleground with everyone stressed and with battle lines drawn. It is understandable how families got here, but how do families find their way out of this uncomfortable place where the whole meal is about *try it, take a bite, why won't you take a bite, tears, anger disappointment, and even gagging or vomiting.* How can you get to peace from there? The whole mealtime has often become focused on the activity that causes you and your child the most stress. Often NO ONE not want to come to meals.

What is mealtime peace?

Feeding is a relationship between the child and the parent. We want to support a positive feeding relationship. To find *mealtime peace*, we ask parents to step back and consider what would it take to have a peaceful mealtime for your family or what would you need to do to find mealtime peace today, now? Can you imagine what a mealtime would look like with no stress, no anger, no pressure, no *take a bite*? With increase calm, for you and your child, might you be able to step back a bit and more clearly look at priorities?

Some parents tell us, *to find mealtime peace, I would feed my child separately* or *I would only feed my child their favored foods"* or *"I would let my child have the phone screen and videos at the table"* or *"I would stop asking him to try something new at the table."* Okay. Of course, the ideal end goal does **not** include feeding children separately, having the videos at the table and not offering new foods at the table, ever. We want variety and mealtime participation, conversation and enjoyment. But, these might be *goals*. They might be your **YET**. Maybe you can find that starting point of mealtime peace and then, with calm and perspective, re-consider how to help your child and family tiptoe into change.

Dear Parents,

What is the starting point to get to mealtime peace in your house?
What small change could you try this week to help you get to mealtime peace?

Mealtime peace is the starting place that allows you to settle, to relax, to breathe for a moment to contemplate the situation. When you are in the middle of such worry and stress, it is hard to think and not just react. From here, if you want to see change, you will need to change things. Your anxious eater has probably felt the stress of mealtime tension for quite a while, as have you. We need to create a new mealtime with new expectations

Your child needs to start by just being able to be at the meal and eat comfortable food without anyone telling him what to eat and how to eat. Not only does he need to experience that, but he has to experience that often and consistently enough to *believe* it, to *trust* it again. He probably won't even know how to react at first with no one prompting him or telling him to eat or try. It will take a while before you notice that he is not as worried about coming to meals, and the pressure to eat at the meal has stopped. The time it takes to get back to *comfortable* will vary with each child depending on how he has perceived the mealtime and how much he believes it is going to change. A hint: If you decide not to push and not to ask and not to pressure and you do that for two weeks and then pressure again, it will be confusing for your child and harder for them to really trust that mealtime pressure is gone. The quicker you can get to peace, and STAY THERE, the better it will make everyone feel.

But many parents tell us they were working so hard to try to get their child to change, to eat more, to eat differently that stopping all that food work feels wrong. Speech pathologist Heidi Moreland, MS, CCC-SLP tells us "sometimes taking a rest from food work feels like you are not doing enough. Remember resting can heal your child's relationship with you and with food."[56]

Mealtime peace reminders

Now that you have decided you will start from today on the best mealtime peace you can create and let your child participate comfortably at the meal with no pressure do you need mealtime peace reminders to help you stay there? To remind you that there will be a different expectation about the meal can you change something? New mealtime peace, new mealtime. Some parents may choose to have a new table cloth, or little quiet background music. Some rearrange the dining room or eating location and others light candles. Some offer new plates or change how food is served.

Dear Parent,

What mealtime peace reminders would help **you** change your mealtime to peace?

Family style

From your place of mealtime peace, can food be served family style so that the food is present and passed around in bowls? Each family member can serve their own food, can take how much they want. The whole family can do this and role model for your worried eater. If he does not want to get near the food (yet) or pass it to start, it is okay. Remember, start with trust. You are still demonstrating the process and the new food exposure is still happening. He can still see the food and the interactions, but from his starting point of a safer distance. It does not need to be up-close and scary, it can just be an observation of YOU doing it. The idea of family style is also important because when parents pre-plate the food, it can be that mountain of pressure and an out-of-balance parent role. If you pre-plate the food, essentially YOU are deciding what the child is eating and the amount. Can your child take on that responsibility or at least help with that?

Food choices

Your starting point may well be that in order for your child to be at all comfortable at the table, there needs to be food choices for him. If you have gotten in the rut where the whole family eats your child's foods every night, you may ALL be tired of the cheese pizza, spaghetti, round waffles and boxed macaroni and cheese.

It is time to celebrate YOUR food choices. Offer what you and the rest of the family want and like but be sure there is a food or two from your child's *List*. SO, if your child only takes his own *List* foods, that is the starting point. If you are trying to find mealtime peace and your child sees nothing at all familiar, the pressure is back. The peace is gone. But vary your family menus for enjoyment for the rest of the family and this will give your child introductions to new foods, from a distance without HAVING to eat them. Research supports our experience that multiple non-threatening and non-pressured exposures to new foods allow them to become less new, less worrisome and gradually, tried.

Have a conversation

We want to give children the opportunity to participate in the togetherness and conversations of the family meals. Invite them back. You may need to be very intentional about NOT talking about food and NOT asking about food in any way. If your conversations have characteristically been around taking bites, stop. Can you talk about something else? Can the focus be on being together with pleasant conversation about what your child likes? *What kind of adventures to each of you have today?* Enlist the help of all the family members to let them know that there will no longer be conversations about trying foods or discussions about what to eat. It may take a while to change the pattern. Some families have even decided to videotape some of their meals so parents can look back on what they are doing and catch themselves when pressure statements inadvertently sneak their way back in.

Once the **pressure** of coming to the mealtime and participating in family meals is stopped, THEN you can focus on teaching your child the skills of eating a variety of foods and participating more directly in the mealtime routine. From the starting point of mealtime peace, we can help build lifelong skills with your child. For many anxious eaters, new food trying time and direct food interactions may not start out at mealtime. Perhaps he needs to learn the skills and confidence of new food trying away from the meal in a quieter interaction. Perhaps he needs to learn the skills, sequence and strategy of new food trying and bring *that skill* to the table when it is a comfortable and established skill. Once he is comfortable and feel less pressure, your child may well be able to find the curiosity and motivation to try YOUR foods.

So, there is lots more to try after mealtime peace is established but, start there. You will ALL feel better during the journey.

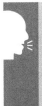

Though it's not always possible, we aim to eat together as a family most nights. Meals work best for us in our dining room, because it helps to be in a room set apart for mealtime and free from other distractions. Teddy's dietitian and therapists have all recommended serving meals family style. We transitioned to this routine somewhat reluctantly because of all the extra dishes and clean up. After trying it, however, I immediately saw the value in having all the food on the table. For one, it almost completely eliminated the need for me to pop up to get anyone anything. It was all right there!

Second, we noticed pretty quickly that even if Teddy opted against a food at the beginning of the meal, he might request some mid-meal once his body settled in and he'd had the chance to observe our enjoyment. When we started family-style meals, I was using pretty serving bowls that all had to be hand-washed. That definitely added to the cleanup time. As we've had practice I've learned to streamline the process.

A few tricks to help are using a larger platter and placing the meat and veggies all on one tray as opposed to lots of bowls that have to be hand washed. I also keep fruit in the fridge in small bowls that I can simply pull out each night. Teddy has the responsibility of placing one or two choices on the table. When we are crunched for time and cannot eat family-style, I still try to have our kids serve themselves — even if I just put a stool in front of the stove and they serve their plates from there. ~Laura Wesp

Change Happens

A central theme of this book is that *change is hard* for very our worried eaters. But, mealtimes are full of change. It is a *change* to transition *from* whatever you are doing **to** the mealtime. Table settings can look different from meal to meal. An empty plate looks different as food is added and different again as food is taken away. Food feels one way as you put it in your mouth and changes as you chew to make it ready to swallow. And foods offered change. The foods you know can even taste or feel different from time to time. It is no wonder many of our anxious eaters have very specific favorite *List* foods. They are predictable. They may have very consistent textures as they are chewed with no surprises. It is no wonder that round, square, or fish shaped crackers, cookies, pretzels, waffles and pancakes, boxed macaroni and cheese, chicken nuggets, boxed juices and smooth yogurts can become favored foods.

Parents so often describe feeling stuck that they can only give those certain foods, certain brands, prepared in a certain way and presented in a certain way. When your child needs a certain colored cup, a sandwich made on certain bread and cut in a certain way, it is hard and very discouraging to change *anything* without your child noticing. When everything about the meal is the same, these anxious eaters *notice* (and probably reject) every change you try. They become visually hypervigilant as they sleuth out what possibly might have changed at their meal. We want to help them experience changes at mealtime starting with the smallest and least significant changes. Likely the first changes will not even be with the food, but with the less worrisome *edge* aspects of the meal. Once your child becomes comfortable in an environment that has occasional changes, **then** the tiny next step food changes may not stand out like such a neon light of *new*.

Start with mealtime peace

In that Circle of Sensitivity, your starting place will, of course, be **mealtime peace**. From that calm place of love, trust and no pressure, you can help your child understand change in tiny steps. In a way your guidance to change will be from that Circle of Sensitivity hug place and not a push place. If you make change too fast, you are pushing too fast toward her worry. Slow down.

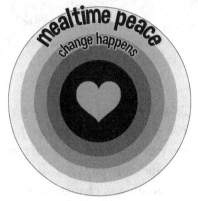

Circle of Sensitivity
Mealtime Peace/*Change Happens*

Change early

Offer change as a part of mealtime from as early as you can when toddlers begin to show their BIG worry about change, *before* the problem becomes huge. Can you change the bowl or the spoon occasionally? Can your baby's food be presented in different containers and, if using commercial baby food, can it be offered *out* of the jar? When the food always comes out of a baby food jar, or certain yogurt container or juice box, children who like SAME grow to expect **that** presentation. Can the mealtime environment change? Grownups can unintentionally enable this rigidity by always presenting foods the same way from the same dishes. Children can grow to expect those presentations and different presentations can be just too new!

Change around the edges first

We need to help our anxious eaters get to a comfortable place where *change happens* at mealtimes and they realize they can survive it! **Change can actually become their normal**. BUT, starting right at the level of changing **their food** can be much too much. It could be pushing DIRECTLY into their most worried place. Change can happen around the edges first before the up-close food change is introduced.

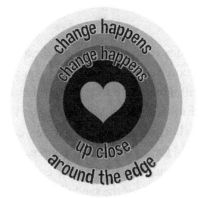

Circle of Sensitivity
Change Happens

In the Circle of Sensitivity *Change Happens*, change will need to become comfortable first around the edges and move toward the up-close food worry. Can we make the tiniest, least stressful changes and tiptoe toward more? We can make a change and watch each child's reaction. Changes around the edges would be non-food changes. Can there be a new table cloth on the table? New place mats? Can there be some quiet music in the background? Napkins folded differently?

Does change need to happen even more distant at first at **someone else's** place setting? Can you change a parent plate or bowl, cup or straw? This helps your child see peripheral change that does not involve her directly so it can be less stressful.

Parents know

What would happen if you offered your child's yogurt from a different bowl or spoon? You know! Some parents tell us you think your child would not worry at all. If that is the case, can the bowl be changed? Can the spoon be changed? The straw or the cup? Grownups can enable *same* in ways you had not thought about by always serving yogurt in the princess bowl, or always using the red spoon. We all get in routines and ruts. If your child is comfortable with changing the bowls, spoons, cups or straws, please do it often. This not only minimizes the creation of ruts and *change worry* about those items, but also can give your child confidence in mealtime change. The idea here is to have *change happen* regularly so change does not become that neon sign of worry alert. Change just happens. In essence changing around the edges like this is a *rehearsal* for later changes with your child's food or drink.

Change your child's foods

What would happen if you changed the presentation of the food your child eats? You know or have a pretty good idea before you even try it! Can you change the sandwich shape? If you say *no way*, then we will think about that differently later in the book. (Could you change it just a little?) If you think it probably will not matter for your child, can you try it? If you always make the peanut butter sandwich in triangles, can you change the sandwich shape regularly? Can your child get used to *change happens* with square and rectangular shaped peanut butter and jelly sandwiches or maybe even a "puzzle sandwich" created with a cookie cutter shape in the middle of the sandwich? Can waffles sometimes be round or square, cut in strips or whole? Can your child help you make it in a new shape?

Recipe

Can *change happen* in the recipe? Many of our anxious eaters learn to like a particular smoothie. Super, but then some parents go on to say that they <u>always</u> make it with exactly half a banana, three strawberries and half a cup of vanilla yogurt. We ask, *would your child be comfortable with a slight variation on that recipe?* Many parents tell us, *I do not know, I just always make it that way.* Well, can you give change a chance? Can you and your child vary the recipe a little? Could you put three quarters of a banana in one day or one extra strawberry? The idea is to use those three familiar ingredients and tip toe into tiny recipe changes to help the worried mouths be comfortable with *change happens*. Of course, we do not recommend pushing right **into** worry, or creating sensory surprises, but if little changes are okay it reinforces the idea that subtle *change happens* and it is still okay.

When you are making homemade waffles and using them to fortify the nutrition with extras, can little recipe changes happen? Some parents will say, they always add one extra egg, or one tablespoon of powdered milk, or one table spoon of applesauce. Can there be an extra tablespoon of applesauce or powdered milk? Maybe your child can help prepare the waffles or smoothie and you can sometimes round the ingredients up with overfilled tablespoons of ingredients? When children help make them they understand that you did not sneak in an extra ingredient for a surprise. You made the recipe together! Homemade recipes are a great place to gently experiment with *change happens*.

Dear Parent,

Are there starting places where *change* could *happen* in your mealtimes?
(Edges, foods, recipes?)

Food Rehearsals

Children need rehearsals. They need to know what is next. When are we eating and what is for dinner? Who are we eating with and what is happening after dinner? Children who are worried about foods seem to do better with new food trying when they know more about the food and expectations ahead of time. They learn a lot from watching others.

Rehearsals are previews of what exactly to expect. When I was worried about trying grasshoppers, I did best when I had more information, rehearsals. Do others actually eat these insects? (I got to watch others show me how to try them.) How did they eat them? (Oh, they hid them in the middle of tortilla and guacamole). What did they feel like? (Oh, they crunched between my fingers.) What did they taste like? (Oh, they smelled like garlic.) Having the preview and being allowed to go at my own pace in my own tiny amounts helped. The rehearsals helped dampen my worry!

Imagine. What if someone said to you, I am going to just put a new food in your mouth (worms?) no warning, close your eyes and trust me. That situation could make a worried eater out of most of us! We **need** to know what to expect. We need rehearsals. We need to minimize the surprise factor. We need to figure out our own trying pace!

Rehearsals provide children with information, a preview, about what to expect in upcoming food interactions. What are THEY going to do with that food? What is that food all about? Think about what children learn as a preview by watching others eat. When young children are at the family mealtime, they learn what grownups do with forks and spoons, how cups work, how straws go in the mouth. They learn from watching others tackle that corn on a cob, dip a chip, use a spoon with soup, and slide their teeth along an artichoke leaf. Children learn a lot about food management and food properties from watching others interact with foods. Watching is a type of distant food rehearsal. What do OTHERS do?

Older babies and young toddlers are notoriously messy in their highchairs. They pick up and drop, pick up and throw, pick up and squish, pat, break, smear and crumble the food we offer. This is absolutely normal and it is a way the child gets a closer rehearsal. They are exploring the food up-close, smelling the food, feeling its texture, its breakability, crunch-ability, melt-ability, squishiness or hardness. They get a rehearsal of what that food might taste like (the smell gives a taste hint) and feel like (from the feel on their fingers and palms) before they even put it in their mouth. And their first tastes might be from fingers or lips and may not be a big in-the-mouth try. This is normal eating development.

At some point many grownups decided to just put the new food in the child's mouth, often over the protestations of the child, in hopes or expectations that they would *just get over it* and probably like it once they tried it. I definitely know adults and children who can try anything and more often than not will enjoy it. They are already going through life with a belief that all or most food is good! But this is often **not** the case for the anxious eaters I know. Their starting point may already be that new food is worrisome, suspect. Their beginning bias may be to **not** want to like the new food. How did we start to believe that just MAKING them try it would teach them to enjoy new foods? When did we stop letting them explore the foods a little ahead of time? When did we strap them in the chair and tell them NOT to touch it? It is my belief and my experience that these children need those rehearsals to gain confidence in new food trying.

We will describe rehearsals in two categories that help children get closer to foods in smaller steps. **Multiple Exposure Rehearsals** give rehearsals about the environment of eating and big picture of family meals. **Sensory Rehearsals** help your child rehearse the *getting closer* part of new food trying and the exploration of the sensory properties of the foods as a preview for what the food might be like in their mouths. Since there are both distant and up-close parts of each of the sensory properties of foods, sensory rehearsals can be further divided into **Distant Sensory Rehearsals** to **Up-Close Sensory Rehearsals**.

Multiple exposure rehearsals

We have learned from research[5,6] that cautious eaters need multiple exposures to foods to be comfortable enough to try them. But this is not a recipe. It is more of a guideline, a concept. Many experts recommend having children at the table and having them around the foods in a non-pressured way to give them the opportunity to try new foods naturally.[21,22,26,27,28,29] Multiple exposure rehearsals are those food interactions that include watching others eat and prepare foods and interacting with foods without the *requirement* to taste or try them. It is *multiple* because children need multiple, repeated positive experiences, not single exposures and not just occasionally. They need exposures, multiple, and often, as a way of life.

Who knows how many interactions it will take with a new food to increase the likelihood of a particular child trying a particular food. Some say five to ten[5] some say ten to twelve. Who knows since each child is unique and this food trying stuff is personal? But we know it is *multiple*! For many people, being around grasshoppers a hundred times may still not increase their interest in trying. Some food may not ever be a good fit, but many might.

The easiest rehearsals tend to be the farther away ones. These are what we are going to label **multiple exposure rehearsals to foods**. This is where we invite children to participate at family meals, to see others eating, and interacting with foods, and to see the foods others eat. This is where anxious eaters learn that others eat foods they do not (**YET**) eat.

Multiple Exposure Rehearsals Teach Children:

What is mealtime like?
What foods are around and what foods do others eat (even though I eat my *LIST* foods)
What do you expect of ME?

What are mealtimes like? Families invite children to the table, to participate in a family meal. Manners happen. Turn taking happens. Food serving happens. Food interactions happen. Mealtime conversation happens. Food eating and mealtime enjoyment happens. Food is offered family style with children participating to their ability in serving themselves and others. Others eat those foods, others enjoy them. Anxious eaters learn to be **at the table**, even if it is while eating their own *List* foods, in a pleasant, non-pressured, non-stressed environment. They learn to enjoy the MEALTIME while they might be gaining the confidence they need to expand their diet later.

Food others eat? When worried eaters are participating in family meals, they see others trying a variety of different foods, family foods. This is important because often, anxious eaters are given only their *List* foods, and sometimes they are eating by themselves away from the family. It is entirely possible that they never get to see others eating other foods. If they are to learn about other foods, these foods need to show up in their lives, as a preview, a rehearsal of foods to come. Think of it. If your anxious eater is never around new foods and then she is in expected to try new foods, she has no rehearsals, no frame of reference for that food.

Just repeatedly being around new foods can increase interest and motivation.

Worried eaters can surprise us. Recently a friend told me her son (who likes six brown and yellow foods) saw her drinking the smoothie she had just made. It had kale, lime, ginger, turmeric, chia seeds, apple juice and a cucumber in it. It was GREEN and did have a BIG ginger smell. Her son leaned over and wanted to taste it. He subsequently amazed her by wanting more and drinking a cup of it! Who would have known? This is exactly the benefit of multiple exposures, of just giving your child the opportunity to be in the same environment as your family foods.

What do you expect of ME? When we want a child to interact with a food, at home or in therapy, we grownups often get directive. It is my philosophy that we find more enjoyment and internal motivation when we offer, not demand. Can we let children see what we are offering, and rehearse our *ask* and give them choices? Can we show them what we are asking of them first? I am passing this to Dad, can you pass this one to Dad? I am going to scoop this food with a spoon, can you do that? Can you show her what YOU do with that food? Can she have some time watching others handle that food before she is expected to jump right in and touch it?

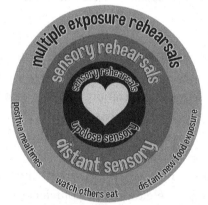

Circle of Sensitivity
Rehearsals

In the Circle of Sensitivity for rehearsals, the multiple exposures outside layer is exposure and opportunity. It can involve distant interaction with food where the child watches others and does not actually touch or interact with the foods or they can involve some interactions with foods, but the child decides. The is no pressure. It is not therapy but a way of life that includes your child in family food preparation or mealtime preparations. We will explore ways to provide multiple exposure rehearsals to foods as a part of a daily family routine in a later chapter and then take closer look at the sensory properties of foods so we can explore the distant and up-close sensory rehearsals.

Multiple exposure rehearsals are the experiences that help your child know about mealtime routines, your foods, and your expectations around foods. But, the starting point is mealtime peace. You first are encouraged to get to a point where you are aware of ways pressure has snuck into your mealtime and are trying to eliminate them. Mealtime peace is the starting point where your child knows you will not push or force or pressure and that just being around the meal is okay. Your child knows your offers can be accepted or NOT. They have choice. They trust that their grownups KNOW this is hard for them and are celebrating that they are just at the table with the family, participating in family mealtime activities as they can. This is not the **YET**, it is the starting point. The multiple exposure rehearsals that follow can be considered a way of life, not a therapy time that is expected as another thing to add to your day.

Model mealtimes

We model mealtimes. We show children that we eat, we interact with food and we enjoy foods. We give natural exposure to food at the family meals as the child sees the sights and sounds of the family eating foods that may not yet be on their *List*. We are looking for what foods your child loves without **requiring** food touching or tasting until the child shows us he is ready and has learned comfortable *new food try*ing strategies. We are looking for those moments when he wants to try that green ginger smoothie.

If your child can be at the table with the looks and smells of foods, great. Maybe she can have the new food on her own plate. Maybe she can pass the food. Passing food can be others passing food around your child, or your child can pass the actual the bowl of food on to someone else. (This gives her a close up look and smell)! The passing can include touching the bowl, the spoon, the tongs or the actual food, depending on your child's readiness. If your child is worried about getting even that close to the food, she can help YOU do the passing and can still be celebrated for that participation.

Mealtime jobs

Children can participate in the taste and smells and textures of mealtimes by participating in the jobs that surround the mealtime, not just in the eating and trying of new foods. Mealtime jobs can include food touching and interaction or ones that do not, depending on readiness. Can she help set the table? Maybe she set the whole place setting, or maybe she can start with just putting napkins around with (or without) adult help. This is a non-food interaction that has your child around the table before the food is there and may give her brief experiences in and out of the kitchen where food is being prepared. They may or may not see what is cooking and may or may not smell it! If being in the kitchen environment with the food smells is even too much sensory exposure for your child, could she decorate the napkins by coloring or with stickers at a non-cooking time?

Can your child help bring family style food to the table, or bring the salt and pepper shakers? (Food will have more obvious smells and different looks, whereas, the salt and pepper shakers will look the same day after day). Can she help pour the drinks or bring the poured drinks to the table? Can she put garnish on each plate (a slice of orange, or piece of green parsley)? Can she spread butter on the bread (maybe not for herself to start, but maybe for a younger sibling)? Can she be a food pass-er or server as she helps give food to others? She could put some food on everyone's plate and maybe even her own (if she is comfortable)? If she is curious, but not yet ready to have a piece of that family food on her own plate, she could serve herself some on a separate plate, near her plate, so the food is there, nearby and under consideration without the requirement to try it? Maybe this time, maybe next time, she might try it? Just like with the grasshoppers, I knew when I was ready.

Sample Mealtime Jobs List

Grocery shopper assistant
Recipe consultant
Food preparer (salad maker, food chopper, food stirrer…)
Appliance turn-er-on-er
Music turn-er-on-er
Table setter (napkin placer, spoon placer)
Garnish-er*
Food passer
Food server
Drink pourer
Plate clearer
Table decorator

With all these mealtime jobs we can grade our *ask* for food interaction to match the place where the child is comfortable and learning, *with* food or *without* food. We can make each job easier, or more challenging.

A word about garnishes

Garnishing is a great bridge to being able to have a food on your plate even though no one expects you to try it. ☺

Food preparation exposures

Food preparation is a nice way to offer multiple exposures to the family foods while getting closer to the rich smells and textures of foods. Again, there is initially no expectation of tasting the foods. Your child can get comfortable with watching you prepare food first, but the smells of foods will begin to enter their experiences. These food preparation exposures can be distant as she watches you from across the room and then closer as she stands near you in the kitchen. She gets closer to the food (and worry) as she can handle it. There are nice kitchen towers or kid friendly kitchen step stools that can be used to help your child be at counter height for closer sights and smells of foods when helping in the kitchen.

Food preparation extends the mealtime past the family table and into the preparation. It involves your child in the big picture family mealtime in a way that changes the subject from *try it, eat it, and finish your food*, to helping in the preparation. When your child is helping make the food, she is contributing to a positive mealtime even if she may not yet be ready to eat the food. Then, many children become so comfortable in the food preparations they find new foods to try and enjoy.

At first your child can do the non-food touching part of the food preparation such as the package opening, measuring, stirring, pouring, the appliance operation, such as turning on the blender, while still seeing and smelling the food. She can participate in food handling up-close smelling and tasting as comfort level allows. It will be easier to touch the food with utensils first. In a continuum of food textures, it will probably be easier for children to touch the drier foods first before the wetter foods. Your child can start farther from his worry, but eventually can help with food preparation and even make recipes that can be shared with the family and friends. He then can be celebrated for his helping!

When preparing foods, can your child add the sugar or measure the vanilla? Can he mash the bananas or open the cake mix? You and he can decide the level of closeness to the food that is comfortable. Opening the cake mix or pouring it may be much easier than interacting directly with the banana, but on the other hand mashing the banana and feeling the texture through the masher and smelling banana smells will also be a great preview for banana trying later! Can your child pick the vegetables from the garden or grocery store and wash them? Can he help pour the cut-up veggies into pan or help make the salad?

The junior chef

Can children help pick out recipes for some family meals? Children's cookbooks with pictures are nice *multiple exposures*. Some children learn to interact with foods first, not by tasting them, but by preparing or cooking them. They eat their *List* food while learning to cook with and for others. Families can get them a Chef hat and apron and teach them to help in food preparation or in particular recipes that get to be the ones they get to cook. (And they then get to be celebrated!)

Our Salad Bar Station

I am a vegetarian, but I cook meat dishes for our family. Night after night I would never quite get to prepping a salad or something for me to eat. At the same time, I really wanted Teddy to learn to love salad, for many reasons. I knew he loved the salad spinner, so I decided to make prepping the salad his kitchen job. We have a small kids' table that I easily move into the kitchen as I'm cooking. I set it up with a cutting board, the veggies, some crunchy topping, and the lettuce. Teddy determines how much lettuce to put in the bowl and then he helps chop some veggies. For the chopping, normally Dad is walking in the door from work and he's able to help supervise that task. It really helps that we've experimented with lots and lots of different dressings. His personal favorite is a classic vinaigrette. ☺ Sometimes I just give him a small bowl of that with a few carrot strips. He often just licks the dressing off his lettuce pieces, but sometimes he'll munch on a few pieces. I try to buy all different shapes and textures of lettuce. He will say that his favorites are the "flat leaves." Teddy is proud that he is helping cook the meal and his creation is on the table. ~ Laura Wesp

Even more distant

Some children are so sensitive that being around actual new food is too worrisome. Their beginning multiple exposures will be need to be **very** distant. So, remember vision is a distant sensory property. Non-real-food interactions can include videos or apps around food themes. Families seem to all have smart phones with entertainment apps for children. The food apps range from watching cartoon foods to watching real photographs and interactions with foods where your child can be an active participate in peeling, stirring and cutting the foods, but on the screen, not in real life (**yet**). These experiences give your child the opportunity to see what is done with foods in a non- threatening way without those pesky smells and uncomfortable touches. It is distant, but it is a starting point.

More distant visual exposures can include reading books about foods together. There are so many common children's books about foods that are colorful and playful. There are books about food vocabulary and naming foods. There are books about trying and learning to like new foods. There are books that describe foods, that describe trying and that learn about hungry caterpillars eating! There are children's cook books with great pictures.

Play food can also be helpful for many worried eaters. There is lots of play food out there that even imitates fast food and commonly appreciated children foods. Children can play games with little play kitchens and have tea parties that appreciate food interactions without the worry. Again, this is not our end goal, but a less worrisome step along the continuum of multiple exposure options along the way.

Grocery shop

Could your child help grocery shop and pick out family foods? The fresh produce section is a great place to be surrounded by a world of fruits and vegetables. Perhaps your child can put the produce on the scale or in the plastic bag? Perhaps your child can help you unload the cart at check out and push the cart to the car? Perhaps your child can help you put the groceries in the car? Perhaps your child can help put the groceries away when you get home (and even wash some fruit to put on the fruit bowl on the table)? OR perhaps there is no way you would even take your child, **yet**, to the grocery store and this is too big of a request, too big of *an ask*. Okay, okay, start where you can, where you both are comfortable.

Food field trips

Can you take your child to the bakery or smoothie shop? Can he watch pizza or donuts being made? Or can he see that bread loaves come in different colors and sizes and shapes? Can he visit farms, pumpkin patches, or orchards? Can he help pick apples or strawberries at farms?

Plant a garden

Some families plant gardens and include their anxious eaters in the whole gardening process. They can help plant, watch the food grow, pick the ripe foods for family meals and try them along the way. It is fascinating how many children will try new foods in gardening that they may not be comfortable at all trying in the kitchen. It is a new environment, maybe one with no previous food worry. For those of us without a green thumb, the Farmer's market can work nicely here.

Have food around

Sometimes children know where to find their *List* food and are allowed to help them-selves. Maybe it is in a low pantry or refrigerator shelf. If their food interaction is to and from that pantry shelf or only the *List* foods, their food world continues to be small. If your child does not *eat* fruits, they still need to be *around* fruits. They need to be around others eating fruits. They need to be around the visual, smell and feel of fruits. Consider how, in your house, you can have food around. Can there be fruit bowls on the table? You might just bite into one of those fruit pieces near your child and model the possibility of trying them.

Food play

Food can be incorporated into play. Children can empty, fill, and stack foods. They play pretend games with fruit and vegetable pieces. Can your child roll a grapefruit back and forth or empty and fill foods in a container? Can food pieces be used for tic tack toe games? Can a piece of food (probably a dry one) be used as a place marker in a board game? These are multiple exposures without the demand to try. (More on this later.)

Food academics

Can food be a regular part of your child's day in academic or homework interactions? Consider using food pieces as manipulatives in math learning. How many is fifteen grapes minus seven grapes? Or how many twos in six pieces of cauliflower or eight cherry tomatoes? Or use the crumbs for writing or a pancake pen for drawing pancake shapes. The act of the counting or drawing helps to dilute the worry as your child has something else to think about. And you get to celebrate something else your child does well! (More on food academics later, too.)

Food art

Most kindergarten school teachers have a thick file of food art? There are so many ways to use food to create artistic projects and the ideas are only a click away on your computer. These projects can be designed to carefully grade the ask so that it meets your child's developmental and sensory needs. You may not start by creating rainbow fruit kebabs for a child who is seriously worried now about the wetness of the food. That child may need to start with dry food and to separate out the colors of a multicolored fruit cereal and use them to make crumbs for coloring a Sand Painting on clear sticky paper.

Thank you-food gifts

Some families begin a family routine where they substitute *thank you-food gifts* for written thank you notes. When there is a need to thank Grandma for babysitting, or a friend for running an errand, the family makes a food gift. This might be cookies, or banana bread or a fruit salad or rainbow-colored fruit kebabs. This becomes a routine. It becomes familiar and your child is celebrated for taking part in these thank you-projects. Your child is then celebrated for the thank you effort (nothing to do with whether she tried the new food or not!)

Be creative

Families find ways to include their children in the food interactions that work for them. The intent here is not to create food therapy time for so many minutes a day, but more to have food interactions as a regular part of the daily or weekly routine. Be creative but do what works for your family. If you both are enjoying it you will do it more often.

It helps in our family to mix things up at mealtimes. This could be as simple as switching plates or cups or possibly rotating who sits where at the dining room table. Additionally, on Friday nights our kids sometimes eat dinner on a blanket in the family room while watching a movie. Just something as simple as moving dinner outside can help. He may not necessarily translate into eating more, but it keeps mealtime fun and fresh. ~Laura Wesp

Food is Sensory!

In order to talk about sensory food rehearsals, distant and up-close, we really need to discuss the sensory properties of foods. So many of our anxious eaters are worried about some sensory aspect mealtime. Food is a sensory experience. There is no way to get around that. The presentation, taste, smell, texture and sound are all sensations that contribute to our enjoyment of food. And these exact sensory variables can be the attractions or roadblocks to trying new foods for anxious eaters. We can look at each sensory variable and discover that we can carefully choose more diluted versions or more concentrated versions of that taste, smell or texture. Let us look at how we can offer a *distant* version of that sensation or an *up-close* version of that sensation to help in more comfortable guidance and support for trying the new food. In other words, we can help *rehearse* the new food by inviting our anxious eaters to *try it from a sensory distance* to start.

Food is Sensory!

It is visual
It has smell
It has sound
It has texture in hands & mouth
It has flavor
It has taste

Vision as a sensory property

Vision is a distant as well as an up-close sense. We see things far away and really close and many places in between. Children learn a great deal about the mealtime by watching others from a distance or watching up-close. They can see how we are using utensils or see us trying different foods. They can see the color and texture and notice its presentation. They can see how much is on the spoon and how fast it is approaching. Vision lets them know if it is a familiar food in a familiar container with a familiar utensil or if something new is on the way. They can feel the pressure of a well-meaning grownup by seeing where they are standing, how they are holding the spoon, how close it is to their face and how intense is the *ask*. Their vision helps them understand the body language of our offer or demand!

We know that the look of food matters. When the octopus was chopped small in a marinated salad, I loved it, but when the whole octopus, suction cup tentacles and all, was offered as a salad, my eyes told me NO, NO, NO!! I could not get THAT food past my eyes! The look matters as we decide whether the dish will be pleasing or worrisome. Many of our anxious eaters DO NOT WANT TO SEE their foods touching on their plate. This can be enough of a turn off for them to reject the whole meal. Children very worried about change who are very worried about new foods become quite specific in their visual understanding of foods. Beth knows that red apple is *her* apple but that green apple is NOT FOOD, or NOT HER APPLE. Or, Don likes a particular square cracker, but once he takes a bite out of one corner, it looks different, so he can no longer eat it. He will eat and entire box of these crackers taking one bite out of one corner of *every* cracker...and then want more new crackers. The look matters.

Many of our anxious eaters become very, VERY observant about mealtimes. Many could actually be called HYPER-VIGILANT about the look of meals. They want the LOOK to be the SAME! No black specks, no color changes and not even a different shaped sandwich! When children are worried about change, they scout out *any* small change visually from a distance and, if need be, protect or prepare themselves from a mouth taste of the food before it even gets near their mouth! Visual changes can be NEON SIGNS to notice, NOTICE, **NOTICE**! Vision is a sensitive check-it-out-from-a-distance sense.

Dear Parent,

Does the look of food matter to your child?

Smell as a sensory variable

Smell is another distant and up-close sense. Smell is 80% of taste.[63] Smell and taste are so interrelated that smell is considered *taste from a distance*. We interpret smells as we breathe IN aromas and they waft through our nose by *oro-nasal smelling*. This type of smelling gives us a preview of what a taste might be before it gets anywhere near our tongue. Imagine peeling an orange. The pleasant, sweet citrus fragrance gives you a good idea of what that orange might taste like before it even gets to your tongue. Or, imagine the smell of brewing coffee or cooking bacon? Can't you almost taste it? You get the *idea* of the flavors way before you put them in your mouth. It is a nice preview because it is giving you a hint of flavor without any worrisome texture.

There is also a closer smell sense called *retro-nasal smell*. This smell information comes from the air you breathe OUT as the food is mixed and broken down in your mouth during chewing. This smell is also interpreted in the nose but comes from within your mouth *up to the nose* as we breath out, rather than coming from a distance. Smell information from both places give us rich information about taste but this retro-nasal smell requires a texture interaction as the smell comes from within your mouth. You can also receive retro-nasal smell from food that is already in your stomach when you burp. Children worried about tasting new foods can gain a preview taste of the food by smelling it from their comfortable distance. Many children will decide to taste a new food on their lips or tongue after repeated pleasant smell interactions with it.

The smell sense is related to our emotions and our memories. We can all usually think of a smell that triggers a memory from the past, a place and time. When I smell dinner rolls baking I think of middle school piano lessons because my piano teacher's mother made white bread rolls every Tuesday and they came out of the oven at the time of my lesson. Or the smell of a certain cheap men's cologne reminds me of my high school boyfriend. Those smells take me right to those memories. Can you think of a smell that takes you to another time and place?

Smells and memories work together in our brain neurology. So, if our anxious eaters have a bad experience with a food at home or in therapy, the smell of that food can take their memory right back to that *bad experience place*. The bottom line is that we want to create good experiences and good memories with the foods we offer. Smells can help motivate children to try new foods or send them running the other direction. Smells matter.

Dear Parent,

Does the smell of food matter to your child?

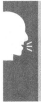

Smell Matters

One night Brady was distressed that the family was having clam chowder for dinner. He did not want to come to the dining room or the table and could not enjoy his own food with that

Sound as a sensory variable

Food has sound. Many children are not worried about the sound of food being chewed for themselves or by others, but others are completely turned off by the sounds. As with smell, the sound sense also has a distant and an up-close version. The distant version, *external sound*, is the sound wave that touches the ear drum turning the wave into vibration for transmission to the inner ear. It is often referred to as *touch from a distance*. Children notice this sound as they hear others chewing. Think of someone chewing an apple or celery nearby. You hear it. You may be able to ignore it, or it may disturb you. Some of our anxious eaters do not want to be in the same room as others eating, and the sound aversion can be a factor. I especially notice the irritating sound of eating as a movie-goer loudly crunches hard candy or potato chips nearby. It can be VERY distracting. Imagine having that kind of distraction when you are trying to eat a meal?

In addition, there is an up-close version of sound called *internal sound* that works by bone conduction through the jaw bones and skull as you *hear and feel* the crunchy food in your mouth during chewing. The sound of crunchy food being chewed is close to the ear where the sound is felt and interpreted. When some children are especially worried about crunchy or loud food, this is sometimes a variable. These children may choose or need *quieter* foods, at least to start.

Dear Parent,

Does the sound of food matter to your child?

Touch as a sensory variable

Touch and texture can be strong factors in liking or not liking foods. Touch relates to *the feel* in our hands as well as *the feel* in our mouths. Sucking and hand movement seem connected. Our hands give us distant touch information that might be considered a preview of how the food texture might feel in our mouth. Finger tips give us some information, but our palms are quite sensitive to texture discrimination. If a we put a new food in our palm, we get a pretty realistic preview of the texture of the food, the fiber, the scatter, the firmness and the density. It can be a beginning way to explore that texture, far from our mouth, with the safeness of distance. Imagine a section of orange in your palm. Explore it. You can tell by the feel that is will be quite fibrous in your mouth. Now contrast that with a bit of baby food pears. The pears feel smooth and you can certainly expect them to be smooth in your mouth! What a nice texture predictor your palm is! Now think about the anxious eaters we know that cannot even touch a food without gagging and vomiting or running to the sink to wash their hands? Why would we expect them to want it in their mouth if they cannot even touch it with their hands??

And food texture *in the mouth* is up-close and complicated. For example, purees theoretically may be easier to manage than mashed, chopped or solid foods as they can be swallowed without chewing. BUT there are so many puree variables. Just because a child likes one puree does not mean he will like all or any other purees. Think about the puree food texture words you know? Smooth, grainy, dense, viscous, thin, thick, lumpy, slimy, slippery and more? Purees are NOT created equal! Because a child likes one puree texture, such as yogurt, does not mean he will be comfortable with other textured puree variations, even if the flavor is the same. The differences in texture are amazing and anxious eaters can *really* notice them! Remember how visual changes can the NEON WARNING SIGNS for change? Up-close texture variation can be a NEON WARNING SIGN for different texture and texture rejection.

Now, think of the other solid food texture words you know. Binder foods (food that stick together in your mouth like mashed potatoes or refried beans), scatter foods (foods that separate or scatter in your mouth like peas or dry rice), chewy foods (foods that require chewing, and that you cannot swallow whole and that do not melt in your mouth), tough, crispy, rubbery, crunchy, and oh, the combinations of textures that are possible! The food can feel like a sensory surprise with every bite.

Dear Parent,
Does the texture of food matter to your child in his hands or mouth?

And brands! It is understandable that many children who are anxious about change would absolutely and vehemently prefer the food that has a particular brand. A certain brand of food, such as boxed macaroni and cheese, has a predictable texture that allows children to anticipate what it will feel like as they bite through it and chew it. There will be no sensory surprises. A certain brand of yogurt may always be smooth. A certain brand of nuggets may always have the same chewiness. A certain brand of juice may never have pulp. Texture is an important consideration when children have brand preferences.

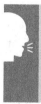 My grandchild recently came to dinner. I fixed him what I thought was the right food, his nugget chicken. My grandson told me, "I am sorry Grandma, I cannot eat this chicken. It is too soggy. I am sorry." It almost broke my heart that he felt he needed to apologize! This is SO hard for him. ~Loving Grammy

Flavor vs. taste

Flavor and taste, what is the difference? You could say they are the same and many people use these terms interchangeably. You could say they are related, but for the purpose of our conversation, let's separate them. Let's consider *flavor* as the taste you get from rubbing your finger on an apple and bringing it to your lips or tongue. This taste has no texture, it's *just flavor*. For a child trying to get to know a new flavor, it is sometimes helpful to separate the flavor from the taste. For our conversation, let's consider *taste as including texture*, as in dipping that same finger in baby food applesauce. There is flavor *and texture*. The whole sensory experience changes when both are combined. When a child needs more distance in early taste tries, flavors can be separated from the texture initially. Rubbing your finger on a piece of bacon then licking it, certainly gives you a bacon flavor, without the much different experience of a bite of bacon in your mouth!

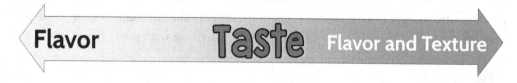

Finger tastes

A sequence to consider when helping your child taste a new food may go from distant to close smell, to finger tastes (flavor first, then texture tastes) on lips then tongue.

You will find that teaching your child FINGER TASTES, where she rubs her finger on a food to make the initial taste try, will become your child's friend! Finger tasting has given so many children more confidence! Think about how this can help your child get familiar with a flavor without having to put too much in her mouth. A slow and gradual introduction! And, your child gets to be in charge of what she puts in her mouth.

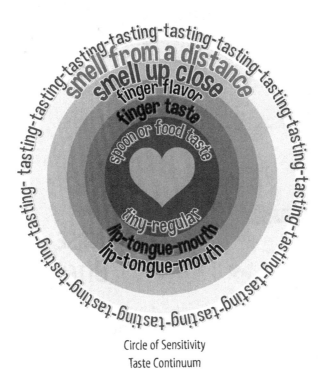

Circle of Sensitivity
Taste Continuum

Little to bigger tastes

And then when your child is comfortable enough to bring a new food to her mouth, the tastes can start out really small as tiny *tastes* or Mouse Bites and work up to bigger and bigger Bird Bites, Kitty Bites, Puppy Bites, Horse Bites or even Elephant Bites, or whatever *size continuum* each child enjoys. Animals size changes are often commonly understood by children, but some children have dinosaur favorites or car and truck favorites small to big! Small somehow can seem like a much smaller worry. This chart not only gives us a progression, a continuum of bite size opportunities, but it is cute and playing with it can dilute the worry.

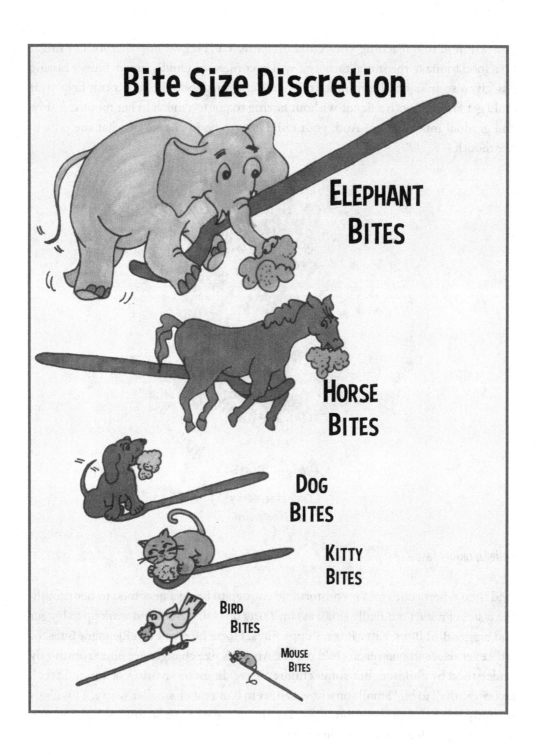

Bite Size Discretion

ELEPHANT BITES

HORSE BITES

DOG BITES

KITTY BITES

BIRD BITES

MOUSE BITES

Sensory properties help

As you learn about the properties of foods, you can modify the way you offer them, or understand why your child might have trouble trying them. You can dilute the big impact of smell and texture by offering them in different ways, or combining the textures, tastes and smells. With careful consideration of the distant and up-close sensory properties of the foods offered, we can give a thoughtful preview or rehearsal of the food your child is going to try. Essentially these become part of your child's food rehearsal that can help him become familiar enough and comfortable enough to want to try them. Remember those grasshoppers? Once I diluted the taste and texture by trying them together with tortilla and guacamole, I could manage the TRY.

We can offer change in one sensory property at a time if we need to make a new food easier for a child to try. For some children we would change the look first and not change the flavor taste or texture or sound. This could be achieved by adding a drip of food coloring to a drink or a yogurt. Color changes slightly but nothing else changes. The color change, of course, can be offered from pale to concentrated to start small.

Some children, on the other hand, will worry so much about the color change, that they may respond better to a small flavor change, no color change and no texture change. This could be achieved by stirring in a tiny amount of a new brand of yogurt, same flavor, same smoothness. For example, stir in a tiny amount of a new brand of vanilla yogurt with your child. The flavor change would be minute but will not be a sensory surprise if your child participated and is anticipating a little difference. Make it a science experiment. *Can you find the new flavor with your tongue? Do you taste the new yogurt, YET?*

Or the flavor change can be a tiny amount of a same *brand* yogurt but new *flavor*, similar color for example, a tiny taste of coconut yogurt added to *their* vanilla yogurt. The colors are so similar, the look will not change perceptibly (for most children). Or on the continuum of flavor change more and more can be added. And texture can be changed within the same flavor and taste. Baby rice cereal or crumbs could be added in a yogurt your child liked changing the texture little by little. There could be a few flakes of cereal or crumbs added as you grade the texture change with him. For the braver new food try-ers you will be able to combine the look and taste and texture change if done carefully in tiny increments and with your child's help to minimize the surprise factor. We will practice these later.

Imagine sensory surprises

We have mentioned sensory surprises before. Let's think about them. We have to be careful not to create sensory surprises. These can worry even the most adventuresome of eaters. Have you ever had that experience where you put a food in your mouth and had such a surprise that you had an overreaction? I remember that time when I was about eight and was sitting at the breakfast table with my brothers. We were chatting and giggling and I did not pay attention as I brought my glass to my mouth. What I grabbed was my purple grape juice. What I thought I grabbed was my milk. My mouth expected milk. What it got was purple grape juice. My immediate response was to make some surprised sound and then spit out the grape juice to get it away from my very confused tongue as quickly as possible. Did I say *spit out*? I meant *spray out*, all over my brothers who angrily had to change clothes before school. That is definitely a *sensory surprise*.

My sensory system was unprepared for the sensory differences between the grape juice and the milk expectation. And from the earlier story about the fish sensory surprises in Hong Kong, I became suspect of new foods. And I am a good eater, an adventurous eater and I am not worried every day about *new*. Imagine if I was a cautious eater to start? Imagine if my starting point was worry? Sensory surprises are dramatic and can make us increase our general food caution and worry. And children remember. When we try to sneak in a new food or taste or texture without warning and they find the surprise, they are on higher alert next time. We can have our children participate, rehearse, food change by helping to create it. We can teach them to smell and examine every aspect of a food before putting it in their mouths to find that hidden surprise ahead of time. They will gain confidence when they have the skills to avoid their own surprises and we do not have to lose their trust by being untrustworthy be offering sensory surprises!

> Dear Parent,
>
> Do you remember a sensory surprise and your reaction to it?
> Can you think of a time when your child reacted to a sensory surprise?

Most parents and therapists who know worried eaters have blown it at times. We just tried to change the flavor a little bit and thought (silly us) that the anxious eater would not mind! But we did not get away with it. The child KNEW it right away! We told him it was *his* cereal, but meanwhile we substituted the generic brand *knowing* he could not possibly *ever notice*. But he DID notice. How did he do that? WE would not be able to tell the difference!! Sensory surprises like this have a way of eroding trust. An unexpected change can put a worried eater on edge every time they eat with us. He wonders what did we do to his food this time? Children often feel the need to protect themselves from our sensory surprises.

And how many of us have inadvertently provided a sensory surprise only to have it soundly rejected. That time we put just a little different yogurt in the bowl? Or the time we bought a new brand of that "O" cereal? Or that time we added just a little jelly to the peanut butter sandwich? That time where we made what we thought was the tiniest change and the child responded with surprise, usually negative surprises, rejection, cough, gag, push the food away or even throw it! And we will also probably remember how they did not trust that food, or us for a while after that. Their hypervigilance increased. Their worry increased and they may have actually dropped that *contaminated* food from their *List*.

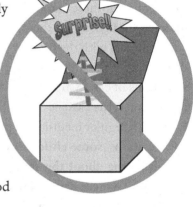

No Sensory Surprises!

Sensory Rehearsals

We have encouraged families to give multiple exposure rehearsals so children can be invited to family meals, food preparation and family food interactions. We offered each child the opportunity to see others interacting with the foods and invited them to interact. In these multiple exposure rehearsals, the focus is being around food interactions in daily life, being around others modeling food interactions. Your child could interact with the sensory properties of the food, or not. If they began to interact directly with the foods, the multiple exposure rehearsals begin to get closer to the sensations of eating and turn into sensory rehearsals. There is overlap here, and the distinction is the closeness the child gets to sensory exploration and eventual tasting. Even with regular inclusion in positive non-pressured family meals, enjoyable family conversations, **some children who are especially anxious eaters need actual support learning about the sensory properties of foods, learning to systematically get closer to these sensations.**

Sensory rehearsals provide a focused and systematic way to help your child explore the sensory properties of the foods so she has a **preview** of what to expect with her food interactions. A sensory rehearsal is one that begins to expose the child to the sensory properties of the foods, first farther away with eyes, smell and touch and the later toward tastes. These rehearsals help her learn about sensations of foods, first from a safer distance with more **distant sensory rehearsal**, and the closer in **up-close sensory rehearsals**.

Of course, we want to create opportunities for children to interact enjoyably with the sensory properties of foods so, with these rehearsals, they are more likely to try the foods. We know from research that interacting or exploring the sensory properties of food can increase the likelihood of a child trying and liking a new food. We know the look has a lot to do with trying. The smell and the touch have a lot to do with trying. We know that smelling and touching foods can make a difference in increasing willingness to try foods for cautious eaters.[64]

A continuum of sensations

Let us look at how each food sensation can be imagined on a continuum of tiny steps from farther away, distant sensations to up-close sensations. Here are some ideas and you will think of others as you consider these sensory sensitivities in the rehearsals you offer.

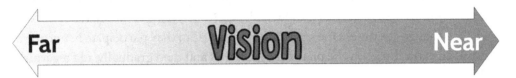

Vision is such a great sensory *rehearsal* because it offers distant previews and then up-close previews about meals and food. But it does not **yet** involve touching tasting and those closer worrisome sensations. The *distant visuals* help children see *others* eating. Children learn from being around the table, watching how others use utensils, try foods, pass foods and put foods on their plates. The *up-close visuals* can help or hinder new food trying as children see food up-close, near them. Many of our worried eaters are hypervigilant about ANY change in the look of a new food. Their up-close visual warning system *notices* new shapes, new colors, tiny specks of a darker color, when apples are not exactly all red or crackers are broken. On the other hand, their visual systems can also be a warning that a small change is happening and allow the child to expect the change and then avoid a sensory surprise.

Many children need to get used to the visual change gradually seeing someone else's food, not their own. This is where we encourage grownups to sit near their child with their new and different food so she can get use to food and presentation changes without the fear that their *List* foods are changing.

As foods are visually closer, we can grade our visual *ask* by helping children get used to visual changes in their food very slowly. We can dilute a color change a tiny bit at a time by including the child in the food preparation. Can the child help drip a drop of food coloring, or diluted colored water into a cup of water to change the look slightly but not change the color dramatically?

We want to **separate out the various sensations** and offer change in one sensation at a time for very worried eaters so they are not having to get used to visual change AND taste or color changes. Can we give the child who only wants his sandwich (crust-less and in triangles) a triangle sandwich that has differently *sized* triangles, or triangles with slightly different shapes and angles? First, they would see us have *our* sandwiches with different triangles near them (as a distant visual). As they get comfortable with our sandwich shape changing, can their triangles (up-close visuals) be slightly different? How small of a visual change needs to be offered that gives the child the idea that *change happens* without too big of a worry? To minimize the visual sensory surprise, can the child be the one who helps cut the sandwich?

Vision also counts with the overall look of the presentation. As the child is given their *List* food on their plate, can the plates change? This changes the look, but not the food. One change at a time? One sensation at a time? Can they participate in putting a garnish, an extra thing, on the plates of others first and then gradually add a garnish to their own plate? The garnish changes the look, but if children get used to that, they can be less worried as they get used to a new food on their plate (that they can try, or not). It can be seen as a garnish that has no pressure attached. The garnish becomes the *rehearsal* for the new family food on the plate later.

By being aware that vision matters for so many worried eaters, we can carefully give them distant previews first on our plates and food before up-close visual changes on theirs.

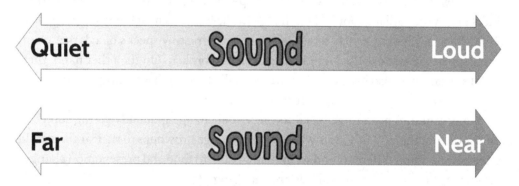

We have talked about how sound can be a factor for children in their new food preferences. The distant sound of others eating crunchy food can be a preview of how the food might sound up-close in their mouths. This is a sensory variation that many children do not worry about at all, a variable they can ignore. Great. No problem. But for the few where the sound of *you* crunching celery or and apple leads them to run out of the room, then maybe you could avoid those experiences directly as you start new food trying with other food opportunities that will be more positive for your child. Maybe you can offer less worrisome, quieter foods when helping him find new foods he can love. Maybe he needs to get more confident in new food trying skills without sound worry. There are LOTS of quieter foods to choose from as we make decisions about what to offer.

We can consider sound variation near to far as we invite children to help us in food preparation. Appliances make noise. Some children need to cover their ears or stand farther away while you turn on the blender. Some need to wear headphones to get closer to the action. We need to do whatever the child needs to get comfortable and not be distracted or turned off by the sound.

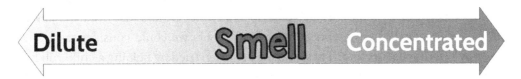

Smell is such a great sensation because it enhances flavor and taste and also has such predictable distant and up-close properties. Remember smell is taste from a distance. It gives the child a pretty good preview of what that food might taste like before it is up-close on his tongue. It gives a taste preview that reduces the *sensory surprise*.

The arrow on this continuum goes in both directions. There are some children that need the smell to be strong and noticeable to even *know* it is there, to attract them to a new food. Think about all the children who absolutely love bacon! Often it is its strong smell that attracts them to it! There are other children who are very worried and hypervigilant about food smells and check every food out initially by smelling it. Acceptance or rejection of any food offered will depend on their smell assessment.

By giving your child opportunities to be around your cooking or food preparation, you can give them smell experiences to decide on the smells, the distant tastes, that attract them. Those smell opportunities can be big concentrated smells or diluted smells. By understanding the power of smell to attract your child to the food or send him running from the food, we can grade our *ask*. For example, think about trying a new drink. You bring the glass to your mouth and your nose is literally inside the cup! Your nose is up-close to the smell of the new drink in a concentrated way. The child is getting a big smell **with** a new taste. For some this is too much. Can we put a lid and a straw on the cup to dilute the concentrated smell? There are lots of cup lids commercially available for children's cups. Some are hard and some are stretchy. Pick the one you and your child both like.

Dilute — **Taste** — **Concentrated**

Taste will have so many sensation variations that are also influenced by the sensations of texture and temperature. As we try to tease out the tiniest of changes, one sensation at a time, we have to remember that we have described *flavor* as the *taste without the texture*. Again, some children can comfortably try new flavors combined with new textures in what we have described as *taste*. Others just need the *flavor,* offered separately. For very worried new food try-ers we could consider taste previews by offering flavors first. These flavors are often tried by helping a child rub his finger on the food and touch his lip. If he is comfortable, he can touch his finger to his tongue or reach his tongue toward the flavor. For children we call these **finger tastes, but we grownups carefully calibrate whether our taste offer is flavor only or taste (with texture).**

Mild — **Taste** — **Spicy**

Mildly Sweet — **Taste** — **Concentrated Sweet**

Mildly Salty — **Taste** — **Concentrated Salty**

Mildly Sour — **Taste** — **Concentrated Sour**

Mildly Bitter — Taste — Concentrated Bitter

Mildly Umami — Taste — Concentrated Umami

These flavors can be diluted or concentrated. When helping your child learn to enjoy a new juice, perhaps it needs to be a tiny diluted flavor change. This might come from using a dropper together to add new flavor drops to a familiar juice, or the flavor change that comes from adding an ice cube of a new juice to their juice. The ice cube can be further diluted by diluting the flavor you put in the ice cube so that change made when it melts in the drink is smaller in a graded way. The child could try the new juice with a sip from the cup, or, as a lesser challenge, by dipping her finger in the juice and having a **finger taste**. The finger taste gives a guaranteed tiny flavor of the new drink, rather than an inadvertent bigger splash.

Another way to dilute a taste might be to combine the new food with a food your child likes already. Remember Marta's story? She diluted the big taste (and texture) of salmon by trying it first with bread. The bread dilutes the salmon taste and gave her the smallest flavor shadow to start. She could add more taste, concentrate it, at her pace.

Consider therapeutic setting foods. Feeding therapists can get stuck with those same tasting *clinic foods* over and over again. Your child may not like the flavor (or taste or texture) of applesauce, or vanilla pudding, or vanilla wafer cookies, pirate crunchies, melt-able veggie snack sticks, the same cheese crackers or the same brand or flavor of yogurt week after week. If we are going to find the flavors that attract them, **we need to think out of the box in the foods we offer**. Maybe she will like chicken broths or miso soup rather than juices? Maybe she will like pickles that can become the familiar food we can use to help her get comfortable with new foods? Maybe instead of sweet pureed yogurt, your child might like spicy Asian or Indian sauces? Or maybe the applesauce will be more appreciated if is berry flavored and red rather than plain? **We encourage parents to *offer all different flavors* at home and to bring interesting flavors from home to therapy sessions for new food trying**

practice. We are looking for what does your child love! So, the flavors we offer should be from all food categories and all flavor categories. Keep offering. Your child may well surprise you with her likes. Give her smell and flavor choices and let **her** decide which ones she is ready for.

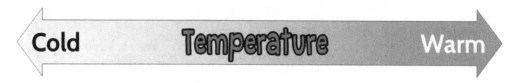

Be aware that this continuum of temperature goes both directions. Some children like their foods hotter and others like room temperature or cooler. And some do not care. For children who care, this is a sensory property **we** can manage in our new food offers. If temperature is really important to your child and you are trying to help him find new foods he likes, it might be better to keep the temperature as he likes it and work on the other flavor, taste, or texture variations first. Why fight this sensation, or any sensations, for that matter? Temperature gradations can be changed very gradually as needed with tiny or bigger ice cubes, or with more stirring or warm foods to cool them. Remember, when changing temperature, do it gradually and do it with your child.

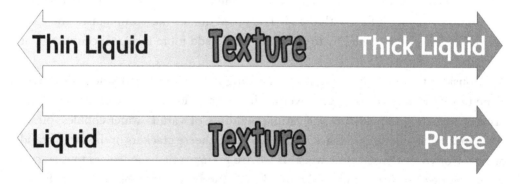

Oh, texture! There are so many textures and worried eaters **notice** texture changes, even the tiniest of changes and even changes you or I might not even notice! Mouths are sensitive! We need to believe them! We need to become texture change detectives and creatively offer the tiniest change in a tiptoe toward texture change. We need to remember that texture influences hand touch as well as mouth touch.

Finger tips and palms are sensitive, too and feel texture and temperature changes as do lips and tongues.

Some children are able to drink thin liquids but need thicker due to swallowing challenges. Others start with thin and just plain worry about changing to anything else. When the challenge is swallowing safety, families need to work with their medical feeding team to determine safety, developmental readiness and a plan to move them toward thinner or thicker liquid. For older children whose swallow is safe but where *change* is the issue, thin liquid might be thickened with nectars gradually to get to a nectar thick drink or thickened with fruit sauces, rice cereals, oatmeal or smoothies to get toward purees. Or, some families need to start with a puree, such as the fruit sauce, and dilute it down toward thin. Remember, though, that the puree thickened as a smoothie will be a different puree texture than the liquid thickened with cereals or applesauce. Texture matters so tread carefully.

Puree ◄ Texture Different Puree ►

We touched on this earlier in the book. All purees are not equal. Imagine the feel in your mouth of baby food apricots in contrast with oatmeal, vanilla yogurt, toothpaste (as a dense and viscous texture), to vegetable puree thickened with quinoa, or blended lasagna or beef stew. They are all so different. Differently thick, differently dense, differently slippery, differently coarse, yet all purees. We still might approach these with a smell first, maybe touching, and then the tiniest taste. Tiny is important because the taste will be flavor and texture combined. Separating out a flavor taste will be somewhat hard to achieve due to the texture component of the puree or sauce. Some children touch the puree with their finger, wipe off the finger and bring the residual flavor to their nose and lips or tongue to get a flavor taste without the texture. This could be a start. Tasting these new purees can be the tiniest taste on the end of a coffee stirrer with more and more added as your child shows he likes the flavor and texture combination.

Smooth pureed foods can be thickened (texture changed) with a variety of foods that have different textures. You and your child can explore these. Baby rice cereal thickening will make a very different texture change than thickening with graham cracker crumbs, saltine cracker crumbs, orzo, quinoa, farro grains, rice, or ground nuts. These all thicken. Some will be a smoother puree and some will be coarser.

Some will be swallowed all at once and others will leave a residual to deal with, like the ground nuts. The texture and amount of the thickener will matter.

The challenge for many children learning texture change is that we assume there is a *usual* texture transition from baby food to solids. But all developmental transitions are not the same. The food choices we offer give different texture opportunities to babies. Though some children transition from breastmilk or formula to commercial baby foods, others transition to homemade baby foods. The textures are different. Think baby food apricots again: somewhat slippery, runny, somewhat creamy? Think homemade baby food peas, less runny, a little textured and still a puree.

And then many babies around the world go from their breast and bottle liquids to a baby version of the family foods. These might be the tiniest careful tastes of plantains, maize, smashed artichoke heart, mashed peas, fish soup or ground nut stew. In some countries the mother chews some of the family food and gives careful, not choke-able amounts of that food to baby, a little at a time, watching for their reaction. Many families give a tiny scraped taste of whole banana or small piece of mashed banana, sweet potato or avocado. Think of all the texture variations in these early baby offerings. The important thing to remember is that babies, when all has gone well and they have the developmental readiness for the introduction of solids, learn to love foods and manage careful small tastes toward bigger tastes. They let us know what works and what they enjoy. Our worried eaters may do well during this these texture transitions, and start their worry later, or they may start their worry at this first sign of texture change.

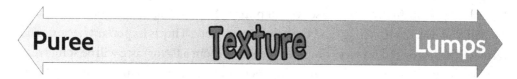

Early on in my career, I believed that *puree to lumps or mashed* was the most usual sequence in texture transition for babies. But, as I work with many families from many different cultures, I realize *usual* differs family to family. Many children today do not specifically hang out at the puree stage. Some get offered baby food purees or differently textured homemade purees. Some start with purees and use them as a foundation to learn soft mashed foods. Some are fed the purees and others learning about feeding themselves by bringing purees to their mouth with their own fingers. Many babies get offered early safe texture tastes and show immediate enjoyment and desire to reach for and bring more of those tastes to their mouths. Some are offered baby food feeders with soft or juicy food inserted and chew on them or mouth them as mouthing toys with flavor and texture. Some get soft foods that they manage to pick up and then actively work to get small morsels of them to their own mouth, gradually increasing skill and volume with maturation and interest. The point here, is that textures vary and most babies manage with careful parental food choices and supervision.

Babies NEED texture variation. All around the world babies get variation from their family food as they are fed carefully off their parents' plates. They learn to enjoy texture and taste variation early. However, we meet many babies who are offered only the smoothest of commercial baby food from the baby food jar, and at a year have not been exposed to family food texture variation. It is no wonder that some of our children who are wired to have more of a worry temperament have some trouble accepting more texture foods or any foods not presented in a jar. This is not to say no babies should have commercial baby food. This is a parental choice. A smooth baby food can be **a part of the careful food tasting options offered babies**. But babies *need variation* to learn to be comfortable with variation. And variation should include the food coming from different containers, such as different bowls, or maybe even little cups.

Texture transition support

The transitions toward textured foods needs an extra step for many children. Instead of purees to mashed solids or lumps, we need to consider carefully giving one puree to another puree offers. Some children need adults to make a concerted effort to offer purees of varying textures to help children gain confidence in puree texture variation. We can offer differently textured purees so the child is not having to make a texture leap from smooth baby food puree to lumps in one giant leap. Children who are comfortable with purees of multiple different textures, will often have an easier time with the texture changes inherent in adding mashed foods and soft lumps because they are already used to variation. The texture leap here is often the reason many children have a harder time with stage three baby foods that have soft solid lumps because they may not have had sufficient experience with puree texture variation.

Texture Transition Support

Smooth puree ➡ Smooth puree from a textured utensil ➡ Textured puree

---

Offering the familiar textured food from a differently textured utensil or mouthing toy can be a very helpful addition to the puree texture change continuum. When children are stuck, really stuck, on a certain textured food and they are highly sensitive to changes in texture, they may refuse all food texture change offered. I remember meeting a child who only ate baby food smooth pears as his wet food. The parents and I tried a standard texture change offer by adding a little bit of baby rice cereal. He was very uncomfortable with the rice cereal change, so I tried again with less cereal. Silly me. He already was worried because I had plowed into his worry, but I just wanted to see what change he would be comfortable with. (Silly me, again). Finally, we went back to offering his favorite baby food pears to find comfort, trust and familiar again. The next time we offered texture change it was NOT in the change in the puree. It was from texture change on the utensil. We started the meal with his familiar puree from his familiar spoon. Then, we offered some alternating mouthfuls from his finger, parent finger, a smooth mouthing toy or textured mouthing toy or textured spoons. He showed us he was comfortable because he KNEW the food. He noticed the spoon texture change as he wrinkled his eyebrows, but the utensil was in his mouth and then out in a flash and what was left in his mouth was HIS familiar food. The **textured tools were the bridge for texture change** for him. Gradually he was able to get comfortable with rice cereal and other careful puree to puree texture changes along a continuum of tiny, tiny changes. Remember the utensils can be fingers and spoons and mouthing toys and therapeutic tools. Each provides yet again, a different experience.

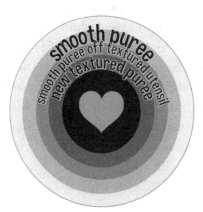

Circle of Sensitivity
Puree Texture Transition

> **This texture transition works because**:
> We started with a FAMILIAR FOOD.
> We changed only the utensil.
> There was a beginning and an end to the new, "different part."
> We followed the child's cues.

Having said all that about the importance of early experiences with puree texture variation, we meet many worried eaters who let us know their *List* preferences are extremes… smooth yogurts or dry foods and solids, but absolutely **do not want** those other purees variations. If that is your starting point, then, okay, that is your starting point! But, we need to help worried eaters transition from their favorite wet food diet (for example, the child who only eats baby food and never got past those smooth textures, or now only eat blended foods). OR We will need to help the worried eaters who like only certain foods (but they must be dry and crunchy) to get comfortable with wet foods. These transitions may need to be eventual transitions, not starting transitions. Remember that if a child likes many purees but needs to add more food groups or more dietary variation, we would do well to celebrate that puree texture and add more foods, more flavors and more recipe **changes to that routine before stressing too much on the texture change.** We start with the sensory variable that work and make new food decisions based on the big picture of their eating comfort and their nutritional needs.

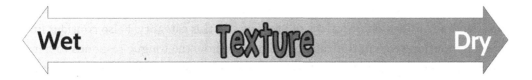

Wet to dry and dry to wet are BIG texture changes! Some children who are very worried about change may need to get comfortable first trying new foods *within their favored food texture range* first before asking them to get closer to a completely different texture. For example, a child who only likes crunchy and who does not like any change from that texture, may need to find ways to add new crunchy foods and learn that new food trying is even possible way before we worry them with purees or wet foods. In my experience, when children understand, really understand the predictability of a new food trying sequence they seem more prepared for exploring sensory changes. They often explore bigger sensory changes because they have strategies to explore the new and trust that we will not push into their worry.

Dry Meltables   Texture   Hard Chewables

Dr. Kay Toomey's SOS (Sequential-Oral-Sensory) Approach[58] has taught pediatric therapists about dry meltables and hard chewables. These are extremes of textures and could be considered in a continuum way. Let's us think about dry meltables. These foods are dry and they mix easily with saliva so that they can be lightly mashed with the tongue or minimally chewed. These tend to be the foods that parents like to give because they tend to offer less of a choking risk. I would put many types of crumbs in this category, too. All the melt-able baby puff-like foods fit in this category. Many parents are very familiar with the little melt-able veggie sticks so frequently available in therapy clinics. Many crackers fit into this category if they crush and melt with saliva. They give the child a texture variation and they are solids, but they melt in the saliva quickly enough to be interpreted as less of a threat or worry. We will discuss crumbs in greater detail later.

Hard chewables are *hard* and can be *chewed*, but do not easily fall apart or break off, offering the flavor and texture but not the requirement to break off a piece and chew. They offer the tongue and mouth experiences to adapt their motor responses. Some clinics consider licorice sticks or beef jerky in this category. I also consider fingers and mouthing toys in this category. Consider how the tongue responds to hard chewable items. Consider a baby finger as a hard "chewable" object that the baby can put in his mouth and not break off a piece (thankfully). Fingers give the mouth an opportunity to adapt its response and get used to different textures from breast nipple, bottle nipples or very smooth purees. When babies mouth their fingers, they are giving themselves early tongue and mouth experiences and these experiences change each time they put them in their mouth. Watch a baby who is mouthing for five minutes. You will be amazed at the different sensory and motor opportunities they give their mouths. One finger on this side, two fingers on that side, a fist in the middle, a fist on the side, three fingers toward the left, or three fingers toward the right. Oops, a gag here, a gag there. They are learning. They are adapting the way their lips and tongue respond to each different opportunity. They are learning about texture. They are learning about gagging and how far is too far to put their fingers in! AND when they are comfortable with their own fingers in their own mouth, we can help them add flavors by rubbing their own fingers on an apple, carrot, pear, or piece of watermelon. We can offer them flavor opportunities from their own fingers and we will learn about how they like (or do not like) this flavor by watching which flavors they come back for more, which flavors they put right back in their mouth.

Children can have these *hard chewable* experiences with mouthing toys also. As they place the toy in their cheek, on their tongues, on one side or the other, their tongue can lean into the toy and experience out-of-the-middle movements that can help prepare them for later chewing. You can flavor mouthing toys by rubbing them on foods. Think, apple, pear or cucumber or bacon. The flavor on the mouthing toy can be the inspiration to continue to explore with it. (Remember the easiest flavors tend to have no texture to start). Some therapy clinics like to add flavor with drops such as vanilla or lemon or mint oils, but I prefer to offer rubs of real foods. I find the oils are often extremely concentrated and a big flavor *ask* for many children. We can also dip fingers or mouthing toys in liquid flavors such as juices, chicken broth, miso soup, or vegetable soups, shake them off to get rid of the excess liquid, and then offer them. In a continuum of flavors, the most dilute flavor is probably water! After the child is used to mouthing the hard chewable of fingers or mouthing toys, they can explore (with supervision) the hard licorice or jerky type food that has very concentrated flavors.

These hard chewables, fingers, mouthing toys, and hard to break foods can be dipped in tastes also. Tastes can be sauces that have flavor and texture. Think broadly in these sauces. They can be yogurts or fruit sauces, marinara sauce or curry sauces, or blended cucumbers or melon. You can introduce many tastes with sauce. We must vary the opportunities we provide to find what children love.

Predictable Lumps ← **Texture** → **Unpredictable Texture**

Textures can be predictable, such as a smooth yogurt, or smoothly mashed sweet potatoes. Adding orzo pasta, star shaped pastas, alphabet pasta, quinoa, farro, rice can all add texture and still be quite predictable. No square lumps or long string spaghetti or round peas are in the mix as a surprise. Unpredictable textures are very different.

They provide the mouth with different shapes, textures, chewiness, or crunch in the same mouthful. I personally love tuna fish salad made with chopped chunks of celery and apples. For me, these add a texture and an interesting crunch experience with each bite. The exact characteristics I love about this salad, the unpredictability, are the characteristics that can lessen interest for others.

The unpredictability of some baby foods that have smooth background sauce and then square carrots, round peas, square chicken and long noodles was what may have led babies to reject them. Baby food companies are striving to unify these texture contrasts more but babies will let us know what they think about this unpredictability when they find it in their mouths. Watch them.

The other factor that is the cause of worry in unpredictability is that the child does not knows what will be in the food offered. By having the child help with the preparation, help with the adding of texture or explaining to them what is in the food can help the texture change be more predictable and less of a surprise.

$$\longleftarrow \text{Binder Foods} \quad \text{Texture} \quad \text{Scatter Foods} \longrightarrow$$

Binder foods stay together in the mouth. They are a texture that feels like the consistency of foods that we have already chewed and are ready to swallow. Think yogurt, guacamole, refried beans, mashed potatoes and blended lasagna. Scatter foods, on the other hand, scatter! They spread apart in the mouth and need to be collected by the tongue and cheek and palate before swallowing is possible. Think peas, crackers, rice (rice that is drier such as basmati rice, in contrast with Spanish rice with tomato sauce which tends to stick together more). Scatter foods need more mature motor skills, more oral organization to collect and chew the food to keep the food over the teeth for chewing and then swallowing.

Some children prefer binder foods. They may have less skill in chewing. They may prefer that texture as the food is presented in a form ready to swallow. Others like the more solid nature of the scatter foods and do not like the wet sauce of the binder foods. We can use tiny steps to help children move in either direction on this continuum. Children who like binder foods may allow a thickener such as crumbs to be added to change the texture gradually. Initially the crumbs might be stirred in and then gradually put on top or under the spoon so the tongue and mouth predominantly feels the binder food with little crumbs on the edges. Gradually more crumbs and less binder can be combined until the child has melt-able crumbs and can chew and swallow them.

This same sequence can be made with a binder food with added mashed food, and then more uneven mashed food and then less mashed food that separates and then soft foods. Think yogurt with mashed banana where the bananas are very mashed, then only slightly mashed and eventually in small soft bits and only a little binder. When mouth organization is a challenge, a feeding therapist can help you help your child to organize her chewing.

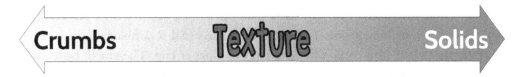

I offer crumbs a lot, crumbs in many forms and calibrated carefully. They can be the bridge from small to large, from wet to dry, from swallowing only to chewing, from quiet to noisier foods, from one food group to others. Crumbs warrant their own chapter later.

Sensory gradation helpful hints

As we are carefully looking at grading our sensory *ask,* we can consider what we know about the sensory properties of foods and the usefulness of crumbs. The structure of sensory gradation is this. **Start with familiar and comfortable (favored *List* foods). Tiptoe. Offer and adjust along the continuum**. Since there are so many sensory variables that influence enjoyment of food, you can offer one sensory change in a careful way. Really, really worried eaters may only be able to try a new change when there is only one change. Braver children may be willing to try a new food with multiple sensory differences. Each child will let their grownups know what works and we need to listen to them. Really, you are just trying to understand where the child has limits and what change is possible. We can help the child experience, *change happens*, and it will be okay. No big sensory surprises. No overwhelming plates of foods, just small changes.

Let's try it. How might you change scrambled egg?

That has a look, a flavor, a texture, a sound. If you aimed directly to change it to a spinach omelet with diced red peppers, you will probably get resistance from your anxious eater. There are way too many sensory variables changed at the same time! So, how could you carefully grade the changes? You could change the distant sensory variable first, the look and the smell and the hand or finger feel. They may be less worrisome than changing the nearer sensory variables of flavor and taste (with mouth feel). However, there is no recipe here. Each child is so very unique that you are *offering* scrambled egg change carefully with your knowledge of your child's sensitivities.

Change the look: You could change the look of YOUR scrambled eggs. You could offer the same scrambled eggs your child likes but served in three little piles on the plate instead of one bigger one. You could offer the usual scrambled eggs in a tiny bowl versus a plate. You could offer the eggs in a paper cup. The smell, taste, and texture are the same. The only variation is the look of the presentation. And what if that is too hard? You could offer your child's scrambled eggs, the ones from the *List*, in the same way on the same plate, but YOU could eat YOUR scrambled eggs from a different plate near them. This is a rehearsal. OR in good Dr. Seuss fashion[65] you could change the color (with them participating in the activity so they know what is happening). Green, maybe? ☺. The plates, taste and texture are all the same. Only the color changed.

Change the smell: If you offer the same textured scrambled eggs from the same plate, you could tiptoe into a smell change. Perhaps you provide the rehearsal by previewing YOUR eggs, near them and you cooked YOURS in a bit of bacon fat rather than the usual butter. The texture and look will be the same but the smell of your eggs, and ultimately the taste when they are ready to try them, will change slightly with the bacon. Since smell is a distant sensory property, it will give a taste from a distance preview and they will get that preview from YOUR food without threatening THEIRS. As the bacon smell attracts them with multiple exposures they may try with limited surprise.

Change the taste: Cooking the scrambled egg in coconut oil, or bacon fat will change the flavor. Cheese will change the flavor if added in small quantities. Neither of these will change the texture much if changed in small amounts. Spices will change the flavor. Be aware that some spices, such as salt, garlic powder, do not change the look much, but green parsley and black pepper may add worrisome little color flecks. Some children will be very worried about the flecks and others will not care.

Change the texture: Texture can vary slightly by making the scrambled eggs slightly wetter or slightly drier with changes in cooking time. Texture can also be changed in varying degrees by adding different amounts of cheese, but this will also change the flavor and will need previews. Cheese has different smells and brands and can be added in tiny amounts or larger amounts along a continuum of change. You can change the texture by adding foods to the scrambled eggs but notice that the look and the flavors will change as you add. Diced peppers, pieces of bacon and ham, broccoli, salsa all change the look and texture and flavor. Perhaps these are not the starting point?

Change the sound: Scrambled eggs are a quiet food to chew. If you want to play with sound, you could combine crushed crackers on top of the eggs or offer them off a crunchy cracker and demonstrate to your child that these eggs sound different. It is a rehearsal for the sound change.

Change the meal: Scrambled eggs could be offered on the usual plate, but maybe another familiar food is offered to go with it. Maybe a familiar cracker is offered with the scrambled egg? You are essentially showing your child that his *List* foods can be combined in different ways. These two usually unrelated foods can be offered together, on the same plate. Something new, *change happens*. If your child will have them on the same plate, great, but the change food may need to be resting on a nearby plate. Or, once your child can accept two familiar foods together, can there be three or four, or can there be a new food on the plate or nearby (without the pressure expectation of trying). Remember these are rehearsals.

Let's try it. How might you change toast?

Change the look: When giving *List* toast, you can change the look. This distant sensory change can be a start for the most worried of eaters. Can the toast be offered on a different plate OR (adjust, adjust) YOU can have the same toast nearby but change YOUR plates? Can the toast be cut in half, or offered as a smaller piece of toast, or be cut into different shapes? OR, (adjust, adjust) if the shape change on his toast is too much, can he help you cut YOUR toast in different shapes and then you eat it near him.

Change the smell: Smell in toast is hard to change without making some changes in the look by toasting different bread, or texture by double toasting it so it smells more toasted.

Change the taste: Toast taste can change with toasting different breads, adding different spreads in various amounts, adding cinnamon sugar which does not change the texture or look too much.

Change the texture: Toast texture can be changed by double toasting so it is crunchier or adding extra butter which makes it wetter and softer. Different breads have a different starting texture. Of course, spreads change the texture, as does the addition of deli meat, cheese (melted or solid) or bacon or spinach when tiptoeing into sandwiches.

Change the sound: More toasting will increase the crunch. Less toasting or plain bread will probably decrease the sound.

Change the meal: And then the meal can change. From toast of one kind of bread you can go to different bread foods, crescents, pizza dough, tortillas, crusty bread, English muffins, bread with raisins, sweet breads, savory breads, yeast breads and breakfast breads. Or how about finding your way to waffles, pancakes or muffins?

Let's try it. How might you change noodles?

We know children who love their spaghetti (plain or with butter or oil only) and who will reject any offer of a new of different noodle. How about if you look at changing fewer sensory variables at first?

Change the look: By now you are thinking, *okay, okay, can I change the plate.* Yes, this keeps the favored food the same but changes a distant sensory variable, the look. Smell and taste and texture are still familiar. OR could you break the spaghetti in half before cooking it? Or (adjust, adjust) can you just break a *few pieces and not all the pieces* in half prior to cooking. Could your child help you break them, or could you just break yours so the change is nearby and NOT on his plate? Once your child is comfortable with eating his noodles broken in half could they be broken in quarters or eights? Could they ultimately be broken small on that continuum of changes and be the one-inch size of tiny fideo noodles or uneven sizes? OR could your child help you crush up the spaghetti prior to cooking so the pieces are so small that you add an orzo type paste to the mix? (These are really small rice shaped pastas). Or can you add a colorful pasta to the mix, his, or even yours first? There are red beet pastas and green spinach pastas, and more! My experience is that the colored pastas often do not have much taste difference. (But, I admit, my tasters for this pasta change may be confused as I often have my red or green pastas with some type of sauce that dilutes the pasta flavor change.

Change the smell: The look of the spaghetti can be the same, but the smell can change. Spice works well here as garlic, cumin, lemon, toasted sesame oil, or lime in the cooking water will change the smell. This smell change can be big or little. OR if your child likes their spaghetti with oil of butter, these flavors can change and that will change the smell. Garlic oil or butter or basil oil, orange or lemon oil will keep the look the same and change the smell. Of course, changing the smell in this way will also change the flavor, so there may need to be a very tiny smell and flavor change or YOU may need to change yours nearby for the smell (taste from a distance) rehearsal.

Change the taste: Tastes changes can come, as mentioned, from spices and butters and oil and of course, from sauces. Red sauces, pesto and white sauces can have great variations in taste and you can start from a familiar sauce and tiptoe toward other brand changes or other variations of flavor. If your child likes cheeses you can tiptoe toward cheese sauces.

Change the texture: Texture changes will come with the shape changes in the spaghetti or as you tip toe toward other pasta shapes, a few at a time. The mistake often made is offering a whole BOWL of a new pasta shape, a mountain of elbow pastas. Yes, the pasta's taste may be the same but the mountain may be overwhelming in its newness. Spaghetti can be more cooked, softer, or al dente, chewier, and places in between on the continuum. This will change the feel of chewing.

Change the sound: Varying the cooking may change the internal sound feel of chewing as the softer noodles may slide down with less chewing and the al dente noodles may make more sound when chewing. You can also practice with sound change by adding crushed crackers to the spaghetti, crumbs to the top of the serving, in the proportions your child is ready for, to add a crunch sound to the bite. Maybe sound changes are absolutely not necessary. Pick your sensations!

Change the meal: From spaghetti, can you get to all different noodles from elbows to farfalle, to rigatoni, to spirals? Can you change up the sauces? Can you get to layered spaghetti and go toward lasagnas? Can you get to rice by shrinking the spaghetti size until it is rice size and bridge from orzo pasta to rice? Can the sauce be on the outside, or gradually in stuffed shells? Can cheese be added to the sauce?

The more you realize that diluting the amount of sensory change can help your child try new foods, the better you will get at it. When feeding anxious eaters, we all usually get lots of practice offering a new food and then having it rejected. Too big of an *ask*! This is the time when we need to get good at quickly adjusting and analyzing or grading the sensory offer we have made. It will become natural. However, to help you think about how these sensory variables relate, I am providing a chart as a framework. It is meant to be an option that might help guide your thinking as you pick variable change. Ignore it if it is too overwhelming or use it as a guide if it helps.

The sensory changes are listed from the look of the food, to the smell, touch on fingers or palm, flavor change (with no texture, finger tastes on lips or tongue), taste change (flavor combined with texture) and sound change. Remember that texture or feel changes can include food texture, temperature, wetness, dryness. Each of those changes can be offered separately without changing other sensations or in combination with other sensation changes. To create some changes, two or three sensations might change too. IS your child ready for that? For example, you can change the presentation look of the food without changing the smell or flavor. You can change the flavor without changing the look.

Dear Parent,
This chart may be more than you would need or use. It probably feels more like a therapy clinic, but it just provides another way to systematically think about these sensory changes. Don't worry. ☺

Change	Without or with these sensory changes	Food choice
Look change (presentation)	Smell change Touch change (fingers, palms) Flavor change (taste but no texture) Taste change (taste with texture) Sound change	
Smell change	Look change Touch change (fingers, palms) Flavor change (taste but no texture) Taste change (taste with texture) Sound change	
Touch change (Fingers/palms)	Look change Smell change Flavor change (taste but no texture) Taste change (taste with texture) Sound change	
Flavor change	Look change Smell change Touch change (fingers, palms) Taste change (taste with texture)	

Change	Without or with these sensory changes	Food choice
Taste change (taste with texture)	Look change Smell change Touch change (fingers, palms,) Sound change	
Sound change	Look change Smell change Touch change (fingers, palms,) Flavor change Taste change (taste with texture)	

Options

Changing sensory variables gives you and your child options. Options for new food trying in tinier steps of worry. Options for systematic de-sensitization rather than flooding. Options for a continuum of tiny steps that offer the smallest change with the bigger possibility of enjoyment. You can think creatively to dilute the up-close sensory challenge, while also providing regular multiple food exploration opportunities for your child to see the foods you are eating. The family foods. These all have looks and smells, flavors, textures and sounds different from the familiar sensations your child usually experiences on his *List*. Even without all this sensation manipulation, children do surprise us when out of the blue, they ask to try your green smoothies, or your shrimp fettucine! The idea is to give lots of exposures to find the ones that work for your child.

Sensory Continuum

	Texture	
Dry Meltables	**Texture**	Hard Chewables
Thin Liquid	**Texture**	Thick Liquid
Liquid	**Texture**	Puree
Puree	**Texture**	Different Puree
Thin Puree	**Texture**	Thick Puree
Wet	**Texture**	Dry
Puree	**Texture**	Lumps
Predictable Lumps	**Texture**	Unpredictable Texture
Binder Foods	**Texture**	Scatter Foods
Crumbs	**Texture**	Solids

Sensory Continuum (cont.)

Far — Sound — Near

Far — Vision — Near

Quiet — Sound — Loud

Dilute — Smell — Concentrated

Dilute — Taste — Concentrated

Mild — Taste — Spicy

Flavor — Taste — Flavor and Texture

Cold — Temperature — Warm

Crumbs are Small

"Crumbs are a game changer!"
~Jake Barnes, parent

As we look at ways to offer small sensory changes, we can consider CRUMBS. When worry is big, our *asks* usually need to be small. Crumbs are small. As we consider tiny *asks* in sensory and motor changes, crumbs can be our friend, and your child's friend. So many of our anxious eaters like some kind of brown and crunchy foods. Right? Chips, crackers, cookies, cereals. Often the favorites are brown and *melt-able* and easy to chew. When a child likes this type of food, crumbs can be a great starting point to bridge to a new food!

We can make most brown *melt-able* foods into crumbs. Remember our adult food *try-er*, Marta? Her idea of *trying* was to put a large mouthful of the new food in her mouth quickly and grimace-faced, wash it down with water. Of course, she was not finding new foods to add to her *List*. The *ask* was too big. She was **flooding** herself! The food sample was too large, the smell too strong, the flavor too new, and the texture too much! This is why we like to start with tiny crumbs, if we can. We involve your child in crumb making and crumb changes so as NOT to give a sensory surprise. Not to give a really big *ask*. Some children are not ready to change their favored foods with crumbs, and others find the smallness of the change possible.

Oh, those crumbs!

Crumbs can be made really small and really fine. Children can learn about crumbs and how to "crumb" with familiar foods they know so the flavor is not new. The smell can be minimized. The texture *ask* can be tiny. The amounts offered can increase gradually to bridge from one texture of food to another. The placement and crumb sizes can be prescribed to make new motor asks in chewing. The volume can be changed as your child is increasing comfort and confidence.

Making crumbs

Children can participate in making crumbs. Let them help as a food exposure, a rehearsal into the crumbs. Crumbs can be made between the finger tips and thumb. They can be put in a clear zipper plastic bag and smashed with spoons, child tool box hammers or rolling pins. They can be stomped on, jumped on or walked on in those bags. They can be made in food processors or blenders, in coffee bean grinders, mortar and pestles, graters and zesters. Each choice changes the crumb consistency depending on starting food and will influence the fineness and coarseness, the evenness and unevenness and the powdery-ness of the offer!

Sensory *asks*

For a child really worried about texture and flavor change, crumbs can help. There is a continuum of crumbs. Each *crumb-able* food has its own characteristics that can be used sensitively to help you find what your child loves. Start safe as you teach the skill. Your child can be given their own familiar foods with a fine dusting of a familiar crumb on top. He can participate in the dusting. In the continuum of sensory changes, *dustings* can become identifiable *crumbs*. There can be lots of crumbs, or a few. They can change in flavor, size, coarseness. We are looking for what flavor and texture attracts your child so you have a crumb starting point. Some children jump right into crumb changes and learn that if the new food is a crumb size it may well be safe to try. Others need a number of steps in between before they are comfortable at all with crumbs. They are a change for them to experience!

Imagine crumbs you might create with your child from these sensory crumb variations. Dry foods crumb foods can be *crumbed* or *solid*. Small, or whole. The small crumbs can be as tiny, as a single particle of crumb, or larger, as a pinch or pile of crumbs. As your child shows skill, confidence and enjoyment with the tiniest crumb, their amounts can be increased for greater sensory and motor challenges. They can become small pieces and eventually bitesize pieces that require organization in the mouth for chewing. Just as we teach new food trying, we *teach* crumbs and crumbing. Once children KNOW crumbs mean small, they can have some more confidence in trying because they have learned small is okay!

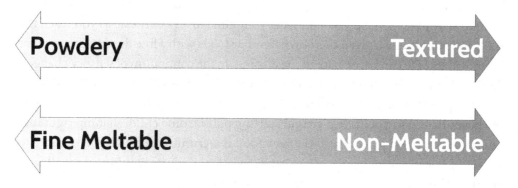

‹ Crumbs   Solids ›

They can be *powdery* or *textured*. Do you know those meringue cookies that turn into powder or dust when crushed or grated? Or if you take a freeze-dried banana chip and grate or zest it, it will be a powder. You and your child can sprinkle or blow a crumb powder on a food! You can blow the powdered crumbs with lips or straws. If powdery is the *here* of the continuum, textured crumbs are the *there*. Textured crumbs would be ANY crumb that is not a powder. As we think in terms of a continuum, powder crumbs or dust would tend to be easier and *any other* crumbs would probably be harder. Crumb texture should be offered in a tiptoe approach from powdery to *everything else*.

‹ Powdery   Textured ›

‹ Fine Meltable   Non-Meltable ›

Crumbs can be *fine meltable* or *non-meltable*. We are familiar with the buttery crackers or cookies and graham type crackers that can be crushed to fine crumbs, bordering on powder. It feels like they melt in your mouth as they mix with your saliva. They *go away* quickly, a beginning and an end. The worry can fade quickly as the crumb melts. Think about fine melt-able crumbs you know.

But, also think about *non-meltable* crumbs? These crumbs do not melt. They stick around and require some mouth movements to organize, chew and swallow them. They linger. We would probably not start with non-melt-able crumbs for a child who has lots of sensory worry about texture changes because they are just too big an *ask* and they hang around too long! But when your child has become comfortable with the smallness of crumbs as a new food trying technique, starting small, starting with just a few "crumbs" can be a great confidence builder and even a way to expand food groups!

For example, nuts grind well in a coffee bean grinder. They become a *non-melt-able* crumb. They might be a great addition to the usual brown or carbohydrates foods that dominate your child's diet. Coconut can be made into crumbs in the food processor or grinder and they do not melt. Beware because both nuts and coconut have big flavors and big smells! These crumbs, though, can be a way to subtly help your child add some extra calories as they are sprinkled on a familiar food or dipped in a smooth food such as yogurt!

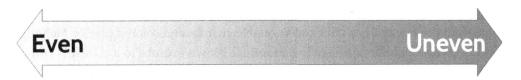

On a continuum of crumbs, there are even and uneven crumbs. Crumbs can be *even* if your child does best with predictable, or *uneven*, if unpredictable is the goal. When crumbs are used as a thickener, *even* will often be the starting point for careful sensory texture changes. There are so many variations of even and uneven that each crumb offer will be unique and a tiptoe process.

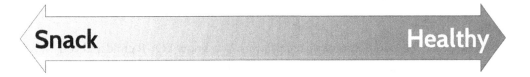

Crumbs can be *snack food* or *healthier* foods. We often think of crumbs as brown and carbohydrate. But think out of that box! Many parents have asked their child's feeding therapist, can we give my child something *other* than those sugary, salty or *snacky* foods? So many clinics have melt-able crunchy *puff* like foods and other snack foods as therapy foods of choice. They are easy to chew and easy for special placement in the mouth. They can be the salty, greasy, cheesy foods that children really like, but parents have said, really, can we do better? Can we think *new food groups* when we are considering crumbs? Freeze-dried fruits and vegetables can be crumbs. They can help add a new food group into the carbohydrate dominated diet and can add color. The color part may be the reason some children are worried about these crumbs. We can adjust. Perhaps we do not start with a new color crumb. Perhaps we start with a crumb that is brown like the familiar food, but we still aim for another food group. For children with wheat dominated snack foods, how about considering a crispy rice cereal as a new crumb? This will add the *rice food group* ☺ ! It is at least a step in the right direction.

Browns ⟷ Mixed Colors

We usually think of crumbs as brown, but they can be *mixed colors*? This can come from the freeze-dried fruit and vegetable crumbs and colored cereals. Helping visually sensitive children bridge from familiar brown crumbs to a colorful crumb can be an important step in learning *change happens*. The color changes can also be an enticement to get involved with crumbs. We can offer various colors (and textures) of sprinkles, colored sugars as a bridge to new crumb colors, flavors and textures. And colored sugars can melt if added to a warm water to change color and flavor.

Quiet Flavor ⟷ Wake-Up Flavor

Crumbs can be *quiet flavors* or *wake-up flavors*. You know YOUR child and you know whether a wake-up flavor is too big of an *ask* to start, but it can be a goal. Quiet flavored crumbs can be plain rice crackers or plain baby rice cracker options. The non-flavored variety have pretty quiet flavors. Lots of crumb foods also come in big, wake-up-your-mouth flavors. Think teriyaki, salty, garlic, ranch, spicy hot and gingersnaps.

Remember as we offer sensory changes for the more worried eater, we want to be careful not to combine too big of a flavor and texture *asks* at the same time. The wake-up aspect of the crumb can be the flavor, texture or sound! Tiptoe!

Sweet ⟷ Savory

Crumbs can be *sweet* or *savory*. Don't get stuck with sweet if you can help it. If that is your starting point, consider little tiny steps toward more varied flavor. Many children are connoisseurs of sweet. We can help them tiptoe toward more savory through more neutral quiet flavors, if needed.

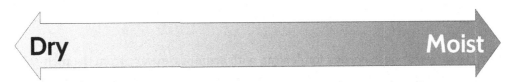

And crumbs can be *dry* or damp or *moist*. We generally think of crumbs as dry. We generally start with dry so your child can learn about crumbs as comfortably as possible from the dry foods he already knows. But the great thing about crumbs is that children learn to trust that **crumbs are small**. Crumbs are safe. Crumbs are comfortable. Crumbs are a way to take a tiny, *tiny* taste. Once your child demonstrates that he is comfortable with helping to make and try crumbs and understands that he can be making choices about how many and how much, we can expand crumb-trying to non-dry crumbs. For example, corn muffins can be made into a crumb. They are crumbly but not as gluey as a banana bread crumb. You can pick the drier type of moist crumb as a starting point. Many breakfast bar crumbs work as a not-too-wet crumb, if you crumb the edges and not the central fruit. Crumbing the edges can be a way toward the more wet (moist) center! Waffle edges can be made into crumbs if double toasted. Then, those edges can be used to tiptoe toward the moister texture waffle center.

Cheeses can be offered as moist or damp-ish crumbs, *cheese crumbs*. Within the cheese category the *crumbs* will be highly variable. Parmesan cheese itself can be powdery, or grated, finely grated, or shredded to change up the texture. Some of the mixed four blend common cheeses are very soft and almost melt-able. Some are cheese sticks, others are waxed cheese balls that can be quite soft. Other cheeses can be offered in the tiniest "crumb" and spread on a familiar cracker with a coffee stirrer. Think of a coffee stirrer as a safer type of toothpick for children to use! Remember with cheese crumbs to factor in that cheeses smells and taste will vary widely.

Once the **crumbs are small** concept is established, anything can be offered as a *crumb*. We have even introduced ground hamburger as a tiny *hamburger crumb* when crumbled or a zested carrot as carrot crumbs!

Motor ask

The chewing response needed for dealing with crumbs can vary from the melt-able powdery crumbs tastes blown on a spoon of yogurt to big crumbs of crackers or nuts that require chewing. The powder is melt-able and easily swallow-able. The bigger crumbs vary in size and melt-ability and require varying different degrees of chewing. Changing the melt-ability and size of crumbs slowly, actually demands a different chewing response. The pieces can gradually be made bigger and bigger as your child demonstrates skill and confidence (and safety) with the sizes and textures. These small crumbs can be placed for your child on her lips, in cheek pouches, or over her teeth to help guide her tongue and chewing responses. Crumbs offered **on** the filled spoon (touching the palate) will be a different sensory experience than those offered **under** the spoon (touching the tongue). Crumbs offered on one side of the spoon (touching the tongue side and cheek) will give your child the sensation input to move this tongue in that direction. This would be an asymmetrical, out-of-the-middle tongue movement. Sucking and swallowing is a center mouth activity. To be a good chewer, children need to be able to notice and interact with texture out of the middle. Crumbs can help.

As crumbs become bigger and more, children need to organize them and chew them small enough to swallow. The amount and strength of chewing needed will vary depending on the crumb choice.

Dear Parent,

Think about *crumb-able* foods your family knows. Can you try crushing or crumbing them? Notice how they feel in your palm as well as in your mouth. Notice how some melt, some don't. Some are uneven and some are even. Some melt and some do not. Some have big flavors and some do not. This activity may help you and your therapy team find foods that are a good new food trying options for your child to explore.

Crumbs can scatter

Too many crumbs too soon can create a storm of scatter for some unsuspecting, unprepared mouths. This is why we start small size and volume, start melt-able to build skills and confidence as the *ask* increases. As amounts are systematically increased, the we use crumbs to actually help the child manage the scatter, little by little.

Crumb rehearsals

As with all new food trying strategies, crumbs need *rehearsals*. The rehearsal can be inviting your child to watch you or sibling make crumbs, or she can be invited to help with the crumb making. Your child can offer crumbs, through her fingers or palms, to others to try them to get familiar with their texture even more. Crumbs can be spread around a sided cookie sheet that serves as a drawing surface for her to practice letters and numbers and get acquainted with crumb feel! Crumbs can be offered as *crumb kisses* with a mirror and silly faces. Just like our continuum of options throughout this book, we do not need to go right to the mouth. When you think about crumbs creatively as a continuum of tiny successes waiting to happen, your imagination will take you all kinds of places!

Crumbs are a game changer

Lucy has always been anxious around food. Anxious to look at it, to touch it, to smell it, and especially anxious about eating food. We tried many different approaches to help her be more comfortable around foods that were unfamiliar or new to her. But no approach helped as much as introducing crumbs. Crumbs were an absolute game changer for Lucy. She just did not like the messiness of wet foods. With crumbs, Lucy was much more in control of the food. Since the crumbs were dry, she knew she could touch them without getting messy. She could touch them, blow them from her hand to the ground, smash them into smaller pieces, kiss them, and eventually taste them. Tasting crumbs was a good step for her because she could feel them in her mouth. She could feel their dry texture, so she was more able to manipulate the crumbs, find them, and move them around in her mouth. Once she figured out one crumb, the sky was the limit! ~Jake Barnes

Crumb Continuum

Crumbs	Solids
Powdery	Textured
Fine Meltable	Non-Meltable
Even	Uneven
Snack	Healthy
Browns	Mixed Colors
Quiet Flavor	Wake-Up Flavor
Sweet	Savory
Dry	Moist
Quiet	Noisy

Food Play

Children learn through play. They learn about the properties of the objects, how they fit together, how to use their own body in relation to the toy, how their hands work, and in the case of food, how their hands and mouths work together. We do not give a child a new puzzle and tell them they have one minute to put it together. We let them check it out, explore it, learn about it, practice with it. And you do not give me a mouthful of grasshoppers that I have never seen before and tell me to "just eat it." We need time to explore, to essentially play with or be introduced to our foods. Yet, there are many different opinions about playing with food. Personally, I like the idea as long as it is in moderation and as long as parents are on board with the idea. When I am cooking, I personally love the food textures and smells, and the exploration of the foods is a part of my enjoyment of cooking. But the exploration of food for exploration-of-foods-sake would never get me to a completed recipe. The food play (interaction, exploration) needs to have a purpose.

I understand that not every family believes playing with or wasting food is okay! That must be respected. However, consider moderation. I am not suggesting the kind of playing with food that has it ending up all over the walls or all over the floor. I am suggesting the kind of supervised, purposive play that allows for another positive food interaction. The goal of this food play is to offer food interactions while we try to relax the general environment around food. For children who have been highly stressed about trying new food, this is a way to take away the pressure to put every food into their mouth. There are some suggestions below of incorporating food in play, but do not let them squelch your imagination! Make it fun!

Ball games

For those at developmental stages where children are rolling balls back and forth, or later when aiming for soccer nets or bean bag toss games are appropriate, can oranges or grapefruits or other fruit shaped balls be used? Why not smell, then hold, then roll a piece of fruit as an introduction to its smell and texture?

Box games

How about using pieces of food as the **play pieces** in board games? Or can checkers be played with stackable cookies or crackers?

Tic tac toe

In Tic Tac Toe you need two different sets of game markers. Could they be different colored cheese cubes, pieces of purple or green cabbage, or fish shaped crackers? Or could you make a large tic tac toe board with laminated construction paper and use small tangerines and plums, a broccoli or cauliflower?

Marbles

When games call for marbles to roll down a trough, could they be exchanged for cherry tomatoes or green or purple grapes, blueberries or peas?

Tea parties

Why not use real food at little tea parties? Children can use cookie cutters and plastic utensils to create the finger food items.

Trucks and trains

For those children who LOVE trucks and trains, vehicles can transport all kinds of foods. They can also drive on roads made out of crumbs. In the excitement of the driving, the worry over the touch of the food may diminish.

Pretend play

For children who enjoy pretend play, carrots can be cow horns and bananas can be elephant tusks or noses or telephones. Lettuce leaves can be hats. String cheese can be a moustache and a wedge of orange skin can be a smile. Any food can be a microphone! Microphones are great way to have the child bring a food NEAR his nose, and mouth. Lips make the first contact so your child can decide if her tongue is ready for a taste.

Arts and crafts

In this time of information explosion, there are so many creative ideas on the internet for food arts and crafts. There are whole books and whole websites devoted to art with food. For children worried about trying new tastes, creating an art piece or design with food can allow food interaction without the requirement of tasting. It is nice to use food art as presents for Grandma and Grandpa or a favored baby sitter. Some families regularly make food designs and make photo books that display this art!!

Perspective

Some families have the time and energy and enthusiasm for food play and food art. Others look at me with glazed over eyes and ask when there could possibly be time for that!!?? You will see this type of activity in therapy clinics and classrooms. Some parents want to save those ideas for those settings, and others decorate their walls in Crumb Art. As in this whole book, a variety of ideas will be shared. I trust you will pick the ones that seem right for you.

Dips and Dippers

Dip and dippers are not just for the party enthusiast. They are a great way to expand food enjoyment. Yes, dips and dippers are a novel way to eat foods. They can be interesting, motivating and fun. They can allow your child to try new foods by **combining new with familiar**. They give "utensil" practice as little hands and wrists figure out how to get the dipper into the dipping bowl and then their mouth. And they can help your child add changing textures and calories by combining the dipping with crumbs.

Child-directed

Children are active participants in dips and dipping. Dips and dipping is not about someone else feeding your child. Actually, you can consider early spoon usage practice as a dipping activity since they are so much more successful if that early practice food is more like a dip. It sticks to the spoon. It is about your child doing the dipping and bringing the filled dipper to his own mouth. Your child is doing the action! Your child makes the choices and goes at his own pace. Your child knows what he is ready for from the dips and dippers offered. Your child knows how much he wants on the dipper and knows whether that dipper can go in his mouth or near it to be licked off by a careful tongue.

Invite interest

Dips and dippers are a novel mealtime activity that can invite your cautious or worried child into the activity. Using different dips, dippers, and bowls can add to the interest. He can watch you dipping and want to imitate. You can create ways to match colors of dips with dippers or dippers with bowl colors. You can practice math by telling him, *I am going to dip one plus one times, how many are you going to dip?* Or *I am going to dip in the red dip, which one will you dip in?* Dips are a buffet line staple so exposure to dips can be lifelong skill training.

Start with familiar

You can start with *familiar*. Children can use a familiar dipper with a familiar dip to learn the activity of dipping. It is also a way to model that your familiar foods can be eaten in a different way, that *change happens*, and it will be okay.

You can offer a familiar dip with multiple kinds of familiar or new dippers. The familiar dip is a good starting point. The new dipper can give your child different looks and textures of foods in or near his mouth. For example, if your child likes strawberry yogurt, can he dip it with a graham cracker or a piece of bagel, which he knows? Or can he dip it with a slice of apple, celery stick, or banana piece to lick the familiar strawberry taste off the new texture of dipper? You would not expect your child to bite the dipper, just lick the dip off it. (Therefore, be careful with the choices you make, and supervise. You do not want to pick dipper textures that could be unsafe, should your child decide to bite through it. Know your child's capabilities first as you make these choices.) This allows your child to get up-close with the dipper to feel apple, celery or banana texture, and get those food smells near his nose. Once he gets the idea that many different dippers can work with his familiar dip, you can vary the dipper options and consider these confidence stretches. Your child can pick the dippers from a bowl of dippers you have provided.

Once your child has learned the concept of dipping, you can change the dips. You can use a familiar dipper to dip in a different dip. Remember you start the skill with a dip your child knows, but you can offer dip variations by changing the color, flavor or texture slightly. The *familiar* becomes the activity of dipping with the familiar dipper. The *new* becomes the dip options. So, that familiar apple slice can be dipped in yogurt, peanut butter, chocolate hazelnut dip. Celebrate when your child becomes comfortable with his finger as a dipper, as he then gets a great sensory experience when dipping his finger in the dips!

Children worried about touching *wet foods* can dip a dipper and hand it to someone else. There is a beginning and end to this activity so it helps the worry. Your child can hand you the apple slice dipped in yogurt and accidentally get a tiny amount on his own hand. He can wipe it off, or maybe even ignore it in the celebration of handing it to you! You can make the initial dippers longer to be farther from the wet dip if need be. When he gets really comfortable with the texture, he can dip his finger in the dip!

Once your child understands dips and dippers, you can add another step in the process, CRUMBS! Crumbs add to the novelty and motivation of the dipping experience. Children can dip the dipped dipper in a bowl of crumbs. This adds another level of interest and novelty and a different utensil practice. It also practices *change happens*. And it can add texture change in as graded a fashion as needed and it adds calories! They can dip their hummus in cracker or crouton crumbs. They can dip their yogurt in dry cereal crumbs, or moist muffin crumbs. They can dip in noisy, crispy rice cereal that can make a little (or more) noise, depending on the amount added thereby grading the sound experience. The crumbs can be even, such as powdered fine crackers, or vary uneven, such as granola. The crumbs can add a new food group by dipping in crumbed freeze-dried fruit. And the crumbs can add calories, such as dipping in crumbed nuts.

Utensil practice

We think of dipper use as utensil training. Dippers can be *held* in a less precise hold than spoons and forks. The *aim* in dipping can be less precise than that required of spoons and forks. The dipper just has to find the bowl, not the precise piece of food in the bowl. One of the motor skills needed for utensil use is the precision of the wrist control needed in bringing the utensil to the mouth and modifying the aim to the mouth to match the length of the utensil and the distance from the mouth. Dips can easily stick to the dipper, providing an easy bowl to mouth experience, or be wetter and need to be scooped and more carefully guided to the mouth. Dippers become great utensil practice.

Sensory expansion

Dips and dipper activities provide the opportunity to offer sensation changes. You can create color, flavor, taste and texture changes. The sensory in-mouth experiences with the differently textured dippers can be graded. Your cautious child may be willing to eat his beloved yogurt from that apple slice, even though he is worried about the apple slice texture. But licking off the familiar yogurt can be quick, so the exposure to the apple texture can be quick initially and, over time, the apple can have more and longer contact with the tongue and lips. A child who likes hummus can use crackers, carrot sticks, bread sticks, or even raw or cooked broccoli dippers. Gradually broccoli can become *familiar* enough to *try*.

Add calories

Dips and dipping can be a way to offer calorie boosters. Dips can be made with cream cheese or nut butters, guacamole, hummus or cheese to add nutritious calories to the dipping activity.

Add a dip to dinner

Consider adding a Dips and Dipper course to the dinner meals where you pick the foods and dippers and family members can then role model this as a typical part of the dinner experience. Everyone does it. Chips and dips, chips and salsa or guacamole, hummus and pita, apple slices and peanut butter, cream cheese and bread sticks, carrots and ranch dressing, yum! It becomes one of the family's routines. It becomes a multiple exposure activity.

We think fondly of Emily. She found that she liked dipping in a chocolate hazelnut spread. She liked it so much that it became her routine way of trying new foods. The spread was her *familiar* dip. It turns out she was willing to dip new foods in it very readily. She would dip the cracker in it a few times and then decide if she wanted to try the cracker. Eventually she learned to eat strawberries, pears, roasted chicken (her choice) and broccoli (again, her choice) by first dipping them in that nut butter spread! The dipping and this spread became her familiar routine AND her bridge to new foods. Whatever works!!

Food Academics

When children have a *List* of preferred foods and they only eat *those* foods, it is easy to inadvertently only be around *those* foods. Why would they want to try anything else? They are not *around* any other foods. We know it helps children to be around food, to see and feel foods as a way to familiarize themselves with food sensory properties. We look for opportunities to incorporate food interactions into everyday activities. Food academics is one way to increase food interactions, give multiple exposures to new foods and provide food rehearsals.

Think of ways food can be incorporated into directed pre-academic or preschool play. If your child has favorite preschool activities, food can be used. Activities can be modified for your child's age and developmental age. You can pick targeted food groups or smells or textures. The activities can require gross motor or fine motor movements. The focus of the activity in these food academics is on the theme, the stacking, the counting, the drawing **not the eating or trying**. This can dilute the worry about the touching or smelling. Remember when children are worried and are stretching into a sensory aspect of the food that makes them a little (or a lot) uncomfortable, it helps to have an activity with a beginning and an end. For example, they can pick up the food knowing they will be able to get rid of it soon by putting it *in or on*. These ideas can be modified for your child's interest level and cognitive skills. Here are some starter ideas.

Emptying and filling

So many foods can be taken *out* or put *into* containers. Think "out of the box" here. Grapes or blueberries, cheese cubes or carrots, broccoli or celery. Foods can be put in and taken out of tall containers and short containers, round containers or square containers, near containers or far containers. Changing the size and shape combinations of containers and foods changes the motor and perceptual tasks. For example, putting frozen peas in a pill sized bottle will be a very different motor activity than putting them in a big bowl. Foods can be put in bowls of water to watch which foods float and which ones dissolve. The foods can be added to containers of familiar toys such as blocks or plastic foods to change up the sensory experiences as they reach to explore.

Stacking

Stacking activities do not just have to be done with blocks. How about stacking crackers, cookies, waffles, bread slices, pancakes or tortillas? Dry may be the place to start, and then you can transition to cheese slices or cubes! And then wet cucumbers and apple slices, or really wet orange slices or watermelon? Stacking can be easier as with bread slices that do not slip, or more challenging with bananas or wet orange slices.

Counting and math

Food is a great hands-on math counting tool, a kind of food abacus! Of course, children can count any food from play food to real foods, from dry to wet, from damp to moist or hard to soft. For children learning to count or those who enjoy math, food can be used in their learning practice. Children can focus their attention on the math answer rather than the food they are touching. The math computation can be a way to dilute the worry. How many are four carrots plus three carrots? Fifteen broccolis minus seven broccolis? Can you divide twenty blueberries by five? For the child who is worried about the texture of the touch, forks, spoons, tongs, and children's adapted chopsticks can be used until the food touch is more comfortable. The great thing about using food as a manipulative in math learning is that your child is concentrating on the math principle or answer and not spending as much time worrying over the food texture. Remember this is not a *food trying activity*, just a *food exposure activity…* just an activity to get comfortable with that food for possible later new food trying.

When working on mouth skills we also have used foods in Mouth Math. We have helped children learn to spit out foods and then practice that skill with mouth math. We might ask your child if he can spit this frozen pea into the green bowl or this frozen square carrot in that orange bowl. We might then ask, *if you have two peas in your mouth and spit ONE into this bowl, how many will be left? Can we do this together?* OR *If you have three frozen carrots in your mouth and spit out one, how many are left?* OR You can work on their oral sensitivity and awareness by placing a frozen pea and frozen carrot in his mouth and asking him to spit the orange carrot in the orange bowl and green pea in the green bowl. This has him concentrate on a higher level perceptual skill of identifying the shape in his mouth without any visual cues. (Stereognosis). Your child is practicing math concepts and trying hard to figure out the math or shape and, by the way, he is also feeling that food in his mouth for longer periods of time as he tries to figure out the math. It is less worrisome because he KNOWS he is on the way to spitting it out. There is a BEGINNING and an END and that helps the worry. NO ONE is forcing him to have these foods in his mouth and he knows he can spit it out as he needs. (Supervise for safety!)

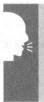
My child liked numbers so much that we would ask him how many tastes he wanted. He would always say eight! He liked eight. He comfortably had eight practice tastes on new foods and this helped him find foods to add to his diet. Numbers helped him get confident with new foods. ~Roy's Mom

Color matching

Foods, especially fruits and vegetables, come in lots of rainbow colors. Children can sort foods by colors into different colored bowls or plates or cups. We can laminate a colored sheet of paper and use it for food color sorting. Children can line up colored foods in rainbow sequences. Let your imagination can go wild.

Shape and size matching

Crackers and cookies come in lots of different shapes and sizes, great for sorting. With the help of a collection of cookie cutters, bread and toast, waffles and tortillas, cheese slices and deli meats can be made into shapes and sizes and sorted accordingly. When bread, cheese and deli meat are all cut into the same shape, they can be matched or lined up into a sandwich. Little cookie cutters can be used for making small shapes in apples, cheese, melon, and lettuce and made into mini sandwiches (which may be a less worrisome size to try)! Oranges and smaller tangerines can be sorted. Big crackers, and little crackers, big pancakes and little ones, round waffles and square ones. Every food has a sortable size or shape! And cupcake or muffin tins are great for the sorting!

Drawing

We think of traditional drawing with pens and crayons on paper. Let's think non-traditionally! First of all, markers come in a variety of smells that can be matched or just experienced. Drawing can be done with a tool in a tray of crumbs or whipped cream or yogurt. The drawing tool can be a paint brush, or chop stick, a carrot, apple, green pepper slice or string cheese. It can also be done with a finger. Children can paint with food purees or puddings with brushes or fingers. These are rich sensory experiences.

When we make crumbs and want to help a child become comfortable with them, usually prior to tasting them, we can make a tray of crumbs together and put them in a sided cookie sheet. We then sift or gently shake it to even out the crumbs and ask the child to draw in them with a finger. They can concentrate on drawing the letter or number or making the happy face and dilute some of the worry about the texture and smell. The drawing becomes the focus and the touching can be come secondary and the familiar part.

Scissors

Who says scissor practice must be done on paper? Children can have increased food interaction experiences by cutting through tortillas, or waffles, cheese slices or string cheese. The resistance of the food will also provide a bit of extra proprioceptive information and might just help with learning wrist stability.

Food science

And lastly, food science. For children, as they get older, you can create opportunities to "study" some aspect of the food. Be a Food Detective, or Food Explorer or Food Scientist. Using food in some type of experiment has the advantage of allowing your child to touch or explore the food, again, with NO EXPECTATION or REQUIREMENT of tasting it. He is just getting more comfortable around it and if he decides to taste it, great! Which of these foods float? Which of these foods melts? Which of these can be made into crumbs?

I remember getting to know an anxious eater years ago. Mom was very worried because her son was going to his first sleep away camp. This was going to be particularly challenging because of his food worries. Mom and he studied the menu ahead of time and knew there would be a lot of hamburgers served. She did not want him to have foods so different from others. She and he went to the grocery store and bought four or five kinds of frozen hamburgers and four or five veggie burgers. (Her thinking was that if she and he found one he liked, that could become familiar and then she could buy a bunch of those to send to camp for him. He could eat burgers with the others, albeit HIS hamburgers. AND if another meal offered was too worrisome, he would know that there were HIS burgers as backups.

We turned this into a grand experiment. We made a list of variables we could compare and a rating system. He judged each on packaging, the inside wrappers, the look when frozen and outside the wrapper, the smell when cooked, the finger taste, and then taste, if he could. He tasted tiny *mouse bites* of six that smelled good enough to try and actually found one of the burgers, a veggie burger, to Mom's surprise, that he liked well enough to take regular bites. Mom and he practiced them at home to establish them as a favored food and went out and bought more. Mom took a bunch to have available in the Camp Kitchen. Those veggie burgers helped him bridge his food worries at camp that first year.

Thinking creatively, food can be incorporated into LOTS of academic preschool type learning activities. These little pre-academics can be incorporated naturally in your food interactions as you ask your child if he can put seven cherry tomatoes in the salad or give you three cubes of cheese. OR If you have more time and energy, you could create a whole little food interaction experience after school at a non-mealtime food interaction or new food trying times.

Dear Parent,

Can you think of a way your child could have more interactions with foods by incorporating food academics into his day or week?

I "get it" that it can be hard to muster the energy to prepare foods that you know aren't even intended to be eaten. It's time consuming enough to make foods for all the meals and snacks. I share this food play story simply as an encouragement. My older son refused to eat pasta for years until I tried making spaghetti noodles in the afternoon and dumping them onto a kids' table (without sauce!). We just played and built sculptures with them. After only two times of noodle sculpturing in a no-stress, playful way, he was willing to try spaghetti at the dinner table. Now pasta night is a regular staple at our house! So, when your therapist suggests playing with food outside of mealtime, consider perhaps that the effort may pay off in the future! ~Laura Wesp

Thoughts About Novelty!

Do I believe novelty helps? Yes, absolutely for many children novelty in presentation invites children into the mealtime in a playful and positive way. I grew up in a family where food was celebrated every day. My mother and grandmother both loved to cook and share their love in the food they offered us. We had adorable salads with halved pineapple rings that turned into butterflies and halved canned pears that turned into bunnies. We had pancakes with happy faces and apples cooked as bowls stuffed with yummy stuff. It was how we did things at our house. Mom did not do these things to *get us to eat*, but to make it enjoyable and to share her love.

Throughout this book we talk about changing the plates or cups or straws to teach children that *change happens*, but also to create some novelty and interest in the meal. We know that we have to be careful about what and when we change, but YES, novelty can be very helpful. It can invite the child into the meal. It can dilute the worry. When we make food art and adorable presentations it can have the effect of inviting to the meal and diluting the worry.

However, the idea of novelty, food art and creative food presentation can be, and has been, taken to an unhelpful extreme. When these presentations come with pressure, overt or subtle, to eat, we defeat the purpose. As we have discussed throughout this book, pressure does NOT HELP. If any strategy is used to *make kids eat*, there is pressure and there will be resistance. Pressure gets the parent child relationship off balance.

So, for me, the bottom line is NOT to take away the novelty or the interesting artful presentation altogether. It is to present pressure free, not judgmental, and above all, loving, presentations of food. If it helps inspire your child to try something new that looks different or especially interesting, great.

As with every strategy mentioned in this book, it is ALWAYS qualified with a need to individualize. To offer and then adjust. Parents need options and therapists need options and I do not think we do a service to either when we throw out a whole category of options. Remember to tip toe carefully. Your child will let you know if it works.

Having said all that, I would like to share some novelty ideas that may be helpful for children learning to try new foods. The qualifier is that we are always careful about change with anxious eaters. For some novelty equals change equals worry. Okay, for those children, we are careful about the change or we may offer change at the *edges*, not really near the worry. We discussed this in the *change happens* chapter.

Dip and dippers

We have mentioned dips and dippers throughout because you can change up the dips, the dippers and the crumb combination to add interest to a meal. We find they can be great utensil practice as wrists need to manage the dippers, and they can be ways to invite increased attention to the task of eating. As children work to manage the dippers, you may well find that they stay interested in the mealtime for longer periods of time. The dips and dipping, for many children, becomes a predictable, routine part of the mealtime.

Bowls

Bowls can be plain colored or themed, tiny or really big. A paper cup can be a bowl as can a tiny medicine cup or shot glass. And we also offer food bowls. Bread can be hollowed out to be a bowl for soup or stew. A carved-out tomato can serve tuna fish or egg salad. (Or a bowl of crumbs or grated cheese, if those are the familiar foods). A carved-out apple or pear or cucumber can be a bowl or cup for drinking. A carefully peeled orange half can be a bowl for dessert. Puff pastry can be a bowl for chicken stew. Of course, we will be careful to pick food textures and combinations that maximize success and minimize worry. Start where it works for your child!

Straws

Once children like straws, they can become an inexpensive way to add novelty to the drinking. Your child can choose the long straw or the short one, the wide milkshake straw of the narrow coffee stirrer straw, the bunny straw or the Halloween straw, the Fourth of July straw or the holiday straw. The *choosing* gives her some control at the mealtime (though YOU were the one in charge of the choices). You can offer a **bouquet of straws** where your child can pick four or five different straws and decide which straw she is drinking from next?

Ronnie was a worried eater who drank one kind of milk. His mother really wanted him to try a new milk. For him, the bouquet of straws helped. He helped Mom pour the new soy milk in the cup. (A small amount). She let him pick a bouquet of straws (several different motivating straws from the straw bin) for his drink and for hers. She picked which straw in her cup she was going to drink from first. A rehearsal. Then it was his turn. They took turns back and forth with him enjoying the picking of the new straw until he had enjoyed four ounces of the new drink that he otherwise would have worried about. The straw bouquet, for him, diluted the worry.

Utensils

Fingers are utensils. Utensils are utensils, and food can be utensils. We love it when children can interact with the food with their fingers because they are getting sensory rehearsals, previews of the food which can prepare them for the mouth tasting. Utensils can be varied in size, shape, texture and theme. These not only add novelty, but often vary the sensory and motor challenge as confidence stretches. Tongs and children's chopsticks add even more novelty and coordination challenges. As your child is playing with the coordination challenge, the new food worry can be diluted.

Popsicles and ice cubes

When you make smoothies with your child, and he is not yet able to drink a significant amount, popsicles and fancy ice cubes can be the solution. You and your child can freeze the leftover drink in the popsicle makers, ring pops, and ice cube shapes and *voila*, a snack for later for your child or another lucky family member. At least the smoothie did not get wasted and the snack is a homemade healthy one! There are so many novel popsicle maker shapes, from rockets to stars, jewel shapes to ring shapes, animal shapes to construction shapes! And ice cube shapes include stars, and hearts, alphabets and numbers to trucks and princess themes. If your child has a favorite movie cartoon character, chances are pretty good that they make popsicle or ice cubes in those shapes. The internet has an expansive array of enticing shapes for children that can add just enough novelty into the offer. Check them out!

One little friend, Eva, recently loved her the Little Pony™ cartoons. She and her mother got a Little Pony™ ice cube tray and they froze different juices and nectars in them. The freezer was full of plastic zipper bags of differently colored and flavored pony ice cubes. These were used to help Eva expand her liquid intake each day and learn to like fruit flavors toward a goal of smoothies. Eva loved her "Pony Water" and asked for it all day. She got past only drinking HER water only from HER special cup this way! She got to juices and smoothies.

Themed meals

As children get older and are more comfortable with change, meals can have themes. Of course, traditions and holidays come with their own themes. Can you bring those back into your family life? Could there be a cartoon character theme one night where everyone has a paper plate or napkin of that character? Or a picnic theme where picnic plates and baskets are present and the meal is on the floor on a sheet?

My dietitian friend tells this story. Whenever she went away to a conference, her husband and two boys would declare a food color night. The Boys would pick a color, orange, for example, and then go to the store and pick out orange drinks, and orange snacks, and orange dinner items and orange desserts and that would be dinner. They sometimes even created their colors with food coloring. Rice and noodles may have been colored with red and yellow coloring. Dad would sheepishly confess that the meal may well not have had all the food groups, but it sure was fun and a treat for the kids! Your anxious eater can participate in whatever part of the shopping, prep or eating that he likes and, most importantly, the meal was enjoyed and, hopefully, a good memory was made.

Invite Your Child Back to the Table

Please invite your child back to the table with emphasis on the *invite* part of that statement. By changing the focus of the mealtime to togetherness, enjoyment and elimination of pressure, the mealtime may well be more inviting for all. Your child will begin to trust that mealtime is a comfortable place that he can be who he is, eat what he can, and be a part of the family meal.

Change up the setting

Some families find that changing the mealtime environment a bit can create a new atmosphere for all and new or different expectations. Some families combine the change in their attitude and approach to mealtime peace with changes in the physical mealtime. Some rearrange the dining room furniture for a new look. Some exchange the placemats for a tablecloth. Some add a quiet background music or candles, or even different plates. New mealtimes, new look and feel! (Of course, these changes will be made carefully, as we do not want the change to be an added stressor. You know YOUR child!)

Create the conversation

Bring back the mealtime conversation. Can you find something to talk about that is not about *take a bite* and *finish your meal*? Some families have their children decorate *talking spoons*. A talking spoon is what we call the prompter for "Your turn to speak." It could be a toy that is passed from speaker to speaker. It could be a little microphone. When holding it, it is your turn. In our house, we called it a talking spoon. We used a wooden spoon. Children paint or personalize them. Each meal, some family member chooses which talking spoon will be used or randomly picks one out of a bag. One family member starts the conversation with or without a prompt. Perhaps each member describes something great that happened that day. Other families talk about each of their ups and downs for the day. Some go online and look for family mealtime conversation starter games or plates that give them ideas for creative ways to have conversations at a meal. There are even conversation starter napkins, each printed with novel children friendly conversation starter questions. These may help families re-think their mealtime conversation until new conversations become natural. Make it work for your family. Make the conversation relevant to family members and absolutely not about *having another bite*.

Mealtime conversation

As my boys think back to growing up in our home, I want them to have fond memories of family dinners despite our feeding challenges. With both a teenager and a Kindergartner in the house the reality is that we are often moving in opposite directions. The most frequent space where we are together is around the table. We have made a conscious decision not to make food and food trying central to our conversation. Rather the focus is on building connection and enjoying one another.

Often, I have to be quite intentional about steering the conversation toward something other than the food. Sometimes we bring a news article or an interesting story from the paper to the table to discuss. Even though the discussion may at times be a bit over Teddy's head, he is still witnessing our family engaging and talking about many interesting topics. Often the news article is a simple means to get the kids talking. Sometimes we pass around a silly comic from the day's newspaper. We have lots and lots of ways to ask about their day in creative ways: What did you do today that was new? What adventures did you have today? Were you kind to someone today? Did you see someone else being kind or doing something funny? ~Laura Wesp

Mealtime jobs

Many families invite their children back to the table by including them more actively in *mealtime jobs*. We described many of these jobs earlier. Even if she is not ready to sit at the table with others, she can get to be celebrated for *coming toward the table* to do her job, for helping with the family meal and for being around food in a way that is *not about the eating of it*. It is about participating, helping, and being celebrated for a food-related interaction that is positive! When your child is placing a napkin at the table, she is coming toward it. When putting the bread basket on the table, she is having a food interaction without needing to worry about tasting it, even if she has to turn around and leave the table after placing the item.

Mealtime jobs can be assigned depending on your child's developmental, cognitive, and responsibility skill level. Some families list the jobs on little folded cards in a jar and let siblings each pick their job of the day or week. Some children are very capable of putting a garnish on each plate, or pouring the milk, and others will be celebrated for distributing the non-food, non-textured, predictable napkins. You are laying the groundwork for that day when your child can help with mealtime jobs without needing to dilute the ask. Remember mealtime jobs are an invitation back into the mealtime atmosphere...even if briefly at first.

Starting point

As we have discussed before, the starting point may be that your child is at the table eating with the family, as usual, but with no *take a bite* or pressure demands. The starting point may be your child eats at the table with the rest of the family, but with at least one food option that is from their favored *List* so she does not need to start from a worried place of all new foods. Or the starting point for mealtime peace, may have been that your child eats in another room or at a table nearby, but not the family table. This depends on the worry level and sensory sensitivities of each child. But the goal will be the invitation back to the table.

When the starting point is farther away

When, in order to achieve mealtime peace, your child is eating away from the family table, we want to help you find a way to tiptoe back *toward* the family meal. This can be done in bigger or smaller steps depending on the level of worry from your child. Of course, while thinking about inviting your child back *toward* the meal, we encourage you to: 1.) start from mealtime peace, 2.) eliminate the pressure and 3.) provide non-mealtime food related interactions or new food trying rehearsals so the looks, smells and textures of food become much more comfortable for your child to be around.

Some families still offer their child's meal separately during mealtimes but make a point of eating family snacks around them to help them get used to foods not currently on their *List*. Can the table your child is eating at be gradually brought closer to the family meal, maybe inch by inch? Or can your child be invited to the family meal for a very short time with that time gradually increasing. Perhaps your child can help to bring the fruit bowl to the table as a way to come *toward* the meal, and then be allowed to leave if necessary? Can these experiences gradually get bigger, and longer as they get more comfortable?

Once fully at the table

Once the anxious eater is fully at the table eating their own foods, they will have regular experiences being around the food of the family. Hopefully this will become more and more comfortable with the child hearing, watching and seeing others eat, smelling the food, and passing and touching the food as they increase their comfort. Many children will then learn to allow themselves to place a piece of the family food on their own plate, or a nearby plate and eventually learn the skills of comfortable new food trying.

Family rules

Okay, sometimes **we need to be parents** and look at rules. Each family has basic rules for their family mealtimes. At a minimum there are probably rules about not throwing food, being polite and staying at the table. It is easy to get out of balance when one or more family member is an anxious eater. It gets so complicated when there are rules for some family members and not for others.

When considering the rules for your family, can you remember the parent jobs and child jobs? Can there still be a way for your child to end her own meal when she is full, not when you decide she should finish all the food on her plate or eat all of *this* before *that*? It is easy to slip into their jobs when we make adult driven rules that step right into the child's job of deciding when she is full or what she is able to eat. Rules of *finish everything before getting up* are pressure.

Family rules

Our family rules are pretty basic. We all come to the table. We eat together. We sit in our chairs and we drink our drinks. We started this last rule as we realized our son just was not getting enough liquid in his day. We tried to find places to expand his water intake. Our son started out with the tiniest amount of water and we've gradually progressed from a baby cup to a juice glass—and by his request—to a normal glass that accommodates a larger volume of water that he wants to drink! We have used a similar principle for more calorie drinks, too. ~ Laura Wesp

Be on the same page

Mom and Dad can take time to have conversations about what they would like their mealtimes to look like. This way, you both can be on the same page of the *rule book*. And as soon as you have agreed on your family rules, there will be a unique situation that you hadn't thought of yet. It is okay, get through it the best you can and have further conversations later, without listening ears. If you have decided that there will be no more *have a bite* or *finish everything that is on your plate*, both parents need to be giving the same feedback to your children. If one of you is not pressuring and the other just needs to say *finish your peas right now* in a frustrated moment, your child get mixed messages and it will take longer to re-establish trust and mealtime peace.

Siblings let us know that it can be hard for them when they have to stay at the table, or they need to have one set of rules and an anxious eater sibling has other rules. Sometimes the rules can be the same, but sometimes they need to be different. In full disclosure, can you have a conversation with the siblings about being a mealtime helper with worried sibling and can they help in the process. Help them understand the different challenges of their sibling and include them in their special place at the mealtime.

You don't *have* to eat it but...

When the pressure to eat is removed and the hover over finishing is eliminated, there needs to be some rules or guidance about how to behave. How about offering the family style foods and letting your child choose? How about, *you do not have to eat the food prepared but...*

~ *You need to politely say no thank you, or politely pass the food on.* (We expect everyone to be polite)
~ *You do not need to comment negatively on the food. No fair saying "EWWWWW, Yuck!"* (Be nice to the chefs, they work hard to prepare family meals).
~ *I would like you to sit at the table while the family eats.* (This is family time).
~ *Eat what you can and until you have had enough.* (Children know when they are full).

Whose Idea is it Anyway?

Many mealtimes for anxious eaters evolve into a sit-down session where the caring and concerned parent has a plan for the amount of food their child should eat. The two will sit together for as long as it might take to finish that certain amount with both parent and child unhappy by the end. Or, in order *to get your child* to take in that amount, you may have added screen time phones or TV, or distractions of toys and books or songs to keep him focused on something else so he will eat without resistance. Okay, this is your starting point. But doesn't the entertainment itself becomes exhausting? And, this is not helping to create an atmosphere where your child can learn to listen to his own appetite cues. Can we help find a way for your child to be a more active mealtime participant?

Is your child an active participant in the meal?

Can we consider how your child is participating in the meal? If your child needs all those puzzles, cheerleading and screen time, then he is participating because of the food motivation YOU provide. A starting point to achieve internal motivation, is to have your child be an active participant. For example, if he is feeding himself and stopping when he is full, (and is growing), he is doing his part. But if he is looking away, watching the screen, not looking at you or the spoon, and requiring you to do all the spoon work, then the responsibility is all on YOU. How do we get HIM to take responsibility or be an active participant?

> Dear Parent,
>
> Does your child need your entertainment to be at the meal?

There is a continuum of self-feeding little steps. The *here* might be that the child is fed, but the *there* is independent self-feeding.

Engage the child

For some worried eaters the starting place is to "check out" during meals and be fed. Mealtime may have been so worrisome that they can only eat *their food* while paying no attention to the process. They use their technology to not *be present.*

Can you pause when the spoon is at his lips to have him look briefly at it or the food *before* placing it in his mouth? Once he can do that and expects that, and is *comfortable* with that, could the pause be lengthened with you getting his attention verbally so he can make a quick glance at you *before* the spoonful is placed in the mouth? Your body language is gradually saying, *Wait, wait, sweetheart, at least show me you are <u>here</u>, that we are doing this together. Show me you <u>want</u> the next mouthful.*

Once he has increased is participation by looking at the food and you, can he begin to help with spoon feeding? Many parents will describe resistance and struggle when trying to hand their child the spoon. When there is resistance, *we need to adjust* or *grade the way we ask.* Perhaps he can briefly touch your forearm as the spoon approaches. We are not initially asking for spoon touching or holding, but merely a brief touch on the grownup arm. He will gradually learn that this favorite food is put in his mouth after he helps by touching your arm. Once he is comfortable with a brief touch, can the touch turn into a longer *hold*? Can he hold your forearm the whole time you are approaching them with the filled spoon, and still keep visual contact with you or the spoon? Can you gradually help him hold your wrist, and then touch the edge of the spoon while you are still feeding him? Then he can hold you *and* the spoon and then just the spoon while you guide it. Can he bring an appropriately sized filled child's spoon to his mouth? Perhaps you can take turns where you feed him a bite then he can feed himself a bite with a spoon you have pre-filled? Then you can guide him to scoop and he can bring the filled spoon to his mouth? Then you can remind him verbally or physically to fill the spoon, scoop and he can do it independently or with you taking turns along the way as needed. This process of active participation does not need to be a battle.

You will gradually, in tiny steps expect more of him. Note that this is not a struggle where there is a battle along the way. You are tiptoeing toward his worry, not pushing right into it. Once you have an idea of this type of sequence you can gradually let it happen as YOUR CHILD lets you know he is ready for next steps. You may need fewer little steps, or many, many more. Make it comfortable for you both along the way. You will gradually, in tiny steps, expect more of him.

To help your child be successful with this, use child-size utensils and a plate or mat that does not slide during the process to maximize success. He may also be more successful when the plate has an edge. Use a food that easily sticks to and stays on the spoon as he is gaining skill and confidence and independence. Here is a general outline of an independence self-feeding continuum.

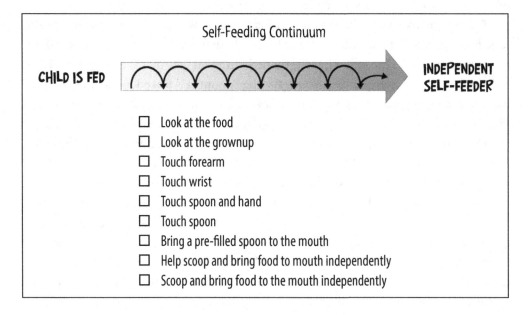

Self-Feeding Continuum

CHILD IS FED → INDEPENDENT SELF-FEEDER

- ☐ Look at the food
- ☐ Look at the grownup
- ☐ Touch forearm
- ☐ Touch wrist
- ☐ Touch spoon and hand
- ☐ Touch spoon
- ☐ Bring a pre-filled spoon to the mouth
- ☐ Help scoop and bring food to mouth independently
- ☐ Scoop and bring food to the mouth independently

Why do they need to engage?

We want children to engage in active participation in the mealtime because whenever they bring food to their own mouth, they are demonstrating internally motivated eating, making their own decisions about foods, pace and volumes. As we teach life-long skills, children need to grow up knowing how to feed themselves and not being dependent on their grownups.

Taking turns

Eating with your child and engaging him in turn taking activities is a great way to build their focus on the self-feeding. He also gets the multiple exposure rehearsals of seeing others eating and participating in a conversation of mealtime interactions. He gets to have a bit of control as HE decides just how fast and when to take the turns. As children are becoming independent in utensil use and parents are trying to reduce their role, the child can feed herself a spoonful and then the parent can offer a spoonful until gradually the child can do several in a row and, eventually, the whole meal.

Choices

A *choice* is the act of selecting, or making a decision when faced with two or more possibilities. To further help your child be present in the mealtime you can offer him choices. This helps him feel the respect of being included and being able to make some of the mealtime choices. This is especially nice for children who have ended up in situations where the parent has had to make all the choices for them regarding foods. This also helps the grownup keep the mealtime going without their making all the pacing decisions. Would you like your nuggets or your mac and cheese first? Would you like your cereal in the cartoon bowl or the yellow bowl? Would you like this curly long straw or this short red one? Would you like your sandwich made into a cookie cutter sandwich puzzle or do you want it cut in squares? Do you want four pieces of this food or six? Remember your offer is a choice. Your child may need to decline your offer and you may need to acknowledge and offer differently.

How NOT to say have another bite!

When grownups are constantly saying *have another bite, eat this,* they *are* the external motivation. We have to find ways to say *have another bite,* without saying *have another bite!* Turn taking and choices can be bridges back to making more internally motivated decisions. Clearly this depends on each child's communication and cognitive skills but consider these. Taking turns keeps the meal going without saying *have a bite. Whose turn is it? Who goes next? Is it your turn or Daddy's turn?*

Choices should be parent driven. If you give a choice, be sure you are okay with whatever choice your child makes. If you ask a child, *do you want salad or potato chips,* do not be upset with the potato chip choice and then try to talk them out of it. ☺ Maybe they get to *choose one potato chip or two? One apple slice or two? An apple from this bowl or that bowl? The yogurt with graham cracker crumbs, or fruit cereal crumbs? The drink with one colorful (new flavored) ice cube or three? Would like to eat this food with this fork or that one? These child chopsticks or these tongs? This silly cup, or Dad's cup?* The choices can add some playfulness and novelty that can also dilute the worry and keep attention into the meal.

What a good idea!

We all know the familiar dread that comes after we've spent time in the kitchen only to be greeted with complaints and grumbling the minute everyone sits down at the table. I wish that I had a magic solution! In addition to always having some familiar foods, one thing that has helped with the grumbling is actively acknowledging Teddy's requests.

When Teddy asks for another food that is not on the table, rather than saying no, I take the time to say Great! What a good idea! Let's have that tomorrow (or Tuesday). I then write it down while he is watching, and I make sure to honor his request. For example, if he asks for spaghetti when I've made chicken, I might say, "What a great idea. Let's make that. We can have it on Tuesday." I then do my best to follow through, and when I serve it I might say, "Thanks Teddy for this great idea to have spaghetti tonight." This reinforces that he has a voice and that his preferences matter. By responding this way, I am fulfilling his request without becoming a short order cook. ~Laura Wesp

Choose Foods Wisely

As you are helping your child learn about new food trying you want to set your child up for success. There are a number of considerations to keep in mind as you are choosing foods wisely.

Perfect may be the enemy of good

Consider your beliefs about what constitutes a healthy diet? Yes, foods do need to fit for you but be aware that "perfect may be the enemy of the good." You may *want* your child to eat fresh, organic and homemade. That may be a great goal, a "perfect" goal. But, your child may eat three processed cereals and two processed crackers and a sweet, sugary yogurt. Her *List* is far from YOUR goal. This is your child's starting point. Your child is not at organic and fresh and homemade, **YET**. On the way to fresh, organic and homemade, there may need to be many small steps, small bridges of "good" on your way to your big goal of "perfect". If your child rejects all fresh or organic options right now and you do not want to try options not completely organic or fresh small step options, it may be hard to see change.

Sometimes foods and used to foods

When we discovered your child has a parentheses diet, we also asked you about her *sometimes foods* and *used to foods*. Many children will add new foods to their diet that they *used to* eat or turn *sometimes foods* into *established* foods on their *List*. Your child has had more experiences with these foods than most other foods. They can be an easier stretch as they have some familiarity. We are encouraged by our dietitian friends to reintroduce foods that have been previously rejected. Just because your child did not eat it last time it was on the menu, try and try again. Keep offering.

Of course, some children will surprise us by finding completely different foods to like. The idea is to give your child multiple exposures, options, opportunities to be around the many family foods and notice those that inspire his interest.

Food Amnesia

Teddy's dietitian, Anna Lutz, RD, gave me wonderful encouragement to keep sending variety in his lunches. She told me to have "**food amnesia**" when I pack. It can be so easy to listen to my inner dialogue of "he won't eat that, so I just won't send it." But, with that mindset, my list of acceptable lunchbox options grows narrower and narrower. Anna encouraged me to keep sending the blueberries, pepperoni, yellow pepper slices, etc. There is no pressure for him to eat them, but if I don't send them, I never offer the opportunity! He has surprised me over and over again by eating a food I would've given up on. ~Laura Wesp

Is this a food your family eats?

You have told us how frustrating it is to be asked by a feeding therapist to give a food to your child that you never eat or have in your home. Food choices need to be personalized to YOUR home, and YOUR family. If you are being asked to have a food available that you hate, or one that your family or culture never eats, is available only at fancy stores, or is wildly expensive, it is not likely to work in the big picture. It is hard to buy it or have long term success with a food if you do not believe in it from the start or if you believe it will just be rejected anyway! You and your child will be more successful if you offer foods you believe will work in your home.

Is this a food worth working on?

You will need to consider, is this food worth the effort? We are clear that progress for really worried eaters is slow. Change takes time. Consider the effort you are going to make to help your child like this food. Is this food worth the time, effort and expense? If, for example, you are picking a crumb for a stretch, could it be a fortified cereal crumb instead of yet another salty or sugary snack? Can there be a way that brown or snack crumbs can become freeze-dried fruit crumbs? Make it worth the effort!

Does this food enhance overall nutrition?

You are well aware that your child is not **yet** eating the perfectly balanced diet. Do your food choices tiptoe toward the food groups that are nowhere to be found on your child's *List*? Are you getting to some vitamin variation, or a new fruit or vegetable or a new kind of protein? Remember, that you may need a few steps, or even many steps, in the stretch toward these foods, but keep an eye on the goal. There need to be frank discussions about nutritional goals with the medical team, but, as we have described, it will not be as easy as "just add more vegetables." Does the food you are choosing contribute somehow to steps toward better nutrition? Parents will need to make nutritional priorities.

Can this food be offered in different ways?

If your child does not like a food you offered, can that food be offered in a less worrisome way? Think about broccoli. It can be plain. This may have a big smell, be bright green and a worrisome texture. Your child may reject it outright. But broccoli can be offered in many ways. You can tiptoe through broccoli cheese soup, Asian food sauces with broccoli, tiny broccoli leaves in rice, broccoli dippers with yummy dips. You do not have to run head on into the scariest form of broccoli.

Do you really need to start with THIS FOOD NOW?

I was recently asked, "how can I get James to eat bananas?" He hates the smell! He gags. My response was, "why bananas and why now?" There are lots of other foods for starters! We want to help our anxious eaters learn to trust new food trying. But, if he cannot even manage the smell of banana without gagging, it is probably too big of an *ask* right now. Certainly, you can have bananas around here and there, but to consciously "work on" eating bananas can be too hard for now. How about picking another food where your child can achieve success without practicing gagging? Bananas can be a later goal, not **yet**. Pick another food that can be successful and build confidence for now.

Can you grade the *ask*?

Did you grade your *ask*? Dilute it! Are you asking your child to interact with a food that is too big of a safety *ask*, developmental *ask*, sensory *ask*, motor *ask*, emotional *ask* or independence *ask*? For example, if you are offering your child a food to pass to a family member at the table and trying to help him get comfortable with that process, you will want to pick the best sensory or emotional *ask*. If he will gag at the smell of that banana, or cringe at the wetness of the watermelon, how about passing dry bread sticks, or allow him to pass the strawberries by touching the bowl and not the fruit? You want him to participate in the meal but be sure your *asks* are not too big. You want him to feel celebrated and successful.

No sensory surprises!

Grading your *ask* will require that there are no sensory surprises. Sensory surprises matter and they diminish trust. To avoid the sensory surprise, offer the tiniest of flavor, smell, texture or taste change and have your child help in the food preparation so he knows what to expect.

Can you pair this food with one your child already likes?

Some children will try new foods if we dilute the *ask* by combining them with another food they already like. In other words, can we pair that new food with something they already like so the smell, taste and texture are diluted. The example here is Marta's salmon in tiny pieces between two pieces of bread. The familiar bread masked the newness of the salmon. This dilution of *ask* works well IF your child knows about it and if there is no sensory surprise. You can say to your child, *one way you could give your tongue an idea about this nut butter is to try a tiny taste on your favorite cracker to see what you think.* OR *One way my friend tried her piece of salmon was to try a tiny, tiny taste in a little bread sandwich. What do you think your tongue would think of that?*

Can you stretch from a familiar food?

Many children have foods they like and are willing to try new ones if the tiniest of flavor change is offered with familiar food. An example would be if your child likes smoothies, can the recipe vary slightly to help you child like a new sensory property? If he likes a smoothie with fruits and yogurt, can banana be offered carefully so he gets used to banana flavor without a big blast of plain banana? OR If he likes yogurt, can you gradually change the flavor or color of the yogurt starting from the *familiar* one? We will call this *stretching* from familiar. Check out stretch ideas later in the book.

Prioritize lifelong skills

Part of parenting is a process of teaching children the skills and confidence of being an adult, so how can we prepare these anxious eaters for adult eating? We need to consider the challenges of mealtimes within the context of lifelong skills. Your child needs to learn to eat in that world where others eat other foods that he does not **YET** eat. He lives in a world where someone will offer him a new food or new food may (heaven forbid!) just show up on his plate at a sleepover with friends.

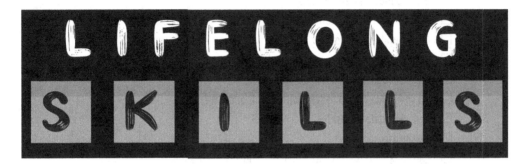

What lifelong mealtime and eating skills are <u>really</u> important? Well, your child may need to learn how to say *no thank you* and politely say *no* without ruining the meal, fleeing from the table or disrupting a family mealtime. He will need to have confidence in how to try new foods and the skill and confidence to spit it out (politely!) if it was not right for him. He will need to learn to manage optimum nutrition and/ or eat enough of a basic food variation to be healthy. Are you teaching strategies for and confidence in new food trying? Are you letting your child learn the internal motivation of eating?

Dear Parent,

What lifelong skills would you like to help your child achieve?

When we consider goals for our anxious eaters, we need to be clear in our priorities. Change is often slow and requires work! Do we want to add yet another snack food to the diet or could we help him add a vitamin? Do we want to work for six months to add one particular food, or do we want to teach new food trying? Do we want to have a goal of adding fifteen new foods for a child who is not even able to touch any new foods without severe distress? Yes, we may aim for fifteen foods, but we may need to get there in carefully designed strategies so there can be enjoyment, and not pressure, along the way. Remember perspective. We need perspective in looking at our priorities.

Choose Foods Wisely

- ☐ Perfect may be an enemy of good.
- ☐ Re-consider *sometimes* foods and *used to* foods.
- ☐ Is this a food your family eats?
- ☐ Is this a food your culture eats?
- ☐ Is this food worth working on?
- ☐ Does this food enhance overall nutrition?
- ☐ Can this food be offered in different ways?
- ☐ Do you REALLY need to start with THIS food NOW?
- ☐ Can you grade the ask?
- ☐ No sensory surprises!
- ☐ Can you pair this food with one your child already likes?
- ☐ Can you help your child stretch from a familiar food?
- ☐ Are you teaching lifelong skills?

Food Waste!

Oh, the food that is left uneaten or thrown into the trash! The pantry shelves overflowing with opened boxes of crackers and bags of snacks. The fridge door packed with sauces and dips. I remember my typically unflappable husband's irritation on a road trip when our son asked for a bagel; we got back in line to order it; and then he refused to touch it because it wasn't toasted to his exact standards. I've come a long way in my thoughts about food "waste". It's admittedly hard not to be annoyed in the moment when food go untouched, but perhaps here are some helpful hints.

First and foremost, I try to reframe "waste". I remind myself of two key principles. The first from the world of economics: once it's on a plate, it's a sunk cost whether or not my child eats the food. Second, and more important, there is value from exposure. Those repeat presentations are the rehearsals that Marsha describes, and even though my sons may not eat a food the first seven times they see it, those exposures may eventually help them adopt that food into their diet. I must think long-term.

But what to do about the cost? And, how do you at least minimize the inevitable food waste? Perhaps one of these tricks will help you, too.

1. The salad bar is your friend! It's totally acceptable to fill a box with one tomato, two cucumber slices, and a tablespoon of pasta salad and then pay by the pound. Depending on where you live, you may have access to an amazing salad bar filled with lots and lots of choices. But, even if you don't, take advantage of the opportunity to buy tiny quantities and benefit from someone else's effort to chop and dice.

2. I half-jokingly say that I should shop for my son's snacks at the gas station where everything comes in single-serving bags! It's honestly not a bad idea.

3. As for dips and dippers, I try to ask for extra sauce or dressing whenever I get take out. It's pretty astounding how many things Teddy is willing to taste with avocado lime ranch!

4. I urge my closest friends not to ditch their leftovers. That soup of which they've grown tired could be a very welcome gift in my kitchen! I remind them that even a few tablespoons of something they've made could be an opportunity for a new food exposure. In that same vein, I try to share, too. This may be a Southern thing, but maybe it could work for you, too.

5. At restaurants sometimes it's fun for kids to have their own meal from the kids' menu, but other times we ask for an extra plate and share from our entrees. ~Laura Wesp

The Art of New Food Trying

"Pretend you are feeding a Lego™ miniature...make it small."
Dawn Winkelmann

When we think about teaching children lifelong skills for interaction with foods, new food trying is a big one! Let's put *New Food Trying* principles all together. It is my experience that many children (and adults) who are worried about trying new foods need *specific guidance* in **how to try a new food**. This is actually an art more than a science. It requires a sensitive blend of strategy and communication. Remember we are always looking for what foods does your child love? We are looking for those foods your child WANTS to add to the *List*. We are looking for enjoyment. To blend those principles requires some careful grading of our offers with careful consideration of your child response.

The mixed-up ideas of forcing yourself (or others) to try a new food is a tough way to build confidence and find new foods to enjoy. (That elevator is going to the top floor of worry pretty fast!) When adults, like Marta, are confused about how to sensitively try new foods, it is hard to expect our worried eaters and worried parents to naturally **know** the continuum of successful and comfortable new food trying steps. OR, children may well have known intuitively that they only wanted to smell or lick a food or only wanted the smallest taste and we well-meaning grownups (both parents and therapists) may have inadvertently vetoed their choices with requirements to try bigger amounts or other pressure-filled techniques that add to new food tasting confusion. This sets the stage for less food enjoyment, less new food trying and more worry.

There are a number of schools of thought that tell us to just let children be around foods and they will ultimately try them. I agree that many, many children will try foods and eventually be *less picky* just by having food experiences. This, "give them time approach" absolutely makes sense for many, if not most, more mildly picky eaters. However, having spent a career helping these **very** anxious eaters and their families, I firmly believe that there are some anxious eaters that just do not feel comfortable enough to try *anything* new. Change is *that* hard for them. They may have no idea how to go about it. They may have no strategies they can believe in. These children need to first trust that the **pressure is gone** and then need to **learn actual tiny steps** that they can manage that help them get closer to the new foods. In some therapeutic settings, new food trying has been filled with pressure and demands. (*Lick this new food three times before you get your favored food* OR *Finish this pile of food before you get that one.*)

I believe these approaches need to be adjusted and the demands turned back into "offers" to help these anxious eaters try new foods. But because some people have misunderstood or misused the *try it* sequence does not mean it has no place in our support of families. We do not need to throw out the tiny step approach because some therapy clinics or families have lost their "offer and demand" balance. Let us look at the components of new food trying in coming chapters and see if these strategies can be used without pressure by sensitively reading your child's cues and going at his pace.

We learned the basics of trying new foods from the grasshopper story. I was *offered* the opportunity to try the grasshoppers. It was not a demand. I *wanted to try* them. We made it a *fun* group activity. I *watched* others eating it to learn how it was done, a rehearsal. I got to *explore* the up-close sensory properties of the grasshoppers. I got to see them from a distance and then had a closer inspection. I got to smell them and notice the taste *from a distance*. It was garlic and I liked garlic. I touched them with fingertips and noticed they were crunchy, crispy, and, I imagined, chewy. (This was where my worry got bigger as I imagined the chewy crunch of an insect in my mouth near my ear!) I got to create my own taste and texture concentration *at the pace* I could handle by grading the *ask* for myself. I did not *ask* myself to try a huge mouthful to start. I did not *ask* myself to eat only grasshoppers, I *diluted the ask* by trying it with guacamole, lots of guacamole. I paired it with something I already knew I liked. I got to increase the *ask* little by little as I was the one who knew how the tasting was going and I was the one who knew when I was *ready for a bigger* try. This strategy will work for many, most, lots of children (and grownups). AND, some particularly worried *food try-ers* may need a few extra steps along the way. We have looked at the parts of new food trying strategies, so let's put them all together.

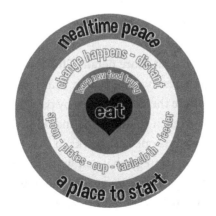

Start with mealtime peace

When your child is comfortable around foods and trusts mealtimes and mealtime partners, it is so much easier for him to want to try foods. Teach him the change can happen around the meal, first change around the edges and then gradually with food properties. And then, it may be time to teach new food trying.

New Food Trying Strategies

First!
> Mealtime Peace
> Change happens
> Rehearsals

Then!
> Sandwich TRY (Pair it with a Familiar)
> Finger Tasting
> S-t-r-e-t-c-h
> Re-Define TRY IT

Children differ in their initial bravery in trying new foods. And different strategies will work for different foods, different moments in each child's new food trying journey. From *it looks good when you are eating it, I will try it,* to *maybe I can eat it with a little of a favorite food to dilute the ask* to *maybe I will put my finger on it to get a little flavor or taste,* to *I really need to re-define TRY it,* there are a number of increasingly diluted new food trying options if needed. We will discuss more on all of these options.

Sandwich TRY-Pair it with familiar

Let's talk about this option in a bit more detail. This is an option to talk about with your child (or adult friend) who is a worried eater. This is an option that is a conscious effort for you and them to dilute the new food try by pairing it with a familiar, known food. It is a strategy that we teach to children (and adults) who WANT to try new foods but are *just not sure how.* It is one that works in a restaurant or at a social event. It is a lifelong new food trying strategy that can work in a variety of settings, and as Marta and I found, it can help your worried eater find new foods.

The rules of a **Sandwich TRY** are simple. Pick a food your child is *motivated* to try.

Figure out together what other food can be tried with that food and at what quantity to DILUTE the taste and texture (and smell). It is called Sandwich TRY because you are sandwiching the tiny taste of a new food with another food that you like so the look, smell, taste and texture are diluted, changed by the presence of the other food.

~ For example, if he wants to try avocado because the whole family eats avocado, what other food can dilute the *ask* for him? Crackers, bread, rice, or even a soup? Start tiny with a larger amount of cracker and the tiniest amount of avocado.

~ If he wants to try regular chicken, what other food can dilute that *ask* for him? Maybe a tiny amount paired on the same fork with a current favorite, chicken nuggets? OR mac and cheese? Or a soup or tortilla? Or maybe a tasty sauce that he already enjoys?

~ If he wants to try rice, what other food can dilute the *ask* for him? Maybe pair it with a cracker or bread or disguise the texture a bit with crumbs or refried beans or mashed potatoes. OR disguise the flavor with a favorite cheese sauce or condiment?

~ If he wants to try a new fruit, what other food can dilute the *ask* for him? Or maybe he can have a *mouse bite* taste of that fruit between to favorite cookies, or as a "jam" with his peanut butter sandwich? Or mixed with some favorite cookie or cracker crumbs?

~ Maybe he likes a tasty blueberry syrup on his round waffles, and this can become the strong flavor used to dilute the *ask* in trying a different brand of waffles, or different homemade variation. The familiar blueberry syrup helps dilute the newness of the visual, taste or texture *ask*.

The known food you pair a new food with will depend on the foods your child enjoys and is willing to consciously try with that new food. The decisions for the Sandwich TRY are made together with your child. No surprises. Dips and dipper tastes could be considered a type of pairing with familiar because there is a known dip and new dipper or known dipper and new dip. They, however, may not be an activity that dilutes the textures and flavors or smells quite enough for some.

An important thing about the Sandwich TRY is that your anxious eater gets to decide the amount of the new food and the amount of the familiar food. Maybe the tiniest *mouse bite* of new with a much larger portion of the familiar? He gets to decide if the tiniest *mouse bite* is okay and if, or when, to add a bigger taste of the new (*bird bite?*) and a lesser amount of the familiar food. You talk about his together and check in *how is that new taste?* You celebrate the trying and respect your child's response. Maybe he likes the tiniest amount of the new food, or maybe not **YET**. Sometimes we remind children that if the food is just okay, *it might take your tongue a few tries to find out if it could actually be a like-able food and one that can be added to your List.*

Teach finger tasting

If actually putting a new food in his mouth is too worrisome, many children (and adults) have discovered that taking a tiny **finger taste** is a nice introduction. The finger is far from the mouth. It allows for an initially distant interaction with the food texture. Remember there are food **flavors** that have only the rub of flavor and not the texture. This may be the easiest place to start as your child rubs his finger on the watermelon as a preview of eating it. If the food is a sauce food or one where there will not be just flavor, but a **taste**, so it also has a texture component, your child can be supported in touching it with the tiniest *mouse bite* of taste on his finger. He can bring the tastes to his lips or directly to his tongue and proceed accordingly.

This technique is a lifelong skill. You could put a food on your plate at a buffet and subtly put your finger on it for a taste to decide if your mouth wants more. I did this just last night. I was at a wedding and at the dinner there were two salad dressings offered. I smelled each but still could not decide which one I wanted to try. They both looked good, but which flavor would I prefer? I subtly put a drip of each on my plate and then did a finger taste of each. I found the Southwestern lime dressing the most appealing. One of the things I like about teaching children this option is that it can be flavor or tiny tastes and does not have to push directly into the worry.

Stretch from a familiar food

We will have a number of chapters about S-T-R-E-T-C-H-E-S to follow. A stretch starts with a familiar food and a new flavor, color, or texture is added ever so slowly so the **change** is NOT BIG. For example, if a child likes a certain smoothie, a stretch would be made if you put a little new food flavor (banana) in it during preparation to help your child get used to banana flavor very slowly. The banana addition could be dime sized and make almost no discernable flavor change. As you note that your child likes that little amount of banana flavor, you and she can add more, little by little, here to there. I prefer to make these flavor offers with the participation of the child because then it is not a sensory surprise. We make stretches from water, from juice toward smoothies. We make stretches from crumbs toward other crumbs and toward moist crumbs and cheese. We make stretches from favorite soup recipes.

It is important to start with a familiar food and tiptoe, stretching toward the new. Some parents will add a tiny bit of a new flavor or color or texture to foods their children like and say that they helped them like lots of new foods this way. It is systematic de-sensitization that helps this work. However, there are some of our very anxious eaters that will interpret the slightest change as a sensory surprise, so know your child, watch, and be careful as we do not want them to lose trust in their grownups. Some children need lots of warning that change will happen (by participating in the recipe) and others are fine with little changes. Most importantly the changes are small.

Re-Define TRY IT

Re-Define TRY IT strategies help children with lots of worry get closer to the look, sound, smell, touch, taste of the food in a here to there, systematic de-sensitization approach as outlined in the next chapter.

Child determines the pace

The pace of new food trying is the child's pace! Not the grownup pace. And many parents tell us how painstakingly slow this can be! But we need to remember that if we push or pressure, the child pulls away, resists, and we can make this journey of lifelong skill teaching even longer. As with the grasshoppers, I took bigger bites with more grasshoppers and less guacamole as I WAS READY and only I knew when I was ready.

Let us look in further detail about how we can re-define what we mean be TRY IT in the tiniest succeed-able steps to help you and your child see progress.

Re-Direct

As someone who loves cooking (or at least used to love it!) and strives to eat a diet rich in plants and whole foods, I've had to let go of many of my expectations. Prior to having children, I imagined my future kiddos happily munching on carrot sticks and hummus and willingly snacking on California rolls. Needless to say, my reality hasn't lived up to that idealized vision.

Although we all, no doubt, want our children to eat a wide variety of nutritious foods, that may simply not be our starting point. And that's okay! I have found that — hard though it may be — letting go of my dreams of "perfect" has led to greater peace and greater variety over time.

For example, after summer camp one day, Teddy came home and exclaimed, "Mommy!! Did you know that some potato chips come in a can!? And do you know what else? There's a man on the front. And he has a mustache!" At this point, I was feeling as if I'd perhaps deprived my sweet son of a slice of American culture! But, later that week, I made a point of taking him to purchase his very own can of stackable potato chips. Now sure, they are not the pinnacle of nutrition, and I'd much prefer to stay away from processed foods almost entirely. But, setting those preferences aside, my child was *excited* about food! We opened the can, and he ate a whole stack of them!! A few weeks later, I noticed he stopped eating them. I didn't think much of it, until he requested the ones in the *green* can. For those of you who may not know, those are the sour cream and onion variety. Thank you, Mr. Stackable Potato Chip for helping expand my son's tastes and prompting him to request variety. A few weeks later when Teddy begged to peel an onion while I was making chili, I had to wonder if Mr. Stackable Potato Chip had played a role in helping us reach that point.

In a similar vein, one night before dinner Teddy exclaimed, "I want a Lunchable™. Apparently, Teddy was enamored with the mini-pizza Lunchable™ that one of his classmates brought to school. It was an easy night, and so I said, "Sure, we have time to get a Lunchable™." (Words, I assure you, that I never dreamed I'd utter.) Anyway, he and Dad went to the grocery down the hill and Teddy came home proudly carrying his Lunchable™. I will add that he didn't actually *like* the prepackaged food, but it was just so refreshing to see him asking for something, manipulating it himself, and happily trying it.

Perhaps if we welcome these "less than perfect" foods into our children's diets they can be stepping stones to greater joy, interest, and variety. ~Laura Wesp

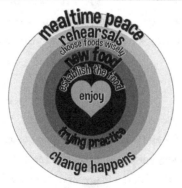

Circle of Sensitivity
Big Picture

Re-Define TRY IT

In a Circle of Sensitivity for New Food TRYING, we could start with mealtime peace, then *change happens*, then rehearsals, then pair with familiar and yet for some, we need to re-define TRY IT.

Think about our notion of **try it** When I make a yummy dessert and offer a taste to my husband and say *try it*, I usually would put a mound, a generous taste, on the spoon and would know he would love it, the *whole mouthful* of it! But for an anxious eater, a mouthful of a new taste or texture, can be way too much. Marta taught us that TRY IT by chugging a glass of water after flooding her mouth with a large piece of new food did not work as TRY IT for her. I learned that TRYING grasshoppers needed a few extra steps along the way to keep me comfortable along the way. We are going to re-define TRY IT in a sequence below.

I hesitant to call this a sequence or a structure. I even hesitant to call this a check-list. Please consider it as an umbrella of ideas. An overview. Guidelines. General tips. Some who see sequences and checklists, might interpret them as rigid, the rules, **THE** sequence. They may want it to be their road map. Their recipe. Their protocol. Their plan. THIS IS NOT THE PLAN. It is just meant to show you a way some of the various steps in new food trying can be broken down for more success so YOU and YOUR child see change. Every child is so different. Some do not need all of these steps at all and others need twenty more steps added to each section for them and you to experience success. Remember I am going to define success as your child getting to his comfortable place in each of these Circle of Sensitivity layers. It is individual and, as we have said before, personal. Re-Define TRY IT will help your child make more progress and help you re-define progress. Offer, get comfortable, and try a little more change.

> **Dear Parent,**
>
> What do you mean when you say TRY IT?

This Re-Define TRY IT Sequence offers examples of what small changes might look like for a child. This process gives parents and children a way to dilute the worry—to lessen it and make it manageable. Remember, when we are using the theory of systematic de-sensitization, we want to start with safe and familiar and then add change little by little to challenge the worry but find *comfortable* before we challenge him again. A sequence for this part of the Re-Define TRY IT list is offered below.

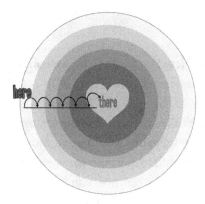

There are a number of options here when it comes to constructing a safe, individualized sequence for a child. Some children need help getting closer to the table and others need help getting closer to the food. These sequences can be worked on simultaneously or separately depending on the child's level of worry. Let's look at a Re-Define TRY IT Sequence and look at the art of new food trying.

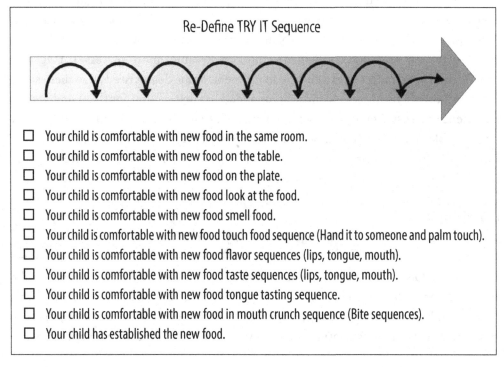

Re-Define TRY IT Sequence

☐ Your child is comfortable with new food in the same room.
☐ Your child is comfortable with new food on the table.
☐ Your child is comfortable with new food on the plate.
☐ Your child is comfortable with new food look at the food.
☐ Your child is comfortable with new food smell food.
☐ Your child is comfortable with new food touch food sequence (Hand it to someone and palm touch).
☐ Your child is comfortable with new food flavor sequences (lips, tongue, mouth).
☐ Your child is comfortable with new food taste sequences (lips, tongue, mouth).
☐ Your child is comfortable with new food tongue tasting sequence.
☐ Your child is comfortable with new food in mouth crunch sequence (Bite sequences).
☐ Your child has established the new food.

In the same room

For some children, being in the same room as a new food is already too scary. Those distant sensations, the senses of vision and smell, and sometimes sound, put them on immediate high alert. How can he actually want to try the food (in his mouth) if his distant sensory feedback says the visual, sound or smell of the food is already too much?

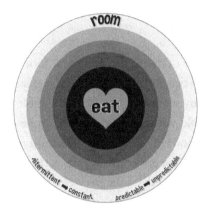

As we tiptoe toward the new food trying in the center of the circles of sensitivity, we start the farthest from the worry. Can the food just be in the same room? Can the child be in the room when the food is presented, just at the doorway…and still be comfortable? OR can the food be brought into the room and then out again…and still be comfortable? OR Can the food be brought just inside the room… and still be comfortable? OR Can the food be anywhere in the same room…and still be comfortable? Can you be interacting with that food in some type of food preparation and have your child even be in the room?

Having food in the room can also incorporate a predictable or not predictable component. A child may have had verbal or sensory rehearsals, warnings that it is going to be there, thereby being predictable, expected. OR A new food may be offered at the table without warning and have an unpredictable component. Life offers unpredictable food exposures, so we will aim to help him be comfortable with foods even if it is unpredictable. And exposure to new foods can be steady, meaning that the food stays in their environment or intermittent exposure, where the food is on the table and then away, or offered then removed.

On the table sequence

Can a child come to the edge of the table when new food is on the table…and can he still be comfortable? We can break this down further by having him come to the table and then leave (for how many seconds) or come to the table and stay. If this is too hard, can he first come to the table without food on it? Can he come to the seat and sit at the table (for increasing periods of time) with new food on the table at the far end… and still get comfortable? Can he get comfortable as the new food is placed nearer to him? (Progress can be seen as the distance between the child and the food gradually decreases until the food is in a bowl or plate nearby…and can he still be comfortable?)

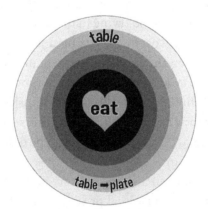

New food on the plate sequence

Some children are not ready to smell other people's foods at the table or nearby and need to learn more about food smells and touch interactions. (Those sequences will come later). But, once a child can sit at the table eating *his food* while others are eating *their own foods,* we can guide him toward allowing new food on his own plate while he still eats only his *List* food. This is a good skill to have as it allows him to have regular exposures to new foods without the requirement of eating them. You are helping *change happen* at the meal without the pressure or offer to taste it, **yet**. Teaching children to regularly help with putting garnish on a plate helps with this one.

New Food on the Plate Sequence

- ☐ Child allows new food on *separate* bowl/plate while eating familiar foods on own plate.
- ☐ Child eats familiar food off *own plate* that has a new food on it.
  - ☐ OR Child is assisted in removing the food to the side plate.
  - ☐ OR Child is able to remove the new food from own plate to the side plate independently.
- ☐ Child is able to try new food on plate.

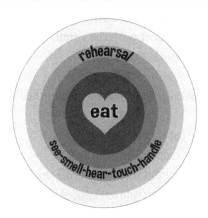

Look at it sequence

Let us look at the **sensory rehearsals** that begin to focus the food interactions on the distant and up-close sensory aspects of the food as new food trying gets closer to the mouth! This section begins the sensory rehearsals layer in the circle of sensitivity toward new food trying. Vision is usually the first distant sensory rehearsal a child can make with a new food. (Though sometimes a strong smell is the first.) A child can visually check out the food without having to touch it or taste it. If he can look at the food and watch others interact with it or eat it, he will be more comfortable exploring it further. Some children need to "practice" looking at foods, watching others, as their first step, before they explore foods further. AND the looking can be distant or up-close.

Look at it Sequence

☐ Child sees other people eating the new food and is comfortable with it. (Distant or up-close)
☐ Child sees the food on the table and is comfortable with it. (Distant or up-close)

Smell it sequence

Remember smell is a distant sensory rehearsal, a way to explore taste from farther away. Since there are strong smells and more diluted smells, the sequence will vary with different foods. Some smells fill the air and others need to be closer to the nose to smell them. Foods can be brought into smell range by the adult or by the child. A child needs to demonstrate a comfort with the smell, his distant taste rehearsal, before he will want to put it to his mouth.

Smelling Sequence (parent directed or child directed)

☐ Child walks in and out of room with food smells.
☐ Child demonstrates comfort with a FAR smell.
☐ Child demonstrates comfort with a quick CLOSE smell.
☐ Child demonstrates comfort with an extended CLOSE smell.

Touch sequences

1. **Hand it to someone sequence**
   Touching food can be a way to get a preview of the texture qualities of new foods with hands, even before having to deal with the texture in their

mouths. Many children who are worried about foods are worried about touching them. We ask ourselves *why would anyone want to put a food in their mouth if they did not even want to touch it?* Touch interactions are really important. We want to use a sequence that guides touching the food but starts at a comfortable place.

One way we can promote comfort in helping a child to handle foods is to help her hand or **pass it to another person.** When she passes a food, the momentum of the food is not directed **at** her but **toward** someone else, away from worry. When she passes a food, there is a clear *beginning and end.* She can touch it and then get rid of it as quickly as she needs. She *knows* there is an end to this activity. She can also gradually become more comfortable with touching or holding it for longer periods or handing it to someone farther away, increasing the length of holding.

For more worried food touchers, initially the adult can hand the food to someone and the child can just hold adult *forearm* and celebrate the hand off… and then can she still be comfortable? The adult is initially doing all the actual touching of the food and the child is just seeing or learning the process of a hand off. Can she touch the adult *hand* while the food is being handed off… and can she still be comfortable? Can she touch the edge of the food with the tips or sides of her fingers during the hand off…and still be comfortable? Can she touch the food with the fingers and palm while helping the adult hand off the food…and can she still be comfortable? Can her adults put the food in her hand and can she take that food and hand it off to another person…and can still be comfortable? When she is comfortable handing food to others and understands the sequence, can her adults vary the distance needed to walk to the other person, thereby increasing the time the food is in the child's hand?

In addition, the adult can vary the touch challenge from dry to moist to wetter foods. Modifications can be made to allow for handing off the food with spoons, tongs, cupcake papers, cups and bowls if direct touching is too worrisome in the beginning. Opportunities to hand food to someone else can be quite easily incorporated into the day so this absolutely does not need to feel like therapy time at home, but more a natural part of your day, your family food interactions and a lifelong skill.

2. **Palm touching sequence**

   Now that the child is willing to touch the food to hand it to someone, can she **explore** it within her palm where sensitive touching takes place? Actively exploring the food in the palm is a texture rehearsal that can give a pretty good idea about what the texture might be like in your mouth. It is a more active exploration than a quicker hand off of the food. The aim is keeping the food in your hand rather than giving it away. (Of course, this is not just a put-the- food-in-their-palm activity. With all these food interactions there is a function. *Could you check this food out? Let's talk about what it looks like? Is it smooth or crunchy? Do you think the one in your hand is the same size as this one? Can you hold this food and walk over to hand it to Dad?*)

We can also look at food touching through a Touching Circle of Sensitivity as we break down the sequence into tinier steps. Some children may initially only be comfortable touching food from a distance. This could be through touching your forearm or hand or could also be through touching tools. They can "touch" food though spoons, forks, tongs, bowls or cups. Still others start their touching through zipper plastic bags or plastic wrap, cupcake papers or even gloves.

The particular food the child is asked to touch **matters**. It is often easier for new food try-ers to touch dry food before wet foods. The dry food touching is farther from the worry on the Circle of Sensitivity than the wetter food. It is pretty easy to define the dry foods as crackers, cookies, pretzels and many snack foods. The wet foods are pretty easy to define as drippy food or foods with considerable water in them such as slices of orange, watermelon, cucumber, pear or popsicles. When cut open, these are wet foods. They drip. You need to wipe off fingers after touching or handling them. However, there are many *in between* foods. Foods such as whole apples, cucumbers, pears, tomatoes are wet/damp on the inside, but not actually dry on the outside. They are a different texture altogether, a dry version of a wet food. And there are moist foods such as muffins, sandwich breads, and breakfast bars that can be made into crumbs, but not dry crumbs. These are wetter, moister crumbs. You can imagine that in a continuum of foods for touching you will need to be thoughtful about food choices. This is especially important in the beginning when a child is LEARNING to hand food or pass foods. In the beginning you absolutely want to pick foods that will be most successful so your child learns she CAN touch and pass foods.

And once your child is comfortable handing food to others or passing food, she can begin to explore the up-close sensory properties of the foods and this will be discussed later. So, a touching Circle of Sensitivity might look like this.

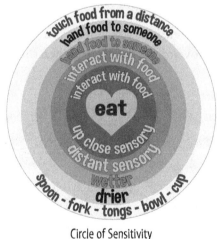

Circle of Sensitivity
Food Touching

Flavor sequence

Let's start with a reminder about differentiating *flavors* versus *tastes*. For the purpose of this book, we are defining flavors as the taste of the food without the texture of the food. By contrast, the taste is flavor AND the texture together. For a flavor of cucumber, you would rub your finger on it and then taste the flavor. The taste would be experienced by putting a piece of cucumber or some pureed cucumber on your tongue, which adds texture to the flavor.

In a flavor sequence, the trajectory of the food interaction is **toward** the lips, mouth and tongue. Of course, the first taste may be that smell taste from a distance. A beginning lip or tongue taste in the flavor sequence may be a **finger flavor taste** to get used to the flavor of the food without the texture. This, requires that the child has become comfortable with the touch of the food with his finger first. He can rub his finger on a food and then rub the flavor to his own lips for the flavor experience. The tongue is not yet involved unless he wants to actively reach out with his own tongue and lick lips. Finger flavor examples might be rubbing a finger on an apple, orange, watermelon, cucumber, piece of cheese, piece of chicken, or even a cracker or cereal and then tasting the flavor on lips. Purees and sauces are *not* used here as we are looking for the flavor only and NOT the residual texture on the lips. The adult can help the child do this with permission or the child can do it himself in imitation of others. Once he is comfortable with the finger flavor placed on his own lips, he can have a finger flavor on his tongue when his tongue reaches out for it, and then when ready on his tongue when it is in his mouth.

Here is a Tasting Circle of Sensitivity that helps you visualize a sequence of tasting from the distance of smell toward the fingers and then the spoon.

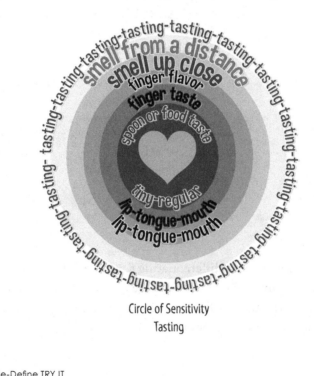

Circle of Sensitivity
Tasting

1. **Finger flavors**

Finger Flavor Sequence
☐ Child can bring a finger flavor to his lips and rub the finger on his own lips.
☐ Child can bring a finger flavor to his tongue and rub the finger on his own tongue when his tongue is *outside* his mouth.
☐ Child can bring a finger flavor to his tongue and rub the finger on his own tongue when his tongue is *inside* his mouth.

2. **Kiss flavor sequence**

    Kissing food can be an interesting game that brings the smell of the food close to the nose and the food close to the lips with a brief texture introduction and a small flavor taste. It can be done initially with a flavor taste, not a taste that leaves texture on the lips. (Ex. Kissing a piece of apple or a carrot.) Kissing can be a tiptoe toward in-the-mouth tasting. The kiss is on the lips and not at the tongue (**yet**). Kissing a food is a kind of invitation to the tongue. *Hey, do you want to try this?*

    Kissing is a way to help your child go from more distant visual, smell and touch exploration to nearer exploration. It continues the trajectory of the food **toward** the mouth rather than keeping it at arm's length. Kissing the food offers the opportunity to bring the food toward his lips, feel it briefly and then take it away. Again, there is that important *beginning and an end*. It is a quick interaction with the lips and then it is gone! Children are often willing to try this quickly and, as they become comfortable, the kiss can be longer and be a more solid touch rather than a quick peck.

    You can initially hold the food and kiss the child's cheek with it. This only works if you are offering, and there is a positive tilt, a leaning in on the part of the child. If your child shows comfort at the cheek, you can hold the food and kiss the child's lateral lip (lip corners) working toward the worried mouth. If there is comfort at the lateral lip, you can briefly touch the central lip, one or both. And, of course, with acceptance there, the kiss can be at central lips for a longer time. If your child is comfortable enough he can bring the food to his own lips from the start or take over at this point imitating the food kisses. Once comfortable with central lip kisses, he can kiss the food multiple times giving the opportunity for repeat tastes.

```
┌─────────────────────────────────────────────────────────────────┐
│                    Kiss Flavor Sequence                           │
│                                                                   │
│  ☐  Adult holds flavor food and kisses child's cheek with it.     │
│  ☐  Adult holds flavor food and kisses child's lateral lip with it.│
│  ☐  Adult holds flavor food and kisses child's central lip with it…briefly. │
│  ☐  Adult holds flavor food and kisses child's central lip with it… longer time. │
│  ☐  Child holds flavor food and kisses it…briefly.                │
│  ☐  Child holds flavor food and kisses the food multiple times.   │
└─────────────────────────────────────────────────────────────────┘
```

When children are learning to kiss foods, put their lips on food briefly, we often play a microphone game where the food is the microphone and we and the child talk, sing, tell jokes with lips onto the food getting more playful flavors on the lips, and sometimes even tongue!

3. **Lip balm or lipstick (extended) flavor sequence**

We call it a *lip balm or lipstick flavor taste* when you or your child rubs the food flavor along his lips, like lip balm or lipstick. This is an extended taste of the flavor. This is a *flavor* sequence so the flavor, not the texture, is left on the lips. This assumes he has comfort already with the smell and touch of the food. You can offer this lip flavor taste, or, preferably your child can provide his own lip flavor taste getting the touch of the food on both fingers and lips with no texture residual.

```
┌─────────────────────────────────────────────────────────────────┐
│            Lip Balm/Lipstick (Extended) Flavor Sequence           │
│                                                                   │
│  ☐  Adult holds flavor food offers it as a lip balm/ lipstick flavor taste, moving along lips. │
│  ☐  Child holds flavor food and puts food on as a lip balm/lipstick. │
│  ☐  Child tastes the lip balm/lipstick flavor with multiple swipes. │
└─────────────────────────────────────────────────────────────────┘
```

With some children we will call these *princess lipstick tastes*. With others we might describe putting the flavor on dinosaur lips, or fish lips to continue to invite the child into the fun of the activity. Flavor tastes can, of course, be practiced with actual flavored lip balm. During different holiday seasons there seem to be multi-packs of lip balm creatively flavored with chocolate chip, or pineapple, or green apple or even soda flavors! These opportunities give more smell and flavor experiences so the child gets used to the idea of bringing flavors toward his own mouth.

Tasting sequences

The tasting sequences will be adding *food texture* to the *flavor tastes*. Some children need these two sequences of flavor and taste separated and others do not. These tastes, again, will go from distant toward close, therefore from lips to tongue to inside the mouth.

1. **Finger taste sequence**

   In a finger *taste* sequence, the child will dip his own finger in the food, puree or sauce and tastes it on his lips, on an outside tongue or an inside tongue. The volume and concentration of the taste will increase, the texture of the taste will vary, and the flavor and texture combinations will change each of these tasting experiences.

   ### Finger Taste Sequence

   ☐ Child can bring a finger taste to his lips and rub the finger on his own lips.
   ☐ Child can bring a finger taste to his tongue and rub the finger on his own outside tongue (when his tongue is outside his mouth).
   ☐ Child can bring a finger taste to his tongue and rub the finger on his own inside tongue (when his tongue is inside his mouth).

   As a guiding adult, you can grade the flavors, smells and textures of the taste to optimize success and enjoyment of this activity.

2. **Kiss tasting sequence**

   This kissing sequence will be much like the flavor kissing sequence but will include texture *with the flavor* to create the taste experience. Some children kiss the food then wipe it off their lips at first. That is okay if that is what he needs to do. (We do not stop the child from doing this. With practice and repetition, the child will become more comfortable. If the wiping off is too upsetting, you likely need to adjust the *ask* to different tastes, or textures, or go back to flavors a bit longer). The kiss tastes may need to start out with the smallest amount of texture and gradually increase toward more texture. If the texture added to the flavor is too fast, stay at flavor level and tiptoe carefully toward taste.

Kiss Tasting Sequence

- ☐ Adult holds flavor food and kisses child's lateral lip with it.
- ☐ Adult holds tasting food and kisses child's central lip with it. Licks it off with tongue or tastes with lip movements.
- ☐ Child holds flavor food and kisses the food multiple kisses and licking off with tongue or tasting lips.

---

3. **Lip balm/lipstick (extended) taste sequences**

These lip balm tastes add texture to the flavor *lip balm/lipstick* tastes above. Whereas kiss tastes are tiny and usually on central lips, lip balm tastes swipe along the whole, or more of the lip. More flavor and more texture are experienced. You and the child can explore just top lip, top and bottom lip, or both.

Lip Balm/Lipstick (extended) Taste Sequence

- ☐ Adult holds tasting food offers it as a lip balm/lipstick taste to lips.
- ☐ Child holds tasting food and puts food lips on as lip balm/lipstick taste. Licks it off with tongue or tastes with lip movements.
- ☐ Child tastes the lip balm/lipstick taste with multiple swipes and licking off with tongue or tasting lips.

Tongue tasting sequences

Hopefully with the multiple exposures to smelling, touching and lip tasting foods, the child begins to show his grownups what foods he is beginning to *enjoy*! What foods does he want to come back to for more? What food flavors does he love? We want to give him the opportunity to *try* many foods in this way, hopefully as a natural and comfortable part of the family food interaction routine.

Tongue tasting can start with flavors as described above, or go right to tastes, depending on the comfort level of the child with each new food. You can hold the food for licking, if needed, but preferably your child will feel less pressure if he can hold it himself and go at his own pace! For children, we call the quick lick a "frog lick" as it is fast--like a frog catching a fly! As he shows enjoyment in the quick lick, we can encourage more licking by what we call noisy licks. He can focus on making silly sounds while licking repeatedly. The focus is on the sounds rather than the multiple taste practices the child is getting. Sometimes in therapy sessions we make a parade with several children licking and making noises on their foods as if in a mini-food licking band!

Tongue Tasting Sequence

- ☐ Child holds flavor food and licks it briefly. (Frog lick?)
- ☐ Child holds flavor food and licks it...Noisily? Musically?...longer?
- ☐ Child holds tasting food and licks it briefly. (Frog lick?)
- ☐ Child holds tasting food and licks it...Noisily? Musically?... longer?

Once your child is comfortable with the distant tastes from smell and the flavor exploration gets closer to his mouth, a Circle of Sensitivity for into-the-mouth-tasting might look like this.

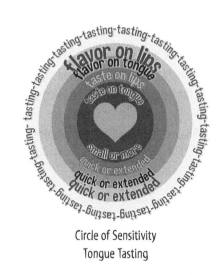

Circle of Sensitivity
Tongue Tasting

Mouth tasting sequence

Once your child has gotten comfortable touching foods (so he has had a rehearsal about what it might feel like in his mouth), and flavor tasting, lip balm/lipstick extended tasting and licking foods, he can put more of a taste into his mouth. Depending on his mouth skills and previous experiences, this may be any texture from puree to solids, from tiny soft wet foods to meltable crumbs or solids.

Safety certainly needs to be accounted for, as well as consideration of whether he has the motor skills to try a beginning taste. It is very important that the *ask* be SMALL and that it is offered in a way that does not push directly into his worry. Minute tastes of liquids or purees can dilute into his saliva and may be less of a worry. When beginning solids, crumbs will require less chewing and a smaller motor response. The offers should be small, careful, and biasing toward success. Sometimes the small taste can be offered on the tongue. Sometime at the cheeks, and sometimes directly over the teeth, depending on the motor or chewing requirements of the food. Note that different children have different starting points for this. Some may start with wet foods, maybe liquids or maybe purees. Others start with dry. Most start with a preferred texture and work toward combination textures. This sequence is one that is hard to predict for children. Each child has his own starting point and could use our creativity in tiptoeing toward mouth tasting changes. (Your child's therapy team can help). In order to help him feel more confidence with tasting actual pieces of actual foods, we give them practice spitting out (with supervision)!

Mouth Tasting Sequence

- ☐ Child tastes a puree that easily mixes with saliva for swallowing.
- ☐ Child tastes a puree of mixed texture that can be swallowed.
- ☐ Child tastes crumbs (on lips then tongue and inside cheeks) that easily mixes with saliva for swallowing.
- ☐ Child tastes a hard melt-able that could be used in biting practice. (Safety first!)

Spitting out sequence

Children need the **option of spitting out**. Remember the grasshoppers! If I had not had the option of spitting out the grasshoppers, I would **not** have tried them! Sometimes we just need to spit out a food and try again later or try again differently in less of an *ask*. Some children need to learn to spit out in a playful non-eating way so they have the skill and confidence to spit out a worrisome food taste. Puppets can help provide rehearsals as they demonstrate spitting out. Also, **we** can demonstrate spitting out. If there is too much spitting out maybe our *asks* are too big we are pushing into a child's worry. We may need to back up and go more slowly with the TRY IT sequence for that food. Remember, we are following their cues and adjusting our asks accordingly.

Either we or your child can put the food in the child's mouth for spitting out practice. But if we do it, it is must be an offer that your child has the option of NOT accepting. Our preference is that your child be an active participant in this part of the trying, but it will be important that we help guide the size of the *ask* so the willing child does not inadvertently get too much in his mouth, even if it is to be spit out. Preferably we help with the sizing and the child puts it in his own mouth himself. (We do not want to create safety worries!)

Spitting food out can also be a way to work on some fun oral perceptual skills at non-mealtimes. As your child gains the ability to direct a spit, you can change the bowls from big bowls, to smaller bowls, to taller bowls, to smaller diameter pill bottle sized containers. Different and more refined oral motor planning skills are required with each smaller container. We have even used spitting out as a way to practice *mouth math*. Check out Food Pre-Academics.

At home visits and at the clinic we go outside and teach children to **feed the birds** by spitting out "O" cereals, or other foods at bushes. We tell them (and the young ones believe us) that we are spitting the cereals to the birds, with love! This becomes a great activity to practice at home. Children love to bring in pictures of their bird feeding at home to celebrate! We often pick "O" cereal because the hole in the center makes grownups a little less worried about a choking hazard, but this activity is done step by step with careful supervision. Once one shape and texture of cereal is efficiently fed to the birds, there are all sort of textures, shapes and flavor of foods that can be put in the mouth and then spit out so the flavor and texture *ask* is brief.

Spitting Out Sequence

- ☐ Adult/child puts food on child's lip and child flicks with finger or pushes with tongue or blows it off lips into big bowl.
- ☐ Adult/child puts food in child's mouth and child spits it out in big bowl.
- ☐ Adult/child puts food in mouth and spits it out in a four inch diameter bowl. (Diameter decreases to pill bottle, medicine cup or shot glass size).
- ☐ Child bites and then spits. (Takes a mouse bite with teeth and spits).
- ☐ Child spits a distance.

Spitting out sequence (variation)

We can play even more spitting out games to help with food tasting with a beginning and an end. Often, a child is more willing to put the new food in his mouth knowing he will be able to spit it out. We can place the food or help him place the food in particular places requiring a particular motor response. We can place the food at the side and ask him to spit it out, or place in the center and move it to the side or place it on one side and ask him to move it to the other side, then spit it out. It is a way to get comfortable with a new food flavor or texture without the requirement (just the option) of chewing it while also helping to build skill, variation, and confidence. Mouth math, as described elsewhere in the book is a great way to practice this type of spitting out.

Spitting Out Sequence (Variation)

- ☐ Adult/child puts food in child's mouth in side......child moves to center and then spits.
- ☐ Adult/child puts food in child's mouth in one side...child moves to other side and then spits.
- ☐ Adult/child puts two items in mouth, child spits out one piece.

In mouth crunch sequence

We sometimes add a step where we place or help the child place a small, melt-able food over the lateral teeth and ask them to crunch or make a noise with it. Of course, we model that activity first, and probably take turns doing it with the child. We are helping him get comfortable with the sound of the food but also ask him to do what it takes to make the noise in his mouth. Once he can do it with noisy crunch food and learns the idea that putting the food over his teeth, it is important and we supervise this skill to softer more varied, less noisy foods. The thing about noisy foods is that they immediately give feedback that they got it right and can feel or hear the *celebration*. Adults can monitor the noise of the crunch and the "melt-ability" of the crunch to optimize success and minimize worry.

In Mouth Crunch Sequence

- ☐ Adult/child puts food in mouth over lateral teeth
- ☐ Child crunches "noisy" food one time…spits out
- ☐ Child crunches "noisy" food …swallows
- ☐ Child crunches "non-noisy" food…swallows

Bite size discretion sequence

We use a visual chart to help worried eaters understand the size progression of new food sizes. The taste or the *try* does not have to be big. We start out with very tiny mouse bites and as the child is comfortable, he can tell us that he wants bigger and bigger tastes sizes. Our usual chart, below, uses animals to size the bite, but you can use whatever the child likes. Some choose dinosaur sizes. Others choose car and truck and construction vehicle sizes. Be creative and make it work for each child. What we have especially liked about the idea of a mouse bite is that mice are small, comparatively *very* small. The *ask* is so much less threatening than the mound of grasshoppers on the spoon! We have offered the tiniest of mouse tastes off tiny coffee stirrers to reinforce how very, very, very small the taste is! We laminate the picture chart below so children can participate in size choice at home and in therapy sessions.

Bite Size Discretion Sequence
(aka Mouse Bite Chart!)

- ☐ Mouse bite
- ☐ Bird bite
- ☐ Kitty bite

	Puppy/Dog bite
	Horse bite
	Elephant bite

Sometimes my son needs help with his bite sizes. Occasionally he will take a bite that is too big, and then because it requires more effort, he will just stop eating. (Of course, if the large bite were a safety hazard, I would act on that immediately). His feeding therapist has helped us with these strategies to prevent the challenging bite from ending the meal. The first approach is to say, "That was a large bite. Sometimes I need sip of water after a large bite." This suggestion reminds him he has a choice to help himself. If he's still reluctant to continue eating, I might propose that he try a mouse bite — acknowledging that his first bite was an elephant bite — or, I may gently direct his attention to another food on his plate. Often giving him something easier to manage can help him resume eating. ~Laura Wesp

How long to work on one food?

Therapists and parents often ask how long do we *work on one* food? *Working on* is a strong phrase. The answer to that questions is that it is very individual and depends on each child's response to the new food and his motivation to add that food. Instead of thinking of this as a protocol or a recipe, think of it as a way of life, an approach, that can used to guide new food interactions.

We do not focus on one food at a time for a number of weeks or months and then pick another. We do offer worried food try-ers interactions with lots of different family foods in the careful ways we have been describing, and with each food interaction we give the child the opportunity to explore it in a comfortable sequence. These are **guidelines** for food trying, **not requirements**. Our ultimate goal is to offer the child experiences with many foods, when they are ready, and THEY will let us know how comfortable they are with that food *that day*. They may get to licking and tasting or they may just be comfortable with touching. We gradually see the child become very comfortable with this routine and they become much more comfortable going directly to lip feel and taste exploration then actual biting. But it takes time for this to be the comfortable sequence. Remember our goal is to find out what tastes your child loves! By offering one food for weeks or months until the child likes that, we are limiting their trying opportunities. What if we picked Brussel sprouts and that was never going to be a favorite? OR what if we picked clinic applesauce and it was not working!? We will waste all that time and may be pushing into worry. But if the child showed interest the day he helped squeeze oranges for juice, or enjoyed handing freeze dried fruit to others, they give us an invitation to offer closer trying opportunities. Follow their lead!

Therapists need to remember that therapy clinics may have really boring foods. Of course, they are chosen for safety or melt-ability, or because they are common children foods, but remember, if you offer experiences week after week with the same snack veggie straws, or licorice, crackers, vanilla cookies, vanilla pudding or yogurt or applesauce, you will not discover that your child loves Indian food sauces, chicken noodle soup, cucumbers and dips, green smoothie, or bacon. Parents and therapists can creatively look at expanding food choices for food exploration. ☺

Below is a Circle of Sensitivity summary that demonstrates the overview of Re-Define TRY IT sequence. It is only a guideline and can be adapted for each child. This Circle of Sensitivity shows the food getting closer to the child from room to table, to interaction with the food in rehearsals, to learning about the sensory properties of the food prior to eating it. It shows tasting from finger tastes to food interactions and from lips to tongue to spitting out. And finally, it encourages skill mastery with the tiniest amounts of in mouth foods, to bigger amounts and the teaching of variation with liquids and solids.

Dear Parent,

What parts of the Re-Define TRY IT sequence might help you
and your child be successful and see progress?

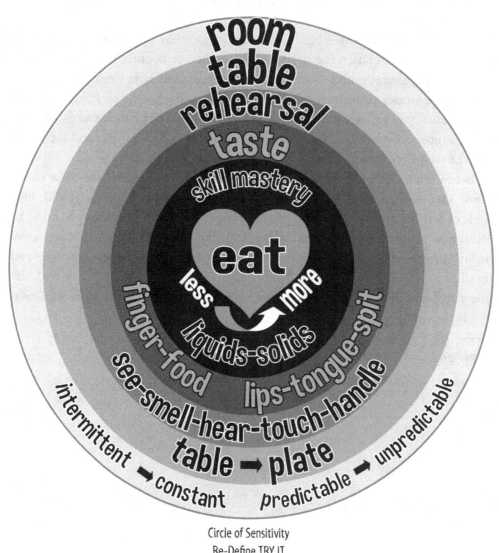

Circle of Sensitivity
Re-Define TRY IT

Adjust! Adjust! Adjust!

"Adults can be the food trying guides, but children determine the pace!"
Get Permission Approach

Adjust the ask

In our *here to there* continuum of tiny steps, we hope each child accepts our offer. We hope we made the perfect *ask* and create a positive tilt. But we may get it wrong and ask too much. Your child may reject it or resist. **He will let us know**. (Remember he has the option of saying *no, thank you* when we offer.) Since we think of resistance as a response to OUR PRESSURE, can we quickly adjust, ask for a response that pushes less into his worry. That is why we grade our *ask*. That is why we are *offering* and not *demanding* and that is why we have *rehearsals*. That is why we observe then **adjust**. We want them to know we are offering support, as we are their Food Partners, their food trying Guides or Helpers, not the Food Police! We are their Circle of Sensitivity Hugger! ☺

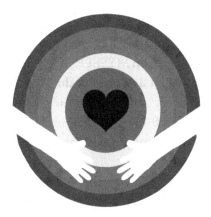

Now for those of you from the **I am and adult and I GET TO MAKE ALL THE RULES** camp I say, wait, read on. You **ARE** making the rules, but they are different rules. We are not being authoritarian. Instead of a rule of *you must do everything I tell you and I am bigger and can make you......* The rule could be *I will offer and you can let*

me know if it is okay or not. If it is not okay, together we can try it again a bit differently so it can be comfortable. (And you must be polite, and I will help you). This works if your child absolutely trusts that you will not force or scare him with too big of an *ask* and if you are starting from trust and mealtime peace. They are just different rules. You still will guide the big picture decisions.

I understand if we offer and the child says NO every time, we need to look at this. Is NO a way to just say *I never want to try anything*? (OR perhaps he does not trust his grownups and is used to everything about mealtime feeling like pressure, perhaps he does not feel well, perhaps his worry is too great? Do we need to back up and reduce the pressure so he quit resisting and rebuild trust? Does he know *how* to try new foods? Can we change the *ask* so it is more comfortable and builds on his skills? OR is NO a way to say, *You are asking too much, I am afraid, teach me and help me*? Is NO a way of saying *your ask is too hard for me*?

Wait! Wait!

An OT fellow made an observation after a couple weeks of shadowing me. *You know, Marsha, you don't let a child tell you No when you make an offer. You hear their No, but then re-direct them to a different place. You just lovingly say Wait, Wait and offer up the activity in a less worrisome way and help him be successful.* It was interesting feedback, as I had not put words to how I respond to *No*. Wait, Wait, gives me a moment to quickly PIVOT to a new *ask*, to wonder what I need to change for the child to **not need to resist**, a moment for me to undo my pressure, a moment to ask differently. In my way of thinking, I turn the questions back on MYSELF. What have I DONE that is pushing too hard at the child's worry? **What do I need to do** (what do we adults need to do) to adjust our *ask* so we can end every activity with the child being successful? It is very important that we help the child find enjoyment in the sensory aspects of eating, is confident with his own oral motor mouth skills and is INTERNALLY MOTIVATED to want to eat.

We adjust!
1. Make the offer
2. The child says YES, GREAT.
3. The child says NO, we do not let **HIM** end the activity. We are going to PIVOT, adjust or step down the *ask* then we end the activity with success.

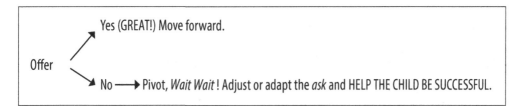

Offer

Yes (GREAT!) Move forward.

No → Pivot, *Wait Wait*! Adjust or adapt the *ask* and HELP THE CHILD BE SUCCESSFUL.

Our *here to there* offer arrow will go back and forth. It will zigzag as we follow the child's cues. Forward, practice, forward, back up, stay there, forward, practice there, forward, back up, try again as we respond to the child's cues. The realistic *here to there* journey is often not direct, but a series of adjustments still ultimately heading in the same direction. Remember it is not a straight line into the worry from here to there. It is a bit of a back and forth, somewhat like a bungee cord stretching a little toward the worry and a little back to find that practice place of comfortable. Layer by layer you tiptoe toward the *there*.

As we continue, we will practice offering and then modifying what we offer if we unintentionally asked TOO BIG an *ask*.

It looks like this.

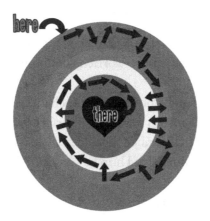

Dear Parent,

Can you think of a time your ask was too big and you might have pivoted, *Wait Wait*, to a more successful ask?

Some days are good days, other are not

We may have in mind that it is a good day for new food trying/offering. But it may not be a good day for your child. What else is going on for him? Is there a lot going on for your child? New school, transition to a new class? Is your child tired, constipated, getting a new tooth, too hungry at this moment? Remember to look at the big picture. *New* can be very hard when there is other stuff to contend with.

If we pick an *ask* and it works, we can help the child have confidence stretches to practice that new food. (Check out Confidence Stretches chapter). But what do we do when we are trying to be careful, to look at tiny steps of re-define TRY IT, and the child says NO or even gags? WE ADJUST OUR ASK. We do not stand our ground and make it a power struggle because we are bigger and we are grownups. Remember we want our worried eaters to understand that we are their guide and helper. Adjusting the *ask* requires the adult to know where the child is at in their new food trying confidence so we readjust appropriately. It could look like this.

Situation #1

> Mom: Owen, can you pass this slice of pear to your brother? (Owen does not want to because he is worried about touching it.)
> Owen: No way!
> Mom: Wait, Wait, you do not need to touch it. You can help me pass it. (As she puts his hand on her forearm or her hand as she does the touching of the wet cucumber slice does the passing. To make this adjustment work, Mom helped him be successful in whatever part of the task he could do)
> Mom: Thanks for helping me.

Note: Mom acknowledges that the ask was a bit big and asked him to help her. He still trusts that she will not push him into his worry. She could have asked him to hand the food to brother or help her do it. That would completely depend on the child, which *ask* backs down a bit to find a less worrisome e place? If she could hand HIM the cucumber and have HIM be comfortable handing it to his brother, that would be optimum. If that went well, she could ask him to then pass one to someone else at the table in the same way and get a little extra practice in at this comfort level. But, if he needed to just touch her arm while she did the passing for today, that is fine. It is today's staring point. But remember, he is learning the passes to others idea. Maybe it would be more successful if the passing was practiced initially with a dry bread stick?

Situation #2

Dad: Karen, would you like to try this smoothie?
Karen: No
Dad: It is okay, can you just smell it and put it right here? (Dad can help her smell it. Dad knows she is pretty comfortable with smell tries OR Dad could say how about a tiny mouse taste on your finger with this coffee stirrer? The *ask* is one you already KNOW will be successful.

Situation #3

Mom: Brennan, I made your new smoothie. Would you like yours with a tall straw or short straw?
Brennan: A short one
Mom: Here, you can pick your favorite.

Note: No adjustment was needed. But if he was worried about the smoothie we could give a bit more rehearsal. Had he said NO to either straw, you could have said, *Wait, wait. you are not ready to try the smoothie yet? (You PIVOT) That is okay, but can you help me pour some for Dad? Do you think HE would like the tall straw of the short one? Now can you pour some for MOM? Do you think I should have the tall straw or the short one?*

Note: The idea here was that the child may have needed more rehearsal time to get toward trying it. He may try to taste it later today, or maybe next time. You ended the activity with him still being involved, him still participating and him being thanked for helping. He got to be celebrated.

Situation #4

Mom: It is fun making a smoothie with you, Jason. Can you put four strawberries into the blender?
Child: I don't want to touch them.
Mom: It is okay. I will help you put them in with the tongs.

Note: Mom could have said, it is okay, *you can put them in with the tongs if you would rather not touch them today* (yet).

Note: Jason will be successful.

Situation #5

> Dad: Thanks for passing me the bread, Emma. Can you smell it?
> Child: (Smells the bread)
> Dad: Smells good, huh? I am going to kiss mine, can you kiss my bread?
> Child: (Kisses the bread)
> Dad: Thanks for kissing my bread. Would you like to taste it with your tongue?
> Child: No thanks.
> Dad: No problem, how about it you kiss it back to me?
> Child: Child kisses it and hands it to Dad.
> Dad: Thanks, sweetheart.

Note: the tasting it was a bit much today. Try again another day.

Situation #6

Mom and child are making peanut butter sandwiches.

> Mom: You are doing such a good job of spreading the peanut butter. Do you like the smell?
> Child: (Smells the peanut butter. Enjoys it)
> Mom: Look, I got some peanut butter on my finger! I am going to lick it. You have some on your finger, can you lick it?
> Child: (Hesitates). And brings the sandwich close to lips.
> Mom: Wait, Wait! Can you just put a tiny taste on your finger and touch your lip? Just a teeny tiny taste?
> Child: (Puts a tiny taste on finger then lip.)
> Mom: How did that taste?
> Child: Good.

Note: If the child likes the peanut butter on her lip, you might ask, I need more on my lip (a rehearsal), can you put some more on yours? Here is the mirror to look at yourself doing that? Or *wait, wait*, which other finger might you try the taste with? Or which of these straws can you use for another taste? (These are activities to build confidence which we will describe further later, but they give the child repetition when he is in a new food trying moment. At any point if he indicates he is done, we could say, have you had enough peanut butter today? Okay, but can you put the lid on the jar and help me put it away. PIVOT)

Situation #7

> Therapist: Don, here is our new drink. Do you want a tiny taste with the big straw or little straw?
> Mom: I would love to try it with the big straw.
> Child: I want the little straw. (Tries it)

OR If the child was too worried, Mom might say, it is okay, can you smell it (or stir it) and then pass it to me? Thanks.

Situation #8

> Mom: Dave, would you like to taste this cucumber? (As Mom offers the cucumber toward him.)
> Dave: No (covers his mouth).
> Mom: *Wait, Wait*, but can you just pass it to Dad and then we can put the rest away?

Note: If Dave passes it, great. We will say thank you. If he pulls away and is not comfortable touching the wet cucumber today we might say, *Wait, wait, can please help me pass it to Dad?* and Mom guides his hand to touch her forearm or hand as they together pass the cucumber to Dad. After the *Wait, Wait* is a reduced ask to go back to a comfortable place in the new food trying sequence, so as not to push Dave into his worry, but to still have the **adult end the activity**, and Dave's involvement is still celebrated. "Thanks for helping me pass it to Dad."

When we get it wrong, and we will…

Okay, sometimes our *ask* it too big. It happens. But with this **Wait, Wait, pivot**, we, essentially give ourselves an out when our *ask* is too big. We step it back down to a more achievable goal and then continue with another interaction. We ask the best *ask* we can, and then adjust. **With this approach we can help a child try anything.** Parents can try home foods or also bring home foods to feeding therapy.

A therapist friend told me recently that a mother she knew wanted to bring a hard-boiled egg to therapy to try. My friend knew that it was a very big *ask* and may not be successful. But, perhaps it was still worth exploring with the parent? Could the child hold the egg with the shell on? Pass it to someone? Or pass it in a cup so as not to touch it? Hard boiled eggs are a big smell and quite a different texture. Could they peel it together, or could the child watch the grownups peel the egg? Could therapist and parent rehearse smelling it as see how that goes? Could they all touch the egg, push on it, and see how it bounces back after being pushed? Could it be sliced in half to find the hard-cooked yolk? Could it be chopped into egg salad sized pieces or even add mayonnaise? Could the child serve it to others? (and be celebrated for that)? Is there a place along the way for a finger taste? Can grownups model that? At any step along the way, it could be rejected by the child, but therapist and Mom are learning together about the child's response and always helping him get to a comfortable place. Mom is learning how to have her child learn a new food trying sequence and how to *ask* or how to back up. ANY food can be a learning opportunity if you do not require the goal of IT MUST BE EATEN TODAY.

Therapists want to be successful too. If getting your child to eat that hard-boiled egg this week was the goal, it may not have been the best choice. But if we can re-define progress, re-define our goals in a different way, this could still be a very successful session. The child had hard-boiled egg rehearsals. Mom got ideas about how her child could explore hard boiled eggs, try a new food. Next time, the group could make scrambled eggs, or fried eggs. How does a finger taste of these compare? How does the smell compare? Is there any more interest in egg in these forms? What about a mouse taste of some type of egg in a Sandwich TRY? OR if this is all too much, can you all go in the direction of finger tastes of other foods to teach the trying sequence? Could you all practice finger tastes of an already favorite food, such as a cracker that the child already knows? Continue new food trying skill learning in more familiar foods, staring maybe with dry toward wet, and someday back to eggs?

Try LOTS of foods, not just foods you think will be volume foods. Find those motivating smells and flavors! Remember in the big picture of new food trying, we want your child to have the skills to confidently approach a new food. With that confidence will come more motivation. In my way of thinking, it is far more helpful to teach children how to approach ANY food, that getting them to eat a certain volume or a certain food on a certain day. When they find the flavors of foods that love, this will motivate their continued interaction with those foods and lead to more tasting then eating volumes.

Dear Parent,   Re: A Swim Story

There is a lot of information in this book. You have probably realized I like to describe the same topic in several different ways. I know each of us learns differently and sometimes it is the story, sometimes it is the picture, and sometimes it is the written description or chart that helps each of us put the information together for our own use. Some of you will relate to the tiny steps in the *here* to *there* image. Others of you will find the *Circle of Sensitivity* a helpful image. *Re-Define TRY IT* can be just the tiptoeing new food trying image that you need. By telling stories and describing the complexities of food interactions in different ways, my hope is that each of you finds information that is meaningful to you, your family and your anxious eater.

I know it can be overwhelming. I know parents and feeding therapists will both be reading this book. I ask you to take the information as an overview and get the Big Picture. Read it again, it you want, discuss it with your child's feeding therapist. Some parents read it and say, I *get it* and others say this is what my child's feeding therapy team is supposed to do! In reality you both will want to know this information. I think of this eating journey with anxious eaters as a partnership not only with you and your child, but also with you and your team. It takes a mealtime village…a committee and lot of sensitivity hugs! Each child's journey toward food enjoyment will look different.

Since there is so much food information in this book and we have just talked about a long Re-Define TRY IT strategy, I want to take you away from food for a bit so you can gain some perspective! Can we think about something else completely? How about swimming? Yes, swimming. Can you see the analogy here?

As a parent in Arizona, we need to teach our children to swim. There are swimming pools every-where. Sadly, children drown every year. I wanted to be a good parent and get this right. I wanted my child to be safe and happy around water. So, to be a responsible parent I felt the need to teach my children to be safe in the water and swim. Our children live in a world where there are lots of swimming pools and they need to be able to safely and comfortably navigate that world.

(As a parent of an anxious eater, you want to teach your child to be safe, and comfortably navigate the world where people eat foods they do not and new foods will happen. As a responsible parent you want to get this right.)

But if your child is scared of the water you approach it carefully. My child had a brief scary incident with water as a one and a half-year old and became terrified of putting his head under the water. He did NOT want his had anywhere near the pool. He did not TRUST the water! What is a parent to do?

(Your child may have had scary food experiences or may be very worried about the look, smell, texture and taste. You want to help him feel confident and curious about foods, to help him expand his diet, but when your child has worry and wants NO change what are you to do? When he does not TRUST food, what is a parent to do?)

If your child is afraid of the water and cries when near it, you have some choices. Some would just throw him in the water to get him used to it (not my choice!) and go from there. But how will that help him TRUST the water if he is already worried about water? OR You can carefully approach the water and teach him skills. (This was my choice, but I needed help because I am NOT a swim expert! I can practice the swimming lessons suggested to me, but I needed help finding a place to start).

(For a child with food worries, new food trying can feel like too much, like they are being thrown in the "deep end" of food sensations. They need to learn the skills of food trying just like beginning swimmers need to learn strokes). It can feel like too much and, as a parent, you probably want some help in teaching that food confidence and new food trying skills. You probably want help finding a place to start and finding trust again.)

The expert swim instructor understood my son was very worried. So, she did not just dunk him the water. She went out to the pool with him and stayed in the pool areas playing with toys. Gradually as he was comfortable, she and he moved the toys a bit closer, and a bit closer until they were right next to the edge of the pool seeing and hearing others have fun in the pool and getting splashed some. They spent two whole sessions there. I PAID to have my son spend two sessions playing at the edge of the pool. Really?! Of course, I just wanted him to learn strokes and be safe, to learn to float and like the water, but MY GOAL was too hard, too fast. SHE was helping him build trust and confidence and learning to tiptoe toward his worry.

*(This is a bit like **Re-Defining TRY IT**. Maybe your child just needs to be in the same room as the food or can get closer and closer to the worry without **going over the edge** of worry. The swim instructor's loving approach was her **Circle of Sensitivity** to help my son get back to a comfortable place around the water, to **trust** again. She was, in essence, getting him to the pool equivalent of **mealtime peace** before teaching the strokes of swimming. The **rehearsals** she provided him were being near others swimming, seeing and hearing others in the pool. She also gave him some **up-close sensory rehearsals** with tiny water splashes, not tsunamis! She was building his trust around water again and following his cues. In a way she was **grading her ask**. Her **ask** was appropriate from a safety point of view (he was not going to drown). It was appropriate developmentally with tiny steps toward the water and eventual swimming. And her **ask** was appropriate emotionally as he had been so worried about the water. She helped him get calm from a distance. He needed two days of playing with toys at the side of the pool. Though my parent worries wanted that to go quicker, she was following **his** lead and watched for **him** to show he was more and more comfortable around the splashes, the sensations of water. With our anxious eaters, we, as parents really want therapy to go quicker, to see changes with eating NOW. But, as with my pool-worried son, the instructor knew she had to build his trust and go at his pace. She knew pressuring him would not help, going too fast would not help, but she knew we **must** teach him to swim just as we MUST teach our worried eaters to learn to manage their interactions with food. Feeding therapists can help in these ways too.*

Next the swim instructor sat on the steps with my son. She and he played with toys that would *happen* to fall on the first step. This was not random play, it was **guided** play. He gradually put his feet on the step to help him balance as he reached for the toy. She gave him little tiny experiences that nudged him gently toward his worry without freaking him out! Once he was comfortable there, she and he would drop toys on that step with lots of repetitions. He got used to reaching, getting his forearm arm in the water and gradually, as the toys *happen* to fall on the next step down, he had to get the water all over his whole arm and get his chin or cheek wet to reach for the toy. He knew the routine, the rehearsals, and continued as he became increasingly comfortable. And then, one time he reached for the toy and got his face wet. She did NOT push him in, but just gave him the opportunity and he took it! (There was a beginning and an end to the water worry). Before I knew it, he put his whole face **in the water** to get the toy, and then sat up happily as he continued to play. He stayed at those steps a while to gain confidence and gradually had his face in and out of the water with ease and tiptoed toward actual swimming skills from there. Whew!

*(The swim instructor taught me, as a parent, to allow my child **to go at his own pace**. He is the one who knows his level of worry just like your anxious eater child knows his own level of worry. She believed my son just as we need to believe our worried eaters. They know their own worry. To learn to swim, my son needed to be at the pool. To learn to eat, our anxious eaters need to be around food and reduce the worry of even being near it. To learn the skills of swimming we need to first reduce our worry about even being near the water. To learn the skills of eating and new food trying we need to get comfortable around the food, to have those rehearsals and multiple exposures. To learn to strokes of swimming you have to get in the water.*

I had struggled with him at the pool because I kept pushing into his worry before I got help. It was a sad experience for both of us. I would take him near water and he would scream. He practiced his worry. If you had asked my son, "do you want to swim?" he would have said NO, **never**. It would have been simpler for me and for my son if we just did not deal with this pool worry, if we could just ignore it. I suppose it is possible to grow up never being around pools, and never face the fear, but, as a parent I then would have worried whenever my child was out of my sight. \What about birthday parties houses with pools? What about class trips near water? What about friends later making fun of him because he did not swim. We parent are so good at the "What-abouts"! He would have been happy never facing a pool and I would not have had to see him in any kind of a worried state near water. But we needed to face it to address the **lifelong** pool safety skill. We HAD to teach him, but it HAD to be done carefully.

It is easier to only give our anxious eaters the food from their List because the worry is eliminated. They are happier and so are we. That is because, as parents, we want our children to be happy and not worried. But, in order to help them navigate the eating world, to be able to learn the "strokes" and skills of eating and not "drown" in the worry, we needed to make a plan. And we worry because of our "what-abouts"! What-about if his nutrition is not good? What-about when he goes to school? What-about if he goes to a friend's house? What-about if friends make fun of him?

So, it may help to think of your child's eating worries in parallel with the swimming pool story. The need for building trust, for tiptoeing, for rehearsals, for a careful introduction to the sensations and then the learning of skills and strokes and just make sense at the pool and at the table. Both need to be careful and proceed at your child's pace. Both need to build trust and both need to support your relationship with your child. Some parents can get past that pool worry to teach their child swimming and some, like me, needed extra help. Some parents will be comfortable with teaching about food and new food trying and some will need help. But in both cases, the practice of swimming at home, the practice of new food interactions at home will be key to the development of lifelong skills. I wish for you to get the help you need for success in your home.

Very sincerely,

Marsha

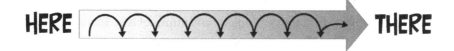

Practical S-t-r-e-t-c-h-e-s

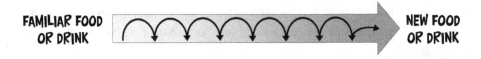

FAMILIAR FOOD OR DRINK → NEW FOOD OR DRINK

Many children tell us they want to try new foods, but just can't or they are willing to try new foods if the changes are really small. We are going to call these S-t-r-e-t-c-h-e-s. As we think of helping a child tiptoe along a continuum of tiny succeed-able, stretch-able steps from a comfortable starting place of *here*, to a new place along a continuum to their *there*, think of a rubber band *stretching* from the familiar starting point. We start a stretch in the direction of change, but we have the option of relaxing, ADJUSTING, that stretch back toward the starting point of *familiar*, if we have made too big of an *ask*. Wait, wait, PIVOT. Remember, we offer, then observe, then adjust! We use *stretches* to help a child get to a new food or help them expand their confidence and enjoyment of the new and familiar foods. We can use stretches to help them get to a new flavor or texture, food group, or a new shape. We use crumb stretches and smoothie stretches so often that they get their own chapters.

S-T-R-E-T-C-H Adjust S-T-R-E-T-C-H Adjust S-T-R-E-T-C-H Adjust S-T-R-E-T-C-H Adjust

The "stretchy part" is the flexibility we have in our *ask* as we *adjust* to help a child move in the direction of worry but not right **into** worry. This is an offer activity, NOT a demand activity. This activity works very well for many anxious eaters. And, it is NOT RIGHT for others. Let's sort this out.

We start with what is working NOW. Remember, if every time you practice any new food trying you are immediately confronted with a NEW food, you will quickly learn NOT to want to do that. Therapy sessions and home practice should both start with familiar, safe, and successful. Calm. **Every** time.

```
S-t-r-e-t-c-h

~Start with a familiar food
~Tiptoe towards adding a tiny amount of new flavor, color, texture change WITH YOUR CHILD
~No Sensory surprises
```

An example: Imagine you are helping your child like a new yogurt. He likes vanilla coconut yogurt. You absolutely start with HIS YOGURT! You might offer change to begin with in utensil or bowls, taking turns and rehearsing. Perhaps you can stir in, or help your child stir in a berry yogurt taste to see how he stretches his enjoyment with that? Maybe your child will try it and like it. You can celebrate that you are helping him toward change through a same texture and very similar food gradually stretching to more and more of the new yogurt mixed with familiar until he likes the berry yogurt. When he learns to enjoy both coconut yogurt and berry yogurt, you and he now have more *List* choices. That would be an easy s-t-r-e-t-c-h. It worked.

But, what if your initial offer was rejected? TOO MUCH CHANGE. What could you do? Maybe the berry yogurt mixed in was too much and he would be fine if the amount of the new yogurt offered was less, much less, diluted. Maybe the change was too concentrated in color change and was, all of a sudden, too red? Maybe it was a surprise and he did not know the change was coming and he might have been more comfortable if HE had helped stir in the change. Maybe he needed a lesser change such as vanilla coconut yogurt, to vanilla dairy yogurt, or vanilla soy yogurt or a different brand of coconut vanilla. Do you see how the *ask* is being adjusted? You start where is seems most comfortable knowing YOUR child and then tiptoe with a readiness to immediately adjust if needed. S-t-r-e-t-c-h-e-s are done with willing children in tiny steps.

Stretch types

Check out the various continua in the Up-Close Sensory Properties chapter. ANY could be s-t-r-e-t-c-h-e-s as each arrow imply tiny steps or s-t-r-e-t-c-h-e-s of change. The most usual s-t-r-e-t-c-h-e-s aim for a gradual *flavor* change, a *texture* change or a *new look* (shape, color) to the food. The child can s-t-r-e-t-c-h from a favored yogurt flavor to a new one, a tiny amount at a time. The s-t-r-e-t-c-h can be from that yogurt texture to a new one by adding the tiniest amount of mashed banana or crumbs. Or the peanut butter sandwich can be presented in the usual four triangles format on the plate with three the usual size and the fourth cut into two triangles for a look change.

The flavor, texture and looks can be changed by tiptoeing along the continuum carefully with child participation to avoid sensory surprises. We also will always be careful that if we made the *ask* too big, that the child is given the option of saying *no thank you*. (This is a lifelong skill to learn).

Within **flavor s-t-r-e-t-c-h-e-s**, a starting s-t-r-e-t-c-h could be a **brand** s-t-r-e-t-c-h or a **complimentary** s-t-r-e-t-c-h. An example of a brand s-t-r-e-t-c-h might be changing from one current brand of vanilla yogurt to another brand of vanilla yogurt or one brand of plain applesauce to another brand of plain applesauce.

This Flavor	That Flavor
This Brand	That Brand
This Food	Complimentary Food

A **complimentary s-t-r-e-t-c-h** pairs a similar flavor with a new, but related similar flavor. An example would be to help a child learn to like a new fruit yogurt if he already likes a fruit yogurt, or slightly different combination of fruits in his smoothie, a slightly new recipe of soup, a slightly new popsicle flavor. The similarities in these flavor changes are fruity and sweet and the s-t-r-e-t-c-h is still within those categories. In all these s-t-r-e-t-c-h-e-s the flavor is the changing component, not flavor and texture.

Within **texture s-t-r-e-t-c-h-e-s** you can s-t-r-e-t-c-h from any one texture to another. From thin liquids to thick liquids, thick liquids to purees, one puree to another, dry to wet, wet to dry, crumbs to pieces, solids to crumbs and from whatever texture starting point the child enjoys to another.

A **look s-t-r-e-t-c-h** offers tiny acceptable changes in shape, color, size of the food, the bowls and presentation. For example, you can get to small noodles by starting a s-t-r-e-t-c-h from familiar full-length spaghetti. Break it in half to start with and cook it and see if that change is ok. (IF not okay, can you just break off an inch or so at the end and then cook it so the overall length is gradually becoming shorter? Can you child help you break it? If halves were okay, then go on to quarters and so on. If the quartered spaghetti is noticeable, but not rejected, can you offer that for a while to help you child get comfortable there, before breaking it down further? Can you see how the pace of your s-t-r-e-t-c-h-e-s depends on EACH child? Some leap past them and others get stuck and need to hang out at one change for a while.

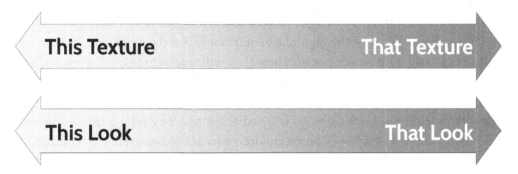

Routine can help

We can create a s-t-r-e-t-c-h-e-s in a way that uses our understanding of the *child's rituals* and routines to be part of the familiar part of the activity. Some examples of routines that may be working for each child. Perhaps our s-t-r-e-t-c-h-e-s can include some of those routines.

~ Billy would try any new smooth food (IF Mom feeds him).
~ Marla would try a new food (IF small enough and offered in a Sandwich TRY).
~ Juan would add a new food (IF it was offered within a smoothie).
~ Oliver would try a new drink (IF it was offered from the blue cup and he got to say "Cheers" first).
~ Justin would eat a new food (IF he was told it was organic).
~ Robyn would eat a new food (IF it was in pureed form and she saw it in the bowl first and rehearsed it).
~ Michael would eat a new food (IF you gave him the choice), *How many tastes would you like, 2 or eight?* He liked the game and the number eight and added a number of new foods to his diet with this learning activity.

Our s-t-r-e-t-c-h-e-s can build on these already okay routines or rules. *Quesadillas are good, I like quesadillas.* OR *I like numbers, eight is my favorite.* OR *When we tap our cups and say 'cheers', I drink some.* OR *I like smoothies. This is a smoothie. I like popsicles, this is a popsicle. I like red, this is red.*

These s-t-r-e-t-c-h-e-s can start out as non-mealtime opportunities of new food trying then later can be brought to the family meal. When they are confident, these s-t-r-e-t-c-h-e-d foods can be more easily added to the *List*. Some children are comfortable enough with s-t-r-e-t-c-h-e-s that they can be a part of the meal. YOU KNOW your child.

We want to bias the s-t-r-e-t-c-h toward success. As we have mentioned earlier, we do not want to change the one central nutritious food the child likes, at least not in the beginning, or if we are not sure how they will react. Often children will allow change in these main foods, but we need to fully understand each child's relationship with change first. We do not want to take the chance they will toss it off their *List*. However, we do not want to be so worried about s-t-r-e-t-c-h-i-n-g that we do not offer the option of a s-t-r-e-t-c-h. Some children start out so completely worried about *any* change in their *List* of foods that they will drop any food from their *List* that we grownups mess with. Oh my! The food *Lists* for these children are narrow enough to begin with that we do not want them eliminating any foods on the *List*, especially the ones where we celebrate the nutritional value! Many parents have had the experience where they cut the waffle in a new shape, or offered their milk in a new cup, or accidentally bought a new brand of peanut butter and the child dropped that waffle, that milk or that sandwich from their *List*. We must be especially careful that we do not inadvertently cause them to drop the s-t-r-e-t-c-h-e-d *foods*.

Have we helped with *change happens* already?

How is your child with the concept of change? Does he *get* that *change happens*? We are careful in changing foods, even with s-t-r-e-t-c-h-e-s, if your child is not even comfortable with *change happens*. Start there and get you and your child comfortable with that first.

S-t-r-e-t-c-h one sensory variable at a time

Depending on the worry level of each child, we may only be able to challenge **one sensory variable** at a time. Though we *can* change the look, flavor and texture, we would probably pick one of these variables to offer an initial s-t-r-e-t-c-h change. In a way, we layer or sequence the s-t-r-e-t-c-h-e-s. Let's look at an applesauce s-t-r-e-t-c-h.

When making an applesauce s-t-r-e-t-c-h, we generally pick one sensory variable to s-t-r-e-t-c-h at a time for our very anxious eaters. We would probably NOT change the color, flavor (brand) and texture at the same time. If your child likes one brand, we might s-t-r-e-t-c-h from that brand first, then gradually change the color/flavor and then lastly change the texture.

The brand s-t-r-e-t-c-h might look like this. First, offer the familiar applesauce brand from her favorite bowl or the container and gradually from different bowls or off different spoons. Once that change can happen, another plain applesauce brand (not flavored with extra cinnamon or berries) might be offered in the side of the bowl for tiny tastes.) OR that new brand can be stirred in the familiar one in the tiniest of amounts. This would be a brand s-t-r-e-t-c-h. Once she can easily dance between the favored and the new brand in different proportions, new same colored flavors (not berry) can be offered and gradually she can stir in a drip of the colored applesauce (mango or berry flavored), adding more and more until she finds enjoyment in the variation. Your child can help make homemade applesauce and experience the texture variation carefully. If texture variation is too worrisome, consider a step along the way where she eats a familiar applesauce off a textured mouthing toy or spoon to give a tiny texture experience to the mouthful of applesauce.

OR This applesauce s-t-r-e-t-c-h might have started with the applesauce in the bowl and with one stirred in drop of a different applesauce brand stirred in. (By stirring it in the difference in favor is diluted). If that is accepted, then two drops and three and so on can be added. There are so many ways to do s-t-r-e-t-c-h-e-s and get to the same enjoyment at the end, we make our best guess of small changes knowing each child and adjusting if our *ask* was too big.

OR Your child who only wants his juice from a certain brand in a certain box will not be as ready for a change in juice color or flavor as one who can already drink his juice from any cup. He may need to tiptoe around change and learn to handle the juice out of the box, before change in juice flavor is offered through a s-t-r-e-t-c-h. Can we help him drink his juice out of a lidded cup with a straw and then use that as the starting point for a s-t-r-e-t-c-h? Once he is comfortable with the new lidded cup, the flavor can be s-t-r-e-t-c-h-e-d gradually. You can start the flavor change as minute as needed for comfort and STAY at the comfort level as long as needed. If he learns to like apple juice with one tablespoon of a new juice in their cup of juice, give him multiple practices with juice that varies between one teaspoon to one tablespoon of the new juice so their mouths get used to *change happens* with the juice so he becomes a bit more flexible wit juice change. If you only offer the juice with one tablespoon of the new, he can quickly get in a rut where THAT becomes his juice for his *List*.

Crumbs can be a great s-t-r-e-t-c-h to a new texture food, but first your child may need to be comfortable with change in the shape of his food. He may need to first get comfortable with broken chips or crackers first before he is willing to crumb them. But once crumbing is a possibility, hang on, because more s-t-r-e-t-c-h-e-s can happen! (Checkout My Cracker is Broken chapter).

Parents KNOW!

"What would happen if we added an ice cube of a new juice to their favored juice drink? Would your child mind?" You **know** your children pretty darn well. Some parents will immediately say, *"Oh, she will reject it completely or throw it at me!"* Others will say, *"I do not think she would even mind, at all, I never thought of that."* When we know a child, we can make an offer of a s-t-r-e-t-c-h with a tiny change and adjust accordingly. If the *ask* inadvertently was too big, we will find that out and try smaller, but it is best to offer the tiniest change first to not push into scary territory.

Tiny changes

Changes along the continuum of change can be miniscule…so tiny that the child needs to be really, **really** worried to notice. A s-t-r-e-t-c-h may be starting from a familiar homemade waffle. We ask the parents *would your child still eat his homemade waffle if you add some extra goodies to it?* Some parents will let us know they have tried this and it did not work! Others will say I do not think my child would even notice as long as their waffle was the right shape and the change is small. (Children who require sameness often pick different parts of the meal to focus on for *same*. Same may be the same feeder, the same shape, the same color, the same cup, or same straw. Can we s-t-r-e-t-c-h to more nutrition for that waffle, by adding an extra egg, or some extra protein powder, or a tiny bit of applesauce, or a little pureed carrot? Once children get used to waffle variation, many parents add fruits, veggies, extra eggs, yogurt, oils and power pack the waffle. That then can become a staple of the diet.

Minimize the surprise

To minimize the sensory surprise, we include children in the process as much as possible. Rehearsal, rehearsal, rehearsal! Can she help make the waffles? Can she make a blender drink? Can she use a special dropper to add a few drops of a new juice to familiar juice and then help stir it? Can the mac and cheese include a bit of extra butter, or cream or extra cheese with her helping in the preparation?

Ice cube meltables s-t-r-e-t-c-h

The *here* is the juice or liquid your child likes. This is the *familiar* part. The *there* is a new juice or liquid flavor (and possible a new look). Say your child likes white grape juice. To help her s-t-r-e-t-c-h from white grape juice to another juice, consider adding ice cubes of a different juice. (Ice Cube Meltables). As the **ice cube melts**, she gets the tiniest amount of flavor change at a time until she can finish the juice with the new flavor added. This is a way to offer change in the tiniest amounts to help find enjoyment in a new flavor, color, or even food group.

To maximize success, consider some assists. Some children need to get used to ice cubes ahead of time with **water ice cubes** or with **familiar juice** such as white grape juice ice cubes in white grape juice so they get used to the ice cube initially **without** a flavor change. Some children will be more comfortable with a lid on the cup so they do not have their nose right into the cup for a big obvious smell change, or obvious visual change. Include your child in picking out the ice cube to make it a rehearsal so they know what is next.

You can use all different **ice cube shapes**. With the internet availability of so many ice cube shapes, it is very possible to find an ice cube shape that will be loved by your child. Flavors can be diluted or concentrated. You could dilute the juice with water so the flavor change is VERY SMALL initially. Or it can be a full-strength concentrated juice.

You can pick the **juice color** carefully. The ice cube juice can start out as a color similar to the familiar juice in the cup or be a bright color change. For example, if the familiar juice is white grape juice, consider picking a similar color juice such as apple juice for the ice cubes. The color contrast is not so different. But eventually, once your child knows this game he may be comfortable enough to offer him choices of ice cubes of red strawberry juice, or orange mango juice, blue blueberry juice or yellow pineapple juice or a green kale smoothie drink. And you and your child can add one ice cube, or two or three after the game becomes trusted. Of course, the ultimate goal is to help your child be comfortable with a variety of different juices, different colors and *get* that *change happens* and it will be okay. Remember that leftover juice s-t-r-e-t-c-h-e-s can be made into popsicles or ice cubes for future s-t-r-e-t-c-h-e-s.

Milk to vitamin-enriched-chocolate-drink s-t-r-e-t-c-h

We have used the ice cube s-t-r-e-t-c-h idea to help children move from the flavor and look of whole milk to a vitamin enriched chocolate drink. Fortifying milk is often one of the recommendations from our dietitians for rounding out the vitamins and perhaps adding calories. We have prepared the vitamin enriched chocolate drink powder in milk and frozen it in an ice cube tray. We help your child add one cube at a time. It can start out fully concentrated or very diluted with a tiny amount of powder as you grade the change. We have known some children who took a week to move from whole milk to a fully fortified chocolate or vanilla milk and others have taken several months. Remember here, though, that if that milk is the only celebrated nutrition in your child's diet, we would probably not start a s-t-r-e-t-c-h there if there is any chance your child will eliminate it as a *List* food because we messed with it. You know your child. Some are okay with the change and others, **not**.

   We have built on this strategy with the supplemental formula drinks that are juice based to help children tiptoe into a fortified juice from the ice cube and juice s-t-r-e-t-c-h-e-s above. Your child's dietitian will make those recommendations. We have also tiptoed toward a Smoothie S-t-r-e-t-c-h, but this has its own chapter.

Puree s-t-r-e-t-c-h for flavor, texture and look

If the puree your child likes is a yogurt, can you s-t-r-e-t-c-h from one brand to another, one complimentary flavor to another and eventually from yogurt texture to different textured meals. Or can you help your child s-t-r-e-t-c-h from yogurt in the container to yogurt from a cup? Or can you s-t-r-e-t-c-h from plain mashed potatoes to cheesy mashed potatoes, or mashed potatoes with mashed cauliflower? Or can you help him s-t-r-e-t-c-h from one pureed vegetable to another since these would be complimentary flavors? If the puree your child likes is a baby food chicken dinner, can you offer that dinner with tiny stirred in tastes of extra baby food chicken, or baby food carrots to get toward a more varied meal?

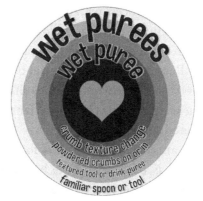

Circle of Sensitivity Puree Texture S-t-r-e-t-c-h

Waffle s-t-r-e-t-c-h

Many children who have narrow diets like waffles or pancakes. They are brown. They are a predictable texture. They have a reasonably predictable look. (And of course, many worried eaters also require that their waffles are a certain brand and a certain shape). We are often quite happy when a child does have a waffle variant on the *List*. It can be a good place to start toward change. The goal will be to help your child learn to like homemade waffles where recipe variation becomes possible. When children already like homemade waffles and are comfortable with the slight variations in flavor and shape, it is the best starting point, but we can help most children get there from *wherever*.

To get to homemade, you need to start at comfortable. A specific brand and round, perhaps? Can he get used to his waffle being cut in different ways? Can others around him have their waffles square? Can your child serve himself cut up waffle pieces that are on a platter that has some round waffles cut up and some square (of one brand and then another)? Can the pieces of cut up round waffle mix with cut up square waffle and can the piece sizes vary a bit. You are helping your child get used to *change happens*. Can you make a similar transition with a commercial waffle versus a homemade waffle so your child sees, then is exposed to, homemade waffles. **Your homemade waffles**, initially, not his. A strong syrup flavor can also help dilute the new waffle flavor (if your child likes syrups). For some children the tiptoeing will start with syrup changes or putting peanut butter or a creamy nut spread that they happen to like on the waffle to, again, dilute the waffle flavor or texture change.

When your child likes homemade waffles, can he help prepare them? Can you first help him get comfortable with the process with no change in flavor or look? Then can he help you add a little variation in the preparation so there are tiny changes in flavor, not big ones? Can you add an extra half teaspoon of vanilla, whipping cream or an extra egg? Can you add a dollop of yogurt, or spoonful of powdered milk? Continue to vary the shapes a bit so your child is learning waffles change. We can help children get comfortable with adding a fruit (scoop of baby food fruit or even baby food carrots) or yogurt, cream cheese grated apple or mashed fruit.

Many parents tell us they are able to make waffles for their children with all kinds of nutritious extras like chia seeds, banana, yogurts, berries or nut butters. When you can vary the recipe and add an extra serving of a new food group or some extra calories it can be a great addition to the day! And yes, it would be best if your child could eat applesauce by itself someday, but meanwhile, as a parent, you can know there are a few extra apple nutrients in the day. You are making these changes *with* your child, not sneaking them in and, when your child is comfortable with waffle changes, you can be quite creative in your new recipes.

Pancake s-t-r-e-t-c-h variations

You can try some of the same ideas to get from commercially available half dollar size pancakes to homemade ones gradually helping your child be comfortable with flavor change, and brand to homemade change. Syrups can help. Cookie cutters can help your child get comfortable with *change happens* in shapes. We make pancake puzzles!

When it comes time for your child to help with making the pancakes, consider using a squeeze bottle as a pen to draw pancakes shapes. (Check out the internet as there are many creative parents making adorable pancake shapes!) Your child can practice his alphabet or numbers or draw happy faces while making the pancake with you and diluting the worry. And gradually, when shape change is comfortable, pancake batter can be put into cupcake papers and made into tiny *pancake muffins*. Now you have a bridge to muffins!

Muffin s-t-r-e-t-c-h

S-t-r-e-t-c-h-i-n-g from homemade pancakes or waffles to muffins can be a terrific change that gives you and your child many more options. Once your child is comfortable with the idea of muffins or cupcakes, he can help make them with small recipe changes that allow him to know *change happens* with cupcakes. Some families we know make a nutritionally packed muffin each day to support basic nutrition and variation. Fruits, vegetables, proteins and oils can add an extra nutritional boost.

Soup s-t-r-e-t-c-h

Many families tell us their child has a very limited diet, but one food on the *List* is a homemade food such as "Grandma's soup". Specifically (Grandma's) soup. The great thing about when a child likes a homemade recipe is that chefs are human and tiny *changes* in recipe, cooking time and look *happen*. We encourage s-t-r-e-t-c-h-e-s from the base recipe. Can Grandma change the proportions a bit without adding a big new flavor or look? Can she add a little extra rice one time, or an extra carrot? Can it be some extra meat or a few differently shaped noodles? Can some extra blended food such as chicken or celery to be mixed into the sauce so it is a small flavor change, but not a big visual change? Some use the soup as a way to add a new vegetable. (The veggie may be added as a blend into the broth, or grated small or chopped, depending on the child). The idea is to subconsciously tell that little worried tongue that subtle changes in recipe are the norm.

Peanut butter s-t-r-e-t-c-h

If a child likes peanut butter, it is often one brand. Can you have him spread peanut butter on his own bread? He could spread a new brand of peanut butter on YOURS. As he demonstrates enjoyment around your peanut butter, can you begin to explore it with him? Which one do you think is yours? Which one do you think is mine? (If the worry over the new is big, of course, adjust). If he starts to worry YOU are going to make them try it, you might lose him. He can try in the way he can when he shows you he is curious and motivated to do so. You may need to have him spread your peanut butter a number of times before he acts ready to take the tiniest of finger tastes or coffee stirrer tastes.

Can you have two medicine cups of peanut butter on the table? (The peanut butter is out of the container so the differences are not obvious). Your child can help spread one peanut butter on the bread (it is the one he knows). We then give him a straw or coffee stirrer (small) to spread a tiny taste of the new one on the same bread (or, if necessary on your bread). He helps with the spreading. The s-t-r-e-t-c-h is from the original flavor of the peanut butter toward the slightly changed new one. But your child helped. If he demonstrates that he is comfortable with the slight new flavor variation, try it again another time to build on this experience. Perhaps more of the *new* one can be added little by little until he likes either peanut butter. You are modeling that tiny taste changes can be possible with diluted tries.

Remember that sometimes the s-t-r-e-t-c-h-i-n-g works better if there is there is a paired food that can dilute the taste, such as the jelly that is on the sandwich.

Sandwich s-t-r-e-t-c-h

Once your child has found a sandwich type he likes, can you help him s-t-r-e-t-c-h to new sandwiches? For example, if your child likes creamy chocolate nut butter sandwiches, can he help make them? Can he make big or little sandwiches? Can he get comfortable with *change happens* in sandwiches? Can he make sandwiches for others on a slightly different bread? As a rehearsal, can you start by helping HIM offer it to others? Can he make that sandwich tiny, like one inch by one inch, or smaller if necessary? Can he make himself a sandwich with one piece of regular bread and one piece of new bread? Can he learn to eat it on a variety of crackers, waffles, pancakes, crescents, English muffins?

Hamburger s-t-r-e-t-c-h

So many children like a particular fast food brand of hamburgers. We want to help them s-t-r-e-t-c-h from this fast food hamburger to frozen brands or homemade because this gives families many more options in meal planning. You can start out exposure to the new homemade burger by having your child in the kitchen when the burger is being made, and then working up to having your child help, as appropriate for developmental and cognitive level. She will need to get comfortable with the smell and look of these burgers before she will want to try them. Once your child enjoys the smell, hamburgers can be quite inviting.

One way to try a new hamburger is to dilute the experience with two pieces of bread or bun and the tiniest crumb size piece of hamburger. A Sandwich TRY. Or condiments can also dilute the flavor of new burger? Or the tiny burger sandwich can have part familiar hamburger and part new. The idea is to include the child and when he is ready *to want to try* we guide him through a way that dilutes the *ask* and increase the chances of success.

Some children will need to get used to *change happens* with the fast food burger first. Can it be served on the wrapper, or in the box, or out of the box or new kind of plate, a paper plate? Can his burger be cut in half, or can yours be cut in half nearby as a rehearsal? Can it be cut into smaller bite size pieces so he learns hamburgers can be small? Once hamburger change is comfortable, homemade ground meat burgers can include ground turkey, sausage, and pork (gradually).

Nugget s-t-r-e-t-c-h

It is common for anxious eaters to enjoy a breaded kind of chicken nugget, one kind, often one brand, one shape. Parents want to celebrate that there is at least one meat group on the *List*. It is understandable why children like these nuggets. They are in the brown group, ground up and easy to chew. Nugget texture is predictable. And then there is that oil, salt and breading yumminess. But it is so complicated when only one type will do. We consciously help children tiptoe toward change s-t-r-e-t-c-h-i-n-g to other shapes and other brands and eventually other ground meats.

In an effort to help with *change happens*, others around your child can start eating their nuggets in different shapes, dinosaurs, stars or alphabet shaped or even cut in halves. These are the rehearsals. Perhaps he can have his nuggets all the "correct" shape, but one piece offered on the platter is cut in half, or a new shape. Perhaps half on the serving platter are one shape and half are different. Your child is welcome to choose only *his* shape but is rehearsing the concept that these nuggets can come in different shapes.

We try to help children experience change around nugget eating. Perhaps it is a rehearsal where they see others cutting nuggets, dipping nuggets, and using forks and small pieces instead of always needing them whole as finger foods. Once they can eat them cut up, they can begin to see YOU eat a new kind of nugget with their nuggets and gradually help them eat some of the new ones, at their pace.

When children get interested in dipping their nuggets, the dipping sauces can become a way to dilute the new flavor *ask* a bit so it is not as intense. Once they like variety in their nuggets, the dipping sauce can also become a bridge in the same tiny transition to chicken patties, hamburgers, sausage patties or even fish sticks.

French fries to potato s-t-r-e-t-c-h

French fries are a favorite. And they are brown, and a predictable texture when eating them. But the fast food fries have a certain look and homemade fries just do not match up. Parents do not want to be stuck having to run out to the fast food restaurants for hot-off-the-grill French fries each noon.

We give rehearsals with *us* eating *their* fries in different ways, broken, two at a time, dipping, etc. These rehearsals demonstrate the possibilities without the pressure. Some children get used to these possibilities quickly and others take a while. Once your child can eat smaller bites of the fries, with and without forks, he has begun to learn *French fry change can happen*. Can we eat new kinds of fries near him, have him pass those fries around without the pressure to try, just for the rehearsal opportunity? Can he try other restaurant fries, frozen fries, or fries in tater tot form, sweet potato fries and even hash browns in different flavor and shapes? Once anxious children learn that hash browns or potato pancakes are safe, there are a multitude of recipes that include a variety of root veggies made into potato pancake forms. Most families find that it is worth their time and wallet to work on a French fry s-t-r-e-t-c-h at least toward a frozen variety that does not require a daily trip to a fast food restaurant.

Mashed potato s-t-r-e-t-c-h

There can be a s-t-r-e-t-c-h from mashed potatoes. The proportion of butter can change slightly, cheeses can be added carefully and increased. Your child can help mash the potatoes and the texture variation can change gradually. He can help you put the mashed potato in cupcake papers and be baked as potato *cupcake*. Other veggies can be added to change the nutritional composition, though this will change color and probably texture. Sweet potatoes, carrots, butternut squash, parsnips and turnips (even celery root) can make interesting changes. Can mashed potatoes be made into patties and fried as potato pancakes? Oh, the places you can go from there!

> Dear Parent,
> Can you think of a s-t-r-e-t-c-h that might be successful for your child to get from here to there?
> Do you need to narrow the s-t-r-e-t-c-h to brand to brand, flavor to
> flavor, or look to look so as not to try to big of an *ask*?
> Can your child participate in the change? (Stirring, cutting, breaking?)

Crumb S-t-r-e-t-c-h-e-s

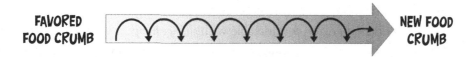

FAVORED FOOD CRUMB → **NEW FOOD CRUMB**

Crumbs can be a great tool in our tool box for helping anxious eaters get comfortable with change. We have discussed the many ways we can grade the sensory and motor *asks* of crumbs. Let us look at some common crumb s-t-r-e-t-c-h-e-s and see how then can bridge to new foods.

The crumb s-t-r-e-t-c-h

To teach children about crumbs we usually start with a dry crunchy food, often a cracker, cereal or chip, that they already enjoy. This is called the **crumb s-t-r-e-t-c-h**. In other words, we use a familiar food to teach the art of crumbing. Once they understand *crumbing*, we can find new dry foods to crumb and add new foods to their *List* of favored foods.

But what if your child is very worried if his favorite cracker gets broken? Chances are you will have to start from a less worrisome place and not go straight to crumbs. If your child is stressed about the whole idea of crumbs, as in broken things, we must adjust, back up and give more rehearsals. (See My Cracker is Broken chapter).

If broken foods do not upset your child you can explore crumbs together. Making them is the rehearsal for the smell and texture of the crumbs. You create them in a plastic bag with a rolling pin or smash them with a spoon.

In continued rehearsals, your child can hand them to you, a sibling, or therapist. In rehearsal, we can ask *others* to try them. We take picture of *others* trying them. We have him look at the pictures of *others* trying them. We may take turns and then ask *whose turn is next to put crumbs on their lips next?* As he becomes comfortable enough, he will want it to be *his* turn! (or not…if today is not the day, okay, not **YET**!)

We can all taste them on our lips. We can put crumbs in our palms and kiss them. We can look at our *crumb kisses* in a mirror. We can tiptoe toward licking and putting them on our tongues, inside our cheeks and in our mouths in varying amounts. As your child shows us he is ready and enjoys the sensory properties of the crumb we are using, we can increase our *ask*. We can transition to utensils by tasting them off fingers and spoons. We can dip other tools (forks, chopsticks, straws, toys) into the crumbs and try them that way. With all the different ways crumbs can be tried, your child gets many different tastes to *get* that crumbs are not threatening. And do not forget the melt-ability and the flavors and colors can all be graded!

After your child has gotten comfortable with *change happens* with a crumb of one of his own *List* foods, you might offer a new crumb food. How about a crispy rice cereal? The advantage here, is that it is not a snack food. It is a real live fortified food that could be celebrated if added to the *List*. We make crumbs of this new food, and together put them on the platter *near his crumbs*. We practice dipping our own fingers in the crumbs and tasting them as tiny amounts of the new crumb mingle with the familiar crumb until he shows a comfort with the new crumb. Some worried eaters have tried 6-8 new foods in the first crumb activity, and others will take a month or so to get comfortable with making their own food into crumbs.

Once your child shows us he is absolutely comfortable with the new crumb we want to establish it as a new *List* food. We give him a bowl of utensils and ask him which one he wants to try the crumbs with next or which one Dad should use? *Do you want to try the crumbs with this red straw or the blue one, the duck spoon or the construction spoon? The fork or the chopstick? The rim of the glass (crumbed like a margarita drink with crumbs…without the liquid).* By giving these choices, you let your child make the decisions and also dilute the worry with the novelty of the game. Though we do not want mealtime to turn into game time, we can use these activities as interesting ways to teach the activity of crumbing so children learn that these small tastes are okay!

Crumbs to new food groups

Once your child understands about crumbs, you can offer crumbs with different flavors and food groups. For the child who has wheat as a main staple in his diet, the addition of that rice cereal may be worth celebrating! For the child who has a very limited diet, the addition of freeze-dried fruit or vegetable crumbs may be a huge step in the right direction of diet diversity. If the fruits and veggies are way too big of a contrasting visual ask from the familiar brown, we can mix them with the browns and tiptoe toward the color. We do this to avoid surprise and dilute the worry.

Dry crumbs to moist

The dry crumbs are the starting place. But, we can then aim for more moist crumbs. Think breakfast bar or soft cookies. When children fully believe that crumbs are small, we can often make crumbs out of a breakfast bar as way to try a tiny taste. Tiny single crumbs can turn into a few crumbs and gradually a pinch of crumbs. Moist crumbs can be cornmeal muffins or even the edges of pancakes or waffles. Double toasting the waffle will make the edges a bit drier so they crumb more like dry crumbs on the edges and you can tiptoe toward the center moister crumbs.

We consider cheese crumbs to be more moist crumbs. And cheeses can be powdered to grated to strings and chunks. You can help your child eat the dry crumbs, such as a cracker, he likes and gradually help him mix together with cheeses to help him get to cheese as a *List* food. The dry crumbs become the bridge to cheese. Children are often successful when they have a dry cracker crumb they enjoy and together we add the tiniest it of grated cheese.

Crumb means small

We offer tiny tastes of new foods as *crumbs* of them. Try offering a taste of new foods off a coffee stirrer, perhaps a *mouse bite* of the new food. (We used to offer tiny tastes off toothpicks until a child tried to eat the toothpick! ☹ Coffee stirrers bend.) The tiny taste can be a *crumb* of cheese, or a *crumb* of scrambled egg. The crumb size for anxious eaters can offer less sensory challenges once the child understands crumbs starting with a familiar food. (We have even offered *crumbs* of hamburgers or *crumbs* of pickles).

Crumbs to the center filling

Sometimes favored foods are crunchy with a filling such as filled peanut butter crackers or cream filled chocolate cookies. We start with the crumbs of the wafer or cracker part. If your child already likes this item, he will be used to the overall flavor so when there is a hint of cream flavor on the cookie or a shadow of a peanut butter flavor on the cracker, it will usually be okay. There can be little bits of the filling mixed with the crumbs as you and your child make more crumbs. Gradually your child can be offered a tiny taste of actual peanut butter filling separately or actual peanut butter.

The crumbed cracker can serve as the bridge to the new peanut butter. We have helped children bridge to cream cheese from the chocolate cookie cream filling and bridge to peanut butter from peanut butter cream cookies in tiny s-t-r-e-t-c-h tastes. Starting with the cookie crumbs dilutes the try.

More crumb tastes!

The breading around favorite nuggets can be considered as *crumbs*. We have helped worried eaters to pick the bread off a breaded chicken nugget piece so they learn about breading, breading crumbs. We have played food detective as they explore the breading of other chicken patties and even popcorn shrimp. Crumbs and crumbing can become the routine for a strategy of trying that can help worried eaters be more confident because they know about crumbs even if they do not know about the new food.

Make *mouse bite* with teeth?

Can you bite a tiny mouse bite crumb, with your teeth? We support children as they transition from crumbs to using their teeth for *mouse bites*. With crumbs, we grownups can initially control the size (and, therefore, the texture). With *mouse bites* your child needs to organize his teeth, lips and tongue to bite off just the right size and NOT a size that would be too scary.

Before asking your child to try to bite a *mouse bite* with his teeth, it is helpful for him to become comfortable with crumbs of varying different sizes and scatter. This helps him gain confidence with uneven and slightly bigger pieces in his mouth before he bites off a little piece with their teeth. We do not want to ask him to try a *mouse bite* if the texture of the crumb scatter in his mouth is going to worry him. Children will usually do better with this if they are comfortable with crumbs first. Then we can help him bite through a bigger melt-able crumb, or small cereal. When we hold these for him or when he holds it himself, any bite through it will be a more comfortable size. He won't be able to accidentally get a half a cracker! We can then guide the size of his bite through a cracker by putting our thumbnail at the edge of the cracker only allowing his bite to be a small one. Gradually he will let us know his readiness for bigger.

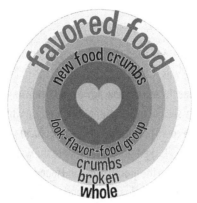

Circle of Sensitivity
Crumb S-t-r-e-t-c-h

A Sample Crumb Continuum

- ☐ Be okay with "broken"
- ☐ Crumb a familiar dry, crunchy food
- ☐ Taste and explore the familiar crumb
- ☐ Crumb a new food
- ☐ Taste and explore the familiar crumb and the new crumb
- ☐ Taste and explore the new crumb
- ☐ Practice with the new crumb in a variety of ways to build confidence
- ☐ Establish the crumb as a new food
- ☐ Crumb a variety of crackers, cereal, freeze dried fruits/veggies
- ☐ Introduce more moist crumbs (breakfast bar textures)
- ☐ Introduce muffin, pancake, waffle textures
- ☐ Crumbs to center filling
- ☐ Crumb cheeses with dry crumbs, then alone
- ☐ Explore breading crumbs
- ☐ Crumbs small to bigger and more scattered
- ☐ Bite a small crumb with teeth
- ☐ Crumb new foods

A Crumb Story

Lucy was worried about new foods. She liked to make crumbs and draw in crumbs. She loved to make crumb drawing happy faces! She was willing to try crumbs in the tiniest amounts and preferred them as powder. She learned to sprinkle the *crumb snow* powder on her favorite pretzels or crackers that used to be just for licking off salt. Now she got to lick crumbs off! It took a while to reduce her worry with the crumbs, but after that while, she could put crumbs on her finger and put some on her lips, then on her tongue then on the inside of her cheek, right side and left. Once she was completely comfortable with her familiar crumbs, we had an excursion to the grocery store and found all the different shapes crackers could come in. She already had a round one so we found oval, and square, rectangular, hexagonal and chicken shaped. We found big ones and little ones, brown ones and yellow ones and we brought them all home. She helped make crumbs of each and spent some time exploring them with grownups and without.

Then we also found a crispy rice cereal that sort of looked like a big crumb. We crushed that into crumbs and by now, crumbs were pretty comfortable. We broke the rice cereal into coarse crumbs until they could be crunched and not crumbed at all! Thinking of them as big crumbs helped.

And then we needed to teach her teeth to bite a crumb bite (or a mouse bite) of a cracker. We started by practicing a mouse bite of a piece of crispy rice cereal. This allowed her grownups to not worry that she would accidentally take too big of a bite. Then we practiced together with her own teeth taking mouse bites of the original cracker. We guided her bite size by putting our thumbnail up to the edge of the cracker so as she bit the cracker she could not get too much. Lucy then explored on her own. She nibbled one whole cracker over an hour. The second one took half an hour and the third, fourth and fifth, about ten minutes each. She practiced with crackers over the next few weeks and became confident with biting and chewing bigger bites.

From cracker crumbs, she got to cereals of all kinds and cheese crumbs with cheese of all kinds, breakfast bars and more. Her parents describe crumbs as the *game changer* toward solids! They were just the bridge she needed.

Juice S-t-r-e-t-c-h-e-s

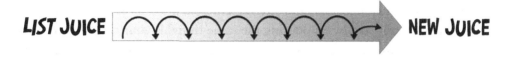

LIST JUICE → NEW JUICE

A juice s-t-r-e-t-c-h is a careful transition from a current familiar juice to a new one. This can teach your child to be comfortable with change and work toward new food and nutrient combinations. For some children it is the foundation of change needed for a later smoothie s-t-r-e-t-c-h.

Out of the box

If your child only likes her juice from the original packaging box she will need help to become comfortable with juice *out of the box* first (see that chapter). It is so hard to change the juice offer from that particular box without creating a sensory surprise. I have sneakily tried to insert a new juice flavor into that box and was dismayed at the sensory surprise I inadvertently created!

Lids

Once your child can drink juice from a cup, you can also help her with straws and lids. Both have the advantage of diluting the strength of the smell. The lids keep her nose out of the open cup that collects lots of the smell! And you will like the spill-proof benefits of the lid! Check out the stretchy lid covers that you can keep handy when on the go at restaurants and in the car too. These lids all have straws as the way to drink the liquid through the lid.

Some children can use a straw without a lid. It is still farther from the drink so her nose is farther from the smell and her eyes are farther from the visual change. For children needing this extra step of support, we can help them get used to straws and lids in gradual achievable steps as a part of their smoothie continuum of experiences.

Juice variation

Some children are used to the same brand and flavor of juice because parents buy and offer that particular brand. Consider does your child NEED that brand? Some families say *"No, I think she just drinks it because it is what we buy."* If that is the case changing the juice, buying different brands and offering different juices so as not to enablers of rigidity inadvertently by always offering the same thing. If your child **expects** that juice can change and cups can change, it helps them be better with knowing *change happens.*

Ice cube melt-able

We use the idea of ice cube melt-ables in many different new drink trying situations. An ice cube melt-able is adding an ice cube to a familiar drink to change the flavor, smell, color or temperature. The change is made in a continuum of concentration changes that occur naturally with the melting of the ice cube while the child is drinking the drink. For some children we can add the new juice ice cube into a familiar juice. The gradual flavor or color change is slow enough from the familiar starting place that many children are fine with it! And there are other worried eaters for whom the placement of even a plain ice cube is too big of a change. Those children will need more steps in their continuum toward change.

They may need to get used to seeing ice cubes in others' drinks or even regularly help put ice cubes in other's drinks. They may need to have the first ice cube be one of the same familiar juice in their drink so when the ice cube melts, there is no flavor or color change. Once ice cubes of the familiar juice are comfortable, some children may need ice cubes made partially with a new juice and partially with the familiar juice so the melting ice cube changes the flavor slightly, but not much. For these worried drinkers, we would probably not pick a juice that is also a concentrated color change, thereby making change in both look and flavor at the same time. So, we pick the juice of a similar color to the familiar juice. Gradually the full-strength ice cubes of the new juice are used and then gradually more than one ice cube can be added to again increase the flavor of color concentration. As your child gets comfortable with ice cubes melting new flavor into the juice, you can offer two ice cubes, one of each new flavor or three ice cubes, two of one flavor and one of the other. There is no particular *recipe* here, but a strategy that goes slowly at each child's pace and that watches his response. It also is helping your child understand *change happens* and the juice will have slight variations and those will be fine. Once she is comfortable with change, we encourage continuing to change up the brands cups or variety so *change* (continues to) *happen*.

Include your child

As we have discussed throughout this book, include your child. If she knows what is about to happen with the rehearsal, there will be less of a sensory surprise. She can anticipate the change rather than fight against it. Can she pick out an ice cube shape to put in her own drink with fingers, spoons or tongs? Can she pick out the ice cube color or number of ice cubes?

Juice to nectars

Once your child is comfortable with juice flavor change, the ice cubes can be made out of juice nectars which tend toward a bit thicker and creamier. These add some flavor change and tiptoe toward texture.

Dip and stir technique

Another way to create juice flavor change is with the stir technique. Take turns stirring the drink with your child. She stirs hers and we stir ours. You can then dip your stirrer or straw in another cup of the same juice then put it in our drinks and stir. Here your child is learning to *dip and stir* and there will be no flavor change. Gradually you can teach her to dip into puree and stir. You can have a discussion with her. "Hmmm, does it taste the same? Does your find tongue a new taste?" This becomes a detective game to determine how many tastes are needed for it to taste differently. Your child can bravely stir in tastes and let you know if the tastes are fine. Many children move from being comfortable s-t-r-e-t-c-h-i-n-g from juice to fruit puree thickened juices this way. The sipping of the tastes can be done with straws to keep the nose a little farther from the smell.

Dropper technique

We can do essentially the same activity with a dropper. Your child can squeeze drops from the dropper to gradually change the flavor or color or texture. The counting of the drops and the stirring can be a way to dilute the worry. She can start with water or with the starting juice and move toward new juices, nectars or purees. The color contrast can be none at first and tiptoe toward color change. We tend to tiptoe from yellows and oranges toward reds and purple but keep the greens until way later. However, we involve each child in the decision making and some children surprise us!

And more

There are great gadgets that can make mealtime fun for the whole family. There are many creative ice cube shapes and very cute popsicle makers. Popsicle makers come in lots of shapes that can coincide with your child's interests. There are slushy makers where the child can make crushed ice and spritz a new favored juice on the ice. There are appliances that add carbonation to favorite drinks. These can all be ways for your child to interact with drinks, and have rehearsals for s-t-r-e-t-c-h-e-s in drink textures, flavors and looks.

Water S-t-r-e-t-c-h-e-s

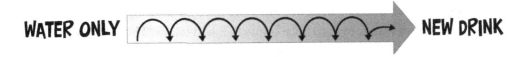

WATER ONLY ➤ **NEW DRINK**

Some children want their water in the *same* bottle. No change. We can help them s-t-r-e-t-c-h to more flexibility in their water drinking to give them and their family more options for offering much needed water. Water flexibility can be the beginning of s-t-r-e-t-c-h-e-s toward new liquids.

Different cups and straws

If your child needs help learning that water can come in different containers, you can drink water next to her with *your* cups or *your* water bottles or *your* straws. Being near you will be the rehearsal for change. Perhaps she can help you pour your drinks into these cups or bottles or choose a straw for you to use?

Perhaps some of her water is offered in *her container* with some of the water poured in front of her into a new cup. The water that has been poured into the new cup can be ignored (or not). You can gradually help your child get used to **her** water being in a new container. (See My Juice Box Must Be Green chapter). Or when a new location, such as outdoors in the play house or at a picnic table, can your child be offered water from a different cup when her special container just does not happen to be around? Thirst and the new environment may lead to the choice of trying the new water container. If not, at least you tried.

Can you and your child pour water into little shot glass sized cups, paper cups of different sizes or plastic cups of different designs? Once she is comfortable with her water from different cups and straws, she is getting the idea that *change happens* around water.

Change the color

You can change the **color** of the water in separate tiptoe steps if your child cannot handle flavor changes first. Use a dropper to drip in various concentrations of food coloring, starting with the most diluted color. Your child can count the drops and do the stirring and play detective to figure out if the taste is the same. (It will be ☺.) The color changes can increase toward juice colors that will follow. The color changes but the flavor is the same minimizing, the sensory challenge.

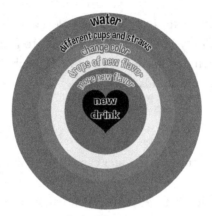

Circle of Sensitivity
Water S-t-r-e-t-c-h

Dip and stir flavor then more flavor

As with other s-t-r-e-t-c-h-e-s we teach children to *dip and stir*. Dipping a straw or spoon or dropper in another colored drink or another flavored drink and then stirring is a nice way to get used to *dip and stir* without a big flavor or color change. Then, can you dip and stir with a dropper, straw, or spoon with a tiny amount of a juice or baby food puree in yours first (with her help) and then do that to hers? Make the amount tiny so the flavor or color change is not big. Will she still drink? And continue dropping drips, then stirring, then drinking so the change of color and flavor gradually changes. If the flavor change and color change are too much to get used to at first, consider going back to putting food color drops in at first to only change the color so she only has to get used to color change and not flavor and color.

You and your child can use droppers to count drops of juice into the water, changing the flavor ever so slightly. This is a rehearsal and can dilute worry. (There are colorful and silly child play droppers on the market to change up this game. The flavor gradually permeates the water and a juice flavor is born! From here, you can look at the juice s-t-r-e-t-c-h toward full strength juices and then other juice flavors.

These water changes can help your child learn *change happen*s. She can learn that drinks come in different colors and that flavors can change. We can use enjoyment of water as a bridge to introduce worried eaters to other foods, such as drinking water out of a carved-out apple or pear or cucumber, or a bell pepper. The goal from the child's perspective is the water drinking, but the child is also getting familiar with a fruit or vegetable along the way.

Dear Parent,

How can you help your child s-t-r-e-t-c-h from water to a different drink?
(Remember to try and then adjust along the way, if necessary)

Smoothie S-t-r-e-t-c-h-e-s

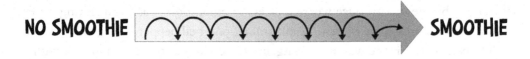

NO SMOOTHIE ➜ **SMOOTHIE**

Imagine a s-t-r-e-t-c-h from a favored liquid to a smoothie made of fruits and veggies or maybe with yogurt added? Then imagine you and your child could actually order a smoothie at a smoothie stand or smoothie restaurant? Many children achieve this goal. It has a continuum of possibilities. In our continuum of worry, some children need a considerable amount of time on the front end of this continuum and then move quite slowly from there. Others take some time at the front end to learn the routine and ritual of *smoothies,* learn to drink these blender-created drinks, but then make lots of change and allow lots of variation later. They need to build up trust and enthusiasm for smoothie making.

Smoothie s-t-r-e-t-c-h-e-s can a part of many children's new food trying, or diet expansion support. Smoothies can be your key to more fruits and veggies and that is a celebration in some many diets.

Smoothies happen

In all the smoothie s-t-r-e-t-c-h-e-s, we will discuss the progress and the smallness of the steps depends on each child. We do not go too fast to push right into their worry. And we, however, should not sit on one goal for months and months with no progress. We must break down the goal into tiny enough steps for the child to experience progress and for each parent to be able to find celebration.

We always want to rehearse, to involve your child in the process of making food whenever it is possible. Actually, if it is not possible, the activity may be too big an *ask.* Often grownups start out leading the whole activity and, once the child is comfortable with the process, he can be included more and more, closer to the smells and textures of smoothie making. In order NOT to push into the worry, parents could start a family routine where *smoothies happen.* Worried eaters like routines. They like to know what is coming next. They like to know the beginning and end. Where does it happen? When does it happen? When will this smoothie activity end? It helps if they see you get out the ingredients, make *your* smoothie, drink *your* smoothie and clean up. They know what is coming next and learn the routine, even if they are not **YET** ready to participate in the smoothie tasting.

In all the steps along the way to making smoothies, grownups can demonstrate and help their child, take on a more active role. Intersperse the activity with choices and turn taking to let your child rehearse the activity and control the pace. And as with juice s-t-r-e-t-c-h-e-s, a lid may help reduce the smell *ask* when children are trying a new drink.

Start with peace

We have discussed the need for mealtime peace. In this case we want peace with smoothie making. If starting at peace means your child just watches from a distance, great, then *that* is the starting place. If your child can help but do no tasting or trying, then *that* is their starting place. If your child is willing to interact with the activity and has been learning new food trying, you can offer him to help put the food in the blender, smell the ingredients or kiss, lick or finger taste, or tongue taste them. Be careful not to start smoothie making with lots of *trying* demands for a child who is worried. He may not even want to make smoothies with you the next time. Remember, you are first teaching that smoothies can be made and invite them to participate. Rehearse! Rehearse! Rehearse! The tasting part can come later.

Ingredients

Smoothies can be a relatively easy way to drink more fruits and vegetables. No chewing required! They can be a predictable texture. The ingredients can be a full rainbow of nutrients and rainbow colors. But you can start with familiar colors. If your child likes an applesauce colored puree, you may need to pick first new fruits to add that are quieter colors, similar to applesauce, such as pears, rather than red or blue berries. You will probably need to wait until farther along the continuum to try those green smoothies. But, as we have said throughout, each child is different. You will know!

Parents add powdered milk, instant breakfast drink powder, chia seeds, and nut butters. These smoothies can be as varied for children as they are for adults, and once smoothies are completely comfortable, offer them regularly and include your child and his creativity in the making of them. For children who start out with no fruits or vegetables in their *List* diet, smoothies are a terrific celebration. But keep them as a part of the family diet so they do not inadvertently get eliminated by being out of the routine.

Some smoothies are a s-t-r-e-t-c-h from juices and move in the direction of varied fruit purees. Some help children move toward yogurt based creamy smoothies with fruits to vary the flavor and color. Some smoothies help reduce dairy by gradually stretching from dairy yogurt toward soy or coconut yogurt. Others can support power packing calories with nut butters and tofu added. You (and your dietitian) will have fun thinking creatively with options to try.

Once a child is fully onboard with flavor variations in fruit smoothies, it is a natural transition to add some veggies. Cucumbers are a nice addition to a fruit smoothie. The flavor blends in well. Avocados blend beautifully with yogurt, orange juice, banana, and strawberry. The drink hardly has a flavor change if half an avocado is used but is a bit creamier. (You may need to start with just a small piece of avocado, though, to tiptoe into that taste change). Carrot juice is sweet and can be part of the base juice. And greens. They are all the rage in healthful smoothies, but for some children the color contrast with familiar smoothies is too much. Many green smoothies taste like a variation on a regular fruit smoothie in their sweetness. See what your child thinks about the gradual change in greenness.

Start with a familiar, non-essential drink

Each child drinks *something*. If the only drink he likes is milk, it could be challenging to start a smoothie s-t-r-e-t-c-h there if your child will not allow change in his milk. (But do know that some children will be fine with a smoothie s-t-r-e-t-c-h from milk. I bet you can already predict your child's response.) We would need to try smoothies for them from a different path, or from their interest in yogurt or pouches. But, if your child drinks several drinks we like to pick the one that is least essential as the smoothie base. If he likes milk, and apple juice, lemonade, and a light-colored soda, we might start with the soda. Or lemonade. Sometimes we start with water.

A water or juice s-t-r-e-t-c-h

If you decide to start this s-t-r-e-t-c-h from water, see the guidelines in the Water S-t-r-e-t-c-h chapter. If you start from a familiar juice, the Juice S-t-r-e-t-c-h chapter can be a guideline. As you move through the juice s-t-r-e-t-c-h-e-s, the nectar s-t-r-e-t-c-h, you can use the *dip and stir technique* to add taste upon taste of a pouch puree or baby food puree to gradually thicken the juice to thin puree thickness.

Puree to smoothie s-t-r-e-t-c-h

If your child likes a commercial baby food, or a fruit pouch, you can use that as the starting point. We help him learn to drink that puree from a cup as a smoothie foundation. Can your child get used to eating the pouch puree or baby food puree off a straw? We use the straw as a spoon. In the case of the pouch, there are actual straw tips that are designed to be screwed onto the opening. Your child can initially get used to that puree that way. You can also just put a regular straw into the opening of the pouch. If the straw fits snuggly, you can squeeze some puree up the straw to get it started or suck the puree up to the tip to prime it for the child. OR, if the straw is not a snug fit you can offer it to your child for them to drink the puree that way. (If your child does not drink from a straw, he will need to start by learning straw drinking separately.)

If you are using baby food puree, you can use a straw as a spoon. We like to cut short straws in half and dip the straw in the puree. Put your fingertip over the end to trap the puree in the straw. Offer that to your child, as a "spoon", pausing at his lips to give him time to suck the puree out of the straw. As he gets used to sucking the puree out of the straw, parents can consider sucking the puree into the straw to prime it or offering it while tipping the angle downward so he has to actively suck up the straw more against some gravity. Then you can dip the tip in the puree and put the other end *in the puree* so your child sucks the puree from the straw. Once he has learned to drink these fruit purees from a straw, he can practice with many different straw lengths and diameters to establish the skill.

Straw in yogurt

For children who already like a smooth yogurt from a cup container or a long yogurt pouch, we can teach them to drink those from a straw and use those as a foundation for smoothies.

Dip and stir s-t-r-e-t-c-h

As with other liquid s-t-r-e-t-c-h-e-s, we can take turns with the child dipping and stirring in differently flavored yogurt, or different baby food flavors with straws or droppers to vary the smoothie flavor or color. We can also use commercially available empty pouches to fill with puree combinations to help children tiptoe toward to new flavors while on the go at the park and on walks. The novelty of the situation often allows an anxious eater to allow some tiny change. You know your child. If that kind of change is too much and will be a sensory surprise…then do not do it that way!

Blender continuum

We want to help worried eaters be confident when participating in smoothie making. This is a **lifelong skill** and one that will allow for great nutritional variation in a drink. The first smoothie we might try would be a smoothie made out of one of the child's already favorite juices or purees (pouch or yogurt). He, then, is learning the smoothie process without a change in flavor or color. He is exposed to the blender, the pouring, and the noise. If he can be the button pusher, great. If the noise is a problem, he can wear headphones, or cover his ears, or stand farther from the noise until he can gradually get close to the blender. After the blended drink is finished, he can help pour the smoothie into cute little tasting cups. These can be paper cups, little disposable shot glass cups or whatever little tasting cups you and they designate. The routine is to pour tastes for everyone, pass them out to everyone and then do *cheers and drink*. *Cheers and drink* becomes the mantra. Just to be clear, **this is not a demand. It is a routine**. If the child happily does *cheers and drink*, great! If he is worried about the tasting part, we follow the Re-define TRY IT strategies with smells, or finger tastes on lips and tongues. Or our initial offers of tastes are tiny *mouse tastes* off coffee stirrers to emphasize smallness.

After your child is comfortable with blenders and with the routine of smoothie making, we can use that familiar base recipe (yogurt or puree) as a starting point. Can he pour the puree? Can he slice a banana and put one slice in, or put a dollup of another yogurt or fruit puree in? A tiny taste change? Run the blender and then try *cheers and drink*. Did your child notice the change? I will often ask a child if his tongue can **find the new flavor**? We ask him if we should add more flavor? One taste more or two, three or five? Some children who are on the less worried side of smoothies will happily add several more tastes and other will stop at the first flavor change. Fine. Do not push into worry. That is the starting point for next time.

Gradually more fruit is added or more puree. Smoothies will change flavor and colors until the idea of smoothies becomes so comfortable that we want to go out and order smoothies from a smoothie restaurant.

Our dietitian friends love to use a smoothie s-t-r-e-t-c-h to help wean a child from a supplementation formula or juice towards a homemade smoothie. Parents could start from the commercial supplement and tiptoe toward adding tiny amounts of other ingredients and gradually reducing the formula volume. This can be a great transition, though, we need to be careful if the specific formula is the ONLY thing the child is taking for nutrition. Sometimes, as we have said before, when we mess with a very anxious eater, a change can cause them to stop eating that food. Caution, tiptoe! Ask your child's dietitian for help.

Change up the recipe

I once worked with a child who was learning smoothies. His mother came to clinic and told me her child now liked a homemade smoothie. She was thrilled that he now liked a smoothie made with exactly half a banana, three strawberries and one container of vanilla yogurt. That was great, it was new. Of course, it is a celebration! However, one of the goals of smoothie making is that recipes can change to help the child fully embrace that *change happens.* This can occur naturally in homemade recipes. So, my question to that parent might be, *can you change up the recipe a bit?* What about ¾ of a banana or pick a really small or really big banana so the banana flavor from half a banana in the final smoothie has banana taste variation. OR can the strawberries be four instead of three? I have said to children, *these strawberries are small, shall we put in four?* We want the child's tastes buds to experience slight flavor changes so they get used to the variation. When children are used to variation, the little changes do not seem like such a neon sign warning of worry.

And, of course, one of the goals of smoothie making is create enjoyment of a lifelong food option. Can you eventually go to a smoothie shop so you and your child can order a smoothie from there? Some families like to go and have everyone order their own different smoothies and then do a family smoothie taste test. (To expand new food trying and possibly find a new one for your worried eater to enjoy!)

> Dear Parents,
>
> Can smoothies be added to your family routine?

Smoothies making

Smoothie making has been a constant source of frustration for me! I know logically that smoothies could be a wonderful solution for Teddy, but he drinks so little of them that I struggle to put in the effort on a consistent basis. It helped to talk with Marsha about fitting smoothies into our life. She asked us to consider a time of day that would work for trying smoothies. What would work for US? Could we consider a smoothie assembly line game on the weekend or think about making them as an after-school activity versus fitting them into our busy mornings. Could one of Teddy's babysitters routinely make smoothies with him? Or, what about big brother? What helped was that she talked with me about our time availability, so we could decide together how this could possibly work at our house. Together we brainstormed not just the "why", but also the who, the where and the when so I could envision actually making the smoothies on a much more regular basis.

In our conversations about smoothies, it also helped to talk about reducing waste. It is sometimes really hard to try new things if I KNOW my son just won't try them or won't eat more than a "mouse bite." She reminded us that leftovers could be made into popsicles or ice cubes for later trying activities or tasty snacks. I now use zipper plastic bags or silicone baby food containers for leftover smoothies. Those leftovers can easily be added to a basic smoothie recipe to increase fruit variety, or even used as ice cubes in a cup of juice. Eliminating the waste helps me be much more willing to experiment. ~ Laura Wesp

Chester Story

Chester was eighteen and going away to college. He had been a lifelong anxious eater. His family has completely accepted him for who he was and never forced him to eat food that worried him. They exposed him to lots of foods but he had his specific favorites. He ate raw carrots as his only vegetable. He liked some juices. Mom was worried as he went off to college that his nutrition might not be the best and that she was not there to hover over it.

Our dietitian and I met with him and discussed his diet. She did a nutrition review and helped him see he had some deficiencies in his diet. We asked him what we would like to do about the diet concern since he was going off on his own to college. He was a very bright young man and we needed to help him take charge of his own diet. She and he decided that he could add a multivitamin which he used to eat and then had since dropped. In addition, he was willing to expand his smoothie intake to add a comfortable regular source of fruits and vegetables. Coincidentally he had recently been offered a particular smoothie he did like so that became his starting point. Needless to say, his parents got him a special blender and sent it off to college with him. Smoothies would be a lifelong skill that was worth the effort.

Vitamin/Medicine S-t-re-t-c-h-e-s

If your child's pediatrician or dietitian recommends a vitamin or medication into your child's day, how will you do that? Let's look at some strategies that might help.

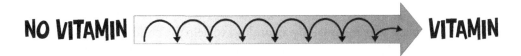

NO VITAMIN ⟶ VITAMIN

Liquid vitamins

Liquid vitamins can have a strong smell that scares away some children. You can try adding the tiniest amount of the liquid vitamin in a drink and gradually increase that amount as your child is able. Remember that lidding the cup and providing a straw can help mask the bigger smell. Chilling the drink with ice sometimes reduces the smell some. (Try it yourself!) Having your child help put in the drops of vitamin or stir it in may help (but also may signal worry too soon.) Consider diluting the vitamin flavor with a stronger background flavor such as a concentrated chocolate milk. Some families say their child will take the liquid vitamin if it is offered with a combination of carbonation and a stronger tasting juice (maybe cranberry, or blueberry, or pomegranate)? You may have to try a few options.

Pills and chewables

Pills are challenging for many children. If your child already knows pills, then adding a vitamin or a halved vitamin to their routine may not be a tall challenge. But, if swallow-able pills are already a challenge, this is not your starting point. Perhaps the pill can be changed in form. We always ask the pharmacist if the particular vitamin or medication will still be effective if we change the properties in any way. First of all, does this medicine come in a different form? And secondly, can we change its current form?

Would crushing the vitamin help? Medicine crumbs can be a less worrisome way to take them. Though, crushed pills can have a strong flavor that is harder to mask. Some children take their crushed pills or sprinkle meds mixed with the creamy white filling of a chocolate sandwich cookie or paired with an enjoyable stronger food flavor such as berry applesauce or yogurt. Crumbs are a bit like sprinkles and some medicines come in sprinkle form. To further rehearse for sprinkle meds, we have practiced with a variety cupcake sprinkles and colored sugars and gradually mixed the medication sprinkles in.

Chewable vitamins can work. There are the gummy textured vitamins and the harder, chewable vitamins. If the child already likes gummy candy, you may well be able to tiptoe toward the gummy vitamin by offering the tiniest of gummy *mouse bites* with the tiniest of gummy candy *mouse bites* to help the child get used to the new gummy vitamin. Remember to avoid sensory surprises by including the child in the cutting of the *mouse bites*, if it is safe to do so.

If the child does not already like the gummy texture, you may have better luck with the standard chewable form of vitamin. This can be broken into smaller pieces for chewing and the pieces can gradually be enlarged as the child is comfortable. But many children need their first vitamins in a crumb stretch sequence, *the vitamin crumb stretch*.

Vitamin crumb s-t-r-e-t-c-h

Think of the chewable vitamin as a crumb possibility. In a vitamin crumb s-t-r-e-t-c-h, we first help your child get used to crumbing in all the ways we have already described: rehearsing crumb making, making crumbs out of favorite foods, feeding crumbs to others. Once your child is comfortable with the routine of *crumbing*, then you and he can make crumbs out of a familiar food and then make crumbs out of the vitamin and gradually mingle them is crumb trying. Consider a colorful fruity cereal as the **s-t-r-e-t-c-h crumb** because of the similarity to the colors and the fruity smells and tastes. Many children take their first vitamins in crumb form with the crumbs gradually getting bigger and more uneven until they are fully comfortable with chewing the vitamin.

Dropper medications

And then there is the medication method. Some families approach the vitamin as a medicine that MUST be taken and they use their *medication offering method* with vitamins. They may offer the vitamin from a dropper and say, *This is a vitamin. The doctor says you need to take it. It will help you. We will put it here in your cheek (rehearsal) and I will count 1-2-3 and then it will be in your mouth. After you swallow it, you can have a drink of (a favorite liquid) to wash it down and then we will* (take a walk, or play a game, or do something distracting.) To dilute the flavor or texture, the dropper liquid can be mixed with a strong liquid such as chocolate milk, nectars, or juices such as pomegranate, cranberry, or orange (if the pharmacists agrees that mixing the medication is an option). OR the crushed vitamin can be offered with a smooth food, such as applesauce, chocolate pudding, peanut butter. Right after your child takes the vitamin, a friendly favorite food or drink is offered to wash it down to mask the residual taste and you are lovingly supportive about, *yes, it is hard*, but it is over quickly and medication is required. *Sorry.* This may work, depending on your child's cognitive and worry level.

Constipation meds

Similar options can be tried when the issue is a constipation medication that needs to be added to liquid. Offer small amounts at first and tiptoe toward full strength. If you offer the medication flavor and texture too quickly and your child gags, it is possible that he will associate a gag with each medication offer and the cycle will continue. Please avoid this by carefully watching your child's cues and grading your *sensory ask*.

Dear Parent,

Do you have a vitamin or medication plan that works for you?

This Cracker is Broken!

Many of you know a child who will only eat his chips or crackers if they are not broken. And many of you are understandably frustrated by this. *These are your crackers! They are the same crackers! They are fine! Broken is fine! Just eat them!* This goes back to the idea that children who have a hard time with change have their own personal logic. It is not logical, at least from our perspective, to only eat one shape of cracker. We know a cracker is a cracker. We know a broken cracker is still a cracker. But can you imagine that your very worried eater may not know that? ☺

What if your child only knows *cracker are supposed to be whole*? Then broken crackers are what? Not crackers, but something else? We know that many children who are anxious eaters become extremely vigilant about looking for change in their food. If the food is not the right look, the right smell, or taste or texture it is not their food. Not only is a cracker not *their* cracker if it is broken, but an apple may not be an apple if it is green (and not red) and a smoothie may not be a smoothie if it is chocolate (and not vanilla) or water is not their water if it is in a different cup!

We can fight them. We can use more and more words to tell them that *this is their food*, that it just looks different. You have tried that, right? For many parents that conversation did not make a difference to their worried eaters. If they do not feel that a cracker is a cracker if it is broken, we are probably not going to change their mind by just telling them and re-telling them. We just reinforce the idea that we grownups cannot be trusted, or they should **not** listen to us!

Kind Dad gave us another example when he shared his story with the feeding support group. He suggested this to us. Imagine that someone gave you a piece of carpet and a glass of kerosene for lunch. YOU KNOW that is NOT lunch. How do you know? What makes you so sure? You are very, very clear that this is not food and you are absolutely not going to eat them. What if your well-meaning parents kept repeating, *it is lunch, eat it now; why aren't you eating it*? Would that make you eat it? No? You just KNOW carpet and kerosene are NOT foods you are supposed to eat. It is personal. We cannot MAKE children like new foods.

Now imagine a child who cannot eat broken crackers. Instead of pushing right into his worry, we can believe him and wonder what do we have to do to help him want to eat this cracker, which we KNOW he likes? We want to help him know that other people eat broken crackers and that he can eat broken crackers. *It will be okay*. It must be debilitating if your crackers cannot even be broken! We want to give children the freedom and flexibility to eat a broken cracker, comfortably and without worry!

Rehearse broken crackers

We do this by *rehearsing* broken crackers with them. We eat their favorite crackers *with* them. We are going to rehearse *broken*. We start by having them serve their crackers to us and themselves. They have theirs. We have ours in front of us. Theirs are theirs. Ours are ours. Ours are in front of us. We do not mess with *theirs*. (When asking a worried eater to make a change, it does help to make change first a bit farther from their foods, so they do not get too worried and then STOP that food).

To start we break *ours* only and eat them in view of the child. We could hand one to another family member. One for them, and one for us. We could break one of *ours* and ask the worried eater to pass that to another person when he is ready. If he becomes worried, we assure him that we are not *making him* eat the broken one, but that they are just passing it on. We do this in a comfortable, not demanding way until he is very comfortable handling the broken crackers. We are rehearsing that *broken may happen*.

We can break them once, or twice. We can put a broken one nonchalantly on his plate observing his reaction. (Remember we offer and then adjust our *ask* depending on their response). If he is comfortable we continue. If he is worried, we can back off to the comfortable place. Maybe that comfortable place is that we sit farther away and break our crackers and eat them without involving him yet. Maybe we help him take the worrisome broken one off his plate to hand it off to someone else.

Gradually we continue this game with quarters, eighths, and so on, until the pieces are small and crumb-like.

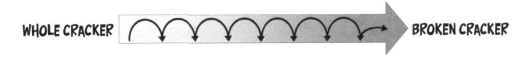

In my experience, a gradual exposure like this helps many children learn, *Oh, MY FOOD, can be small and it is still MY FOOD*. Children learn that broken crackers can be eaten, that they can be on the child's plate, and often the child will pick them up and eat them when distracted and eventually with full attention. Teaching that crackers can be eaten if broken is a requirement, a bridge, for many children learning that change can happen at mealtimes and they can be okay. It may need to be a prerequisite for making crumbs!

This is a summary of the ideas but is **not a checklist** that works for every child. It just shows you a general sequence that includes the importance of not breaking the child's crackers. We break ours to start farther from their worry. And it shows the sequence of demonstrating near the child until he demonstrates he *gets* that his crackers can be broken and he can still eat them. I like to dilute the experience by having conversations about anything NOT CRACKER. NO pressure.

A Sample Broken Cracker Continuum

☐ Child serves non-broken favorite crackers to himself and grownup
☐ Both grownup and child eat the crackers in front of them.
☐ Grownup breaks a cracker in half and eats it in view of the child. Repeats.
☐ Grownup breaks several crackers on her plate. Eats them.
☐ Grownup offers broken cracker to the child to pass on to someone else.
☐ Grownup puts a broken cracker on child's plate. (NO pressure to eat it. It is just there.)
☐ Grown up keeps eating broken crackers and repeats these interactions
☐ Grownup hands child a broken cracker and so on until the child seems comfortable with broken.
☐ Child eats a broken cracker.
☐ Have some more. Enjoy!

My Juice Box Must be Green

When children worry about change, sometimes they determine that a food is safe for them ONLY when very particular variables are present. *My water needs to be in a certain straw cup, or my apples must be red and sliced a certain way and my waffles must be round.* Their personal logic escapes us, but it is absolutely real to them. Parents find themselves saying, but it is just the *same* waffle, it is just *square!* Or it is the *same* water, just a different container! For children very worried about change, the presentation can become part of the food or their *perception* of the food. They are unable to eat that new food that we presented differently. It is **NOT** *their* food. When the presentation needs to be highly specific, it can make it hard for the caring adults around the child to figure out HOW to help them eat that food in any other way.

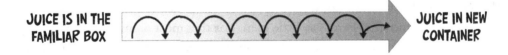

JUICE IS IN THE FAMILIAR BOX → **JUICE IN NEW CONTAINER**

Green juice box

Many of us know children who like juice (but it MUST be a certain brand of apple juice in the certain green box and the child MUST open the straw and put it in himself). Where can you go from here? We know if we change the box, the child might reject the juice altogether, and when diets are limited, no one want the child to eliminate a food from his *List*.

Remember we are offering change slowly in a careful and systematically desensitized way. Here are some ideas that have helped some children. Some children will happily transition to another container if they can use the same straw. It becomes the ridge to new. Great, if it works.

But others are more worried. Another option might be to sit near your child and have your own juice box. YOU open YOUR juice box and squeeze some of the juice into a cup, then drink YOUR juice from that cup. This is a rehearsal. You are showing your child, *"Here, sweetie, see the juice comes out of the box? Then I can drink it."* You can do this several times in a row, gradually putting more juice in your cup from your juice box. Rehearsals.

We will ask parents, *would your child let you pour some of his juice in a cup and then still drink HIS juice?*

If the answer is *no*, maybe the child needs more time watching you or helping YOU take juice out or YOUR box in front of them. More rehearsals.

If the answer is *yes*, can you (or your child) squeeze the juice into a cup so he is not stuck on *needing* the juice in *that* box. It is harder to make change from *that* box. If he is, in fact, comfortable with different presentations please make the presentations different regularly so he continues to believe and be comfortable with *change happens*.

If the answer is *"I am not sure"* or *"maybe"*, then we can tiptoe into offering change. (Remember you have YOURS and the child has HIS? Rehearsals still help.) On the first day or the first offer, could we help your child squeeze a little from the box into a cup? And could he still drink the rest from the box? This can happen a number of times until your child is fully comfortable with the idea of squeezing some juice from the box. Gradually, you both squeeze more and more from the box offering him the rest of the box to drink. But, the volume in his box becomes smaller as more juice is poured into his cup. Eventually there is so little in his box that most of his juice is in his cup. Then you model drinking your cupful and offer him his cup. You are hoping that the repetitive rehearsals have helped him understand that the juice in the cup is actually his juice. They have seen that *change happens* without pressure, multiple times. Once he will comfortably drink the juice from the cup, give them lots of practice and alternate cups if you can, so they can build confidence. A child who is a confident drinker can drink their green juice box juice out of a red cup, a blue cup, or a straw cup.

Yogurt container

The same sequence can be offered for the child who MUST have the yogurt from a particular container.

Consider, *would your child <u>let you take a scoopful</u> of yogurt from his container and put it in a nearby bowl and then still eat his yogurt from his container?*

If the answer is *no*, maybe your child needs more time watching you or helping YOU take a scoop of yogurt out of YOUR container into a bowl in front of them. More rehearsals.

If the answer is *yes*, then can you ask him, *can you (or your child) scoop a spoonful of yogurt from the container into a bowl before eating the container contents?* It is harder to make any change from *that* exact yogurt container so helping him change first to bowls from that container could be a step along the way.

If the answer is *"I am not sure"* or *"maybe"*, then we tiptoe into offering change. Remember you have YOURS and the child has HIS? Rehearsals still help. He sees you practice taking yogurt from YOUR container into your bowl until he no longer needs that. Could you help him scoop a spoonful from his yogurt container into his bowl? And could he still eat the rest from the container? This can happen a number of times until he is fully comfortable with the idea of scooping out some yogurt from his container. Gradually, you both scoop more and more from his (and your?) container offering him the rest from the container. But, the volume in the yogurt container is reducing. Eventually there is so little yogurt left in his container and most of his yogurt is in his bowl. Then you model eating your yogurt from your bowl and offer the child his bowl. You are hoping that the repetitive rehearsals have helped him understand (and believe) that the yogurt in the bowl is actually his yogurt. He has seen that happen without pressure multiple times. Once he will comfortably eat the yogurt from the bowl, you can give him lots of practice and alternate bowls if you can do so without worry.

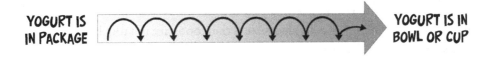

YOGURT IS IN PACKAGE → **YOGURT IS IN BOWL OR CUP**

As in all the suggestions in this book, you are tiptoeing toward the change and following your child's cues. Depending on your child's language and cognitive understanding, you can do lots of explaining in your rehearsals, but remember that simply *saying* it is the same juice or yogurt in the cup or bowl may not make your child believe it initially. Some children zip through this process and believe it quickly and others need lots and lots of little supported steps.

Dear Parent,

If you child is stuck with a preference for a certain cup or container, how could you rehearse and then tip toe toward change?

I Do Not Like My Foods to Touch!

How many times have you heard that? This is a common challenge for worried eaters, and many not so worried eaters, too! Since we know children try to control the foods they eat to be the ones they absolutely know and expect, it makes sense that they want each food pure, not blemished or changed by the sauce on a nearby French fry or the yolk of a nearby runny egg yolk.

Pick your battles carefully. You can work through all the issues of food touching while offering all the food on the same plate. But, why add that stress of needing to place the food just right on the plate knowing the food may just touch accidentally and create a BIG WORRY! And, really you are probably not the one putting the food on the plate if your child is capable of doing it himself but touching may still happen. Remember serving is supposed to be his job, but food placement without getting anywhere near another food is a big responsibility. If touching foods can ruin a meal, maybe starting with less worry is better! This is what divided plates are for!

Of course, if there is no worry about food touching, use whatever plates work. But, it you are trying to reduce your battles and the worry, consider the divided plate. The immediate advantage of a divided plate is that foods are not touching. Whew! But once that stress is gone, the other advantage is that there are three, sometimes four sections. We often get used to offering one favored food in a bowl. The same bowl. By offering a divided plate, you are reminded to offer a couple of familiar foods, and then, hopefully, a new "exposure" food in the third or fourth compartment. This exposure food can be just for the experience and not the pressure to try it. It may end up being a trying food, but, bottom line, it is an opportunity to be around a food other that the usual favored mac and cheese!

Change them up

But, be careful. Many families go right out and buy a divided plate. They serve food on that plate every day, every meal. The child is happy and the mealtime is calm. But, one day the plate breaks, or it is dirty and you offer a new plate and …fireworks and return of the WORRY! The divided plate is a good idea and you will like it, but can you get two or three plates and alternate them (and not in a predictable way)? It is so easy to enable a routine that becomes rigid before you know it.

Make a plan

Children who need divided plates to manage their meal, will still need the opportunity to carefully learn, in tiptoe continuum steps, to have food touch. This is a very important lifelong skill that will serve the child well out there in the world of eating! We try to help worried eaters by offering the familiar food they know as a starting point. If these foods start out separated, it is okay. If *separated* helps them add and establish new foods, great.

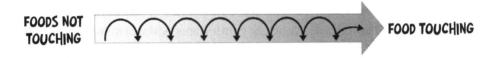

FOODS NOT TOUCHING   **FOOD TOUCHING**

But to help them get to touching, there may need to be multiple tiny steps along the continuum. Can we mix up which section the foods are offer in? Can we help them have a new food in one of the divided plate sections? Or does the new food just need to be visible nearby in a separate bowl? Can that separate bowl be placed closer and closer to their plate? Can the child put a new food that was served family style on her own plate? Or can a parent offer that new food? What would happen if the parent offered the new food and it barely touched the other food? *Here* to *there* can be a continuum of tiny steps.

If the touching foods are dry, the concept of touching may be less worrisome. For some children we start with two foods the child already knows. How about two different crackers or crackers and cereal or chips and crackers? Can they be offered as a snack touching in the bag or the container? This can be a start to touching foods. Dry food touching is often easier than wet food touching.

As we continue to think about the sensory properties of the foods there are many foods that are not actually dry like crackers, but not actually wet like a slice of orange or watermelon, or a wet sauce like hummus or spaghetti sauce. Perhaps it will be easier for the dry familiar crackers to be offered in a bowl WITH a slice of apple (a moist food, but not a wet food?) or a grape or hunk of cheese. If your child is comfortable enough to eat the dry crackers anyway, eating around the fruit can be your starting point for touching exposure. If your child would prefer to pick up that fruit (a sensory rehearsal) and remove it to the side of the bowl or plate, or to the table, that is okay also because he got to touch the food and manage their own worry by removing it. (A lifelong skill!)

What if your child really likes a particular macaroni and cheese? Can you make it with one or two peas in it? Can your child learn that she can eat around the pea, or remove the pea to the side if necessary, or take it out of the dish and put it in a separate nearby dish?

Planned touching

As children get a bit more comfortable with different foods, we tend to consciously put them together. As Ryan learned to like different foods, we worked with him on confidence s-t-r-e-t-c-h-e-s where once he liked pasta and black beans, we offered them in the same bowl, a few of each. As he got comfortable with them in the same bowl, they could be offered together. As grated cheese became an established food, we helped him sprinkle grated cheese crumbs nearby and eventually on the pasta. When he learned to like his crackers in crumbs, he learned he could make recipes adding them to his bowl. He eventually liked different salad dressing as dips and learned to dip cucumbers and carrots. His parents made sure they offered him the opportunity to have a bowl for dinner with different family style foods offered, and as he served himself in his bowl, things touched.

Garnishes

Garnish placement on the dinner plate can be a family routine that can become very familiar and also be an opportunity to place a new food on the plate, that may just touch another food, a little. Garnishes can be bright colors and give early orange or wet experiences with orange slices, or green experiences with parsley! When they are initially seen as a decoration to the plate, it takes away any stress about trying it while your child just gets used to a new food nearby. (A rehearsal for later tasting.)

Dips offer sauce touching opportunities

Any sauce can be a dip. One of the ways we help worried eaters get used to the idea of dipping is by blending up a casserole type food. For example, lasagna blends well. Pizza sauce and toppings blend well. Pick a flavor that the child already enjoys and blend it smooth into a dip. The wet sauce then touches the dipper long enough for the child to get it to her mouth. Children can dip pasta tubes, or lasagna noodles in the lasagna sauce and pretty soon can dip several of the tubes in sauce and put them on her own plate and she will have tiny steps toward pasta and sauce. You can do the same type of sequence with pesto, and cheese sauce, and hummus, and guacamole and refried beans. Start with the dip then make a plate of dipped items.

Dipping is also a way to accidentally do more food touching. If your child does not want to dip her own food, she can dip for *your* tasting enjoyment, and possibly get a little dip on her own fingers along the way. A rehearsal! (See Dips and Dippers chapter.)

Divided plate

We love divided plates not only because they keep foods separate, but also because they visually suggest variety. We are beginning to talk to Teddy about nutrition and food groups and remind him that different foods do different jobs in his body. He now expects there will be a food in each section of the plate and knows where each food group goes. He may not always eat his veggies, but he will add some to that section of his plate as we pass foods at the table. "Here's the veggie spot." It is nice that he gets exposure that is dictated by the PLATE and not Mom. The plate helps reinforce that veggies should always be a part of the meal.
~Laura Wesp

Worry Diluters

In order to reduce the worry at mealtimes, parents discover that there are ways that worry can be diluted. One way many parents have resorted to is to let their child watch TV or actively engage with the computer or phone in a way that takes the child to *another place* while eating. The child concentrates on the screen distraction, movie or game and *zones out*. When focusing on the screen, she is not as directly engaged in the meal or the mealtime worry. She may open her mouth and allow you to place the food in it. You may well be able to get a number of bites, and larger bites in over in a shorter time, more efficiently and with less worry all around. Not only is she less worried but she is also less of a participant. The worry diluters turn the responsibility of the mealtime back in the parent's court and unbalance the division of responsibility. However, many parents say it does reduce the stress. Think about how you got there and where do we go from here?

Of course, it will be a goal to try to tiptoe back toward the internally motivated version of the mealtime, to hand back the responsibility of eating to your child. However, parents describe being overwhelmed when a feeding team member says to *just take away* the screen time. *Just take it away? All at once? No way!!* Parents have used screen time because it has worked. Their mealtimes are more peaceful. It is a worry diluter that may have helped create mealtime peace, but, it is not where you want to be down the line. It is **not the end goal**. It should only be thought of as a transition. There needs to be an exit plan. We are not saying here that parents should run out and connect their screens to reduce the worry. We are saying, if it is already part of the meal, breathe. It is a starting point, but let's work toward removing it as we help your child increase mealtime comfort and participation. And of course, if we meet younger children without this routine, we encourage those families not to start it as a worry diluter if they can help it.

Dear Parent.

What dilutes the worry for your child at mealtimes?

Distractions

Other distractions can be worry diluters. Eat a bite or a serving, turn the page. Eat a bite, your turn playing the game. Eat a bite, play with the toy. The distraction (and the reinforcement of these toys) can dilute the worry (as well as give a bribe), but we are not helping the child focus on the meal in a way that develops lifelong internally motivated skills. These distractions may well be a step along the way for some children, but they are NOT THE END GOAL. We would like to create a mealtime that is more comfortable to attend. Less pressure, more familiarity with the foods offered, more skill at new food interactions and trying. The goal is to not need those outside distractions and have the food interaction, the meal itself and the family togetherness be invitation enough. Tiptoe in that direction.

The big picture

As you are thinking about reducing the mealtime distractions, remember that you will also be reducing the pressure and making the mealtime a safe and trusted place for your child. You are giving multiple positive exposures to foods. It will be a multi-pronged approach to change the whole face of this mealtime. As you are working on reducing overall pressures and helping your child become comfortable eating at the table, you might consider the role screen time is playing and see if it can be reduced gradually. Can the screen be given for a few minutes then removed? Can the sound gradually be turned down or off? Can it be moved farther from the table? Can it be given after a part of the meal is done to allow time to focus on the food? The goal is gradual removal of the screen itself so your child learns to play with it after or between meals. The same thing can happen when eating is done in front of the TV for dilution of the mealtime. Can the TV gradually be turned down? Can the distance from the highchair to the TV be gradually increased? Can the TV be on after a portion of the food is eaten, and gradually after the meals is done and eventually have nothing at all to do with the meal? Can these diluters be consciously removed step by step?

The worry diluters helped, but please have a conversation about tiptoeing away from them. Using the same strategies that we have discussed throughout the book might help you think about a number of tiny succeed-able steps toward less worry diluters.

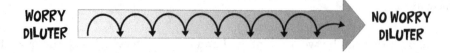

WORRY DILUTER → **NO WORRY DILUTER**

Some children next extra help

Some children have sufficient anxiety that medications can help. Since we know that worried eaters tend to run in families and have discussed their worry temperament and wiring, there are some children for whom some medication just might make sense. These might be children where the worry is so absolutely great, the wall is so high, that they are just a ball of worry in every part of their lives. We know when anxiety is that great, it can interfere with learning and daily life experiences. When all these techniques and strategies for new food trying that we have described throughout are just are not working to help your child feel more comfortable at meals, his doctor may recommend a trial of medication to reduce overall anxiety. It may well be a help. It may just take enough of the edge off for your child to be able to learn and find some increased comfort and enjoyment at meals. Check with your child's medical team, pediatrician, psychologist or psychiatrist to see if a trial of medication might be helpful for your child's learning.

Establish the Foods

In the Big Picture chapter, the foundation of the triangle is *mealtime peace* and the top of the triangle is *establish the food*. In my experience, it is very helpful to have a place along the journey with new foods to consciously focus on giving the worried eater experiences establishing the food as a regular part of the current diet, or *List*. **Pretty soon you will notice there is still a generally preferred list with not so many parentheses.**

An established food is one that your child has added to her *List* of favored foods. It is a food that your child will eat most anytime it is served. It is a food that you, as a parent, can count on. It is a food you are glad is on the *List* because it helps you move in the direction of healthier nutrition for your child. But, unfortunately, experience tells us just because your child tried it once or in a certain place with a certain person does not mean that food is generalized. We can find tiny steps along the way to purposively get there. Here are some considerations when trying to establish foods. Can we help your child get from here to there?

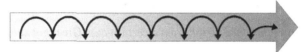

Your child has just tried a new food. Great, but how can we teach her confident new food trying?

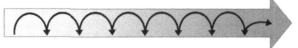

Your child ate that brand of yogurt with you. Great, but how can we help her eat it for other parent or Grandma or sitter?

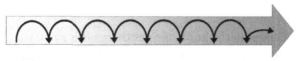

*Your child ate a new food at therapy clinic. Great, but how can
we help her eat that at home, in the park, in the car?*

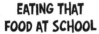
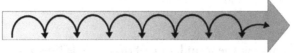

EATING THAT
FOOD AT SCHOOL

EATING THAT
FOOD AT HOME

*Your child ate that new food at school. Great but how
can we help her eat it with you at home?*

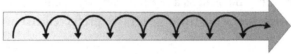

EATING THAT
FOOD AT HOME

EATING THAT
FOOD AT SCHOOL

Your child eats that food at home. Great, but how can we help her eat it at school?

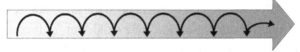

EATING THAT
FOOD AT HOME

EATING THAT
FOOD OUT AT A
RESTAURANT

*Your child eats that food at home. Great, but how can we
help her find a way to eat it at a restaurant?*

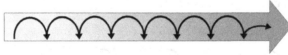

EATING THAT
FOOD FROM A
CERTAIN CUP

EATING THE FOOD
FROM DIFFERENT
CUPS/TOOLS

*Your child eats that food/drink from a certain cup. Great but can she eat/
drink it from a variety of different cups or utensils or therapy tools?*

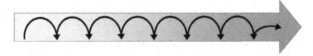

EATING THE
FOOD IN ONE
PREPARATION

EATING THAT
FOOD IN
DIFFERENT
PREPARATIONS

*Your child eats one preparation of that food. Great, but can
she eat that food presented in different ways?*

How to get there or there or there?

As with all the challenges in the book, we get there with small steps. We get there by
starting where it is working and tiptoeing. We get there by guiding your child in that
direction. We will be discussing Bridging Foods Home and Confidence S-t-r-e-t-c-h-e-s

in upcoming chapters that will focus on those aspects of transition. The purpose of this chapter was to get you started on thinking about creating specific goals, specific ideas to purposively establish those foods. When change is hard and when there is WORRY, we cannot assume these transitions will just happen on their own.

Dear Parent,
Can you think of a way to help your child establish a new food in one of these ways?

Change Up the Mealtimes

We encourage families to offer mealtime change as the child is comfortable. First of all, when *change happens* and your child is comfortable with multiple little changes, it can reduce his high-alert-flashing- NEON-SIGN indicating change is near! When they get that *change happens*, children to do not get into such a rut of expectations. And sometimes children are more willing to try new foods in new situations where there are less expectations. In the *Change Happens* chapter we discussed the importance of little tiny changes around the edges of mealtime as a starting point. As children get comfortable with the concept that *change happens*, use that to your and his advantage. As soon as you always serve that cereal in the same bowl, or you always buy that same brand of on sale yogurt, or you always cut the sandwich in the same way, then that can quickly become a requirement, a need for your child. Then you have to work to undo that pattern. If it is possible to avoid that pattern from being established in the first place, it helps.

Feeder diversity

Can you change up who eats with your child or who feeds them? The feeder can accidently become part of the rigidity of the mealtime. *Mom ALWAYS feeds me. I do not want to eat for anyone else!* These ruts happen. Often times it is one parent who has the success of feeding or *getting more food in* the child, but looking at the big picture, this can be a problem. First of all, the responsibility for the mealtime is off balance. (It is the child's job to determine how much to eat.) Secondly, it is a huge pressure on one parent when the child will ONLY eat for and with *that* parent. It is exhausting when you are the only one who can feed your child. We encourage diversity of feeders, rotate through feeders so your child does not *require* one feeder. Can Moms and Dads, or even siblings take turns? Can Grandma and Grandpa or babysitters get good at eating with your child? You and your child need options.

Mealtime novelty

Once children are used to multiple feeders, and lots of little mealtime change, it is easier to introduce novelty. I have heard it said that novelty can be pressure. It can be if the novelty is used as a bribe to eat new, differently or more, in other words, pressure! So, do not make it pressure. Novelty can also be an invitation into the meal. It can be what attracts the child to the food that is a new shape, or the utensil that is different and interesting. How about themed meals, or napkins? How about breakfast for dinner? How about Orange food Night, or Yellow food night? These can be interesting themes that make the meal different and a bit of fun for all. (See Thoughts about Novelty chapter.)

Manners Night

We don't do it every Sunday night, but I try to have at least a few nights when we pull out our nicer things and focus a bit more intentionally on table time manners. After years of feeding therapy and playing with food. It is a nice balance to talk about "hostess" manners. We may spend a bit more time setting the table, cutting flowers for a centerpiece, and selecting pretty napkins. ~Laura Wesp

New environments can HELP!

Sometimes it is easier to try new foods in new environments. Children may know what mealtimes are *supposed* to be like at home. Mom feeds me *this* way and Dad feeds me *that* way. There may be particular feeder, utensil, and food expectations at home. But your child may not have the same expectations away from home, or even in the car. We often hear the story about how an anxious eater ate a crazy new food at Grandma's house, at the birthday party, or at school. When you think *novelty*, consider changing the location of a meal to change your child's expectation. For example, he may expect screen time to accompany the meal at home, but maybe not at Grandma's house. The new environment may allow for new and creative changes to be accepted.

Why does this happen?

When you are a creature of habit, when you like things a certain way, change is so hard. We have described worried eaters as hypervigilant observers of the tiniest change in presentation of foods. But, when they are hungry and eating somewhere else, their worry can get much worse, OR, they may well let down that wall of protection a bit. There are different variables at Grandma's house. The dishes are different, the table cloth is different, the food may be a bit different. Some children may actually be more flexible as they may have different expectations. Grandma may have a different expectation, a different emotional need for the child to eat. She may offer a new food that she is eating and to her amazement, your worried eater may try that new food. Your child may be more confused about the rules and rituals here and might just try the food. And might just like it. Now, just because your child tried it once does not mean she will try it again. And it does not mean she will try that food at home, even if Grandma sent home a take home container of the exact food that she ate there. But it is a start. Your child tried a new food and lived through it. It was okay and *okay* is a place to build upon. There is still the **yet**!

New environment

We often suggest giving new food trying opportunities in new places. We know a family that has a beautiful play fort in their back yard. Mom decided she would offer her child, and the siblings a new kind of snack when they were outside playing. To her surprise her anxious eaters tried a new food in the fort, then another and then another. It became the *new food trying place* until that food became comfortable enough to offer as one of the foods at the family meal. Other families create snack themed play groups at various homes or in the park and are surprised that their anxious eaters try food in these environments. These are not demands they are offers, but the new place seems to change up the ritual rules some for the anxious eaters.

Breakfast changes, maybe?

Maybe mealtimes started getting better at our house when we were at the breakfast table. By nature, breakfast is a smaller meal with fewer foods, sometimes just biscuits and choice of honey or jam. That is a LOT lower ask than is dinner in the dining room with meat and veggies and side dishes and salad and condiments ... We tried making mealtime changes at both meals, but I wonder if the simplicity of breakfast helped him do better with dinner? ~ Laura Wesp

Confidence S-t-r-e-t-c-h-e-s

One of the strategies you have seen throughout this book is *enjoyment*. We want your child to find new foods to enjoy that can then be part of an ever expanding, and perhaps more flexible *List*. The sensory part of eating certainly contributes to the enjoyment. It includes the smell and taste and texture. In addition to this enjoyment, we will also try to help each child find *confidence* with that new food. It is one thing to find a new food to like. It is another to have the **confidence** that *that food* can be eaten flexibly, in different ways, in different places and from different eating partners.

Lose the parentheses

Confidence s-t-r-e-t-c-h-e-s allow foods not on the *List* become newly incorporated into the *List*. And, to take this one step further, **this is where foods the child enjoys lose their parentheses**. In other words, the qualifiers settle down and the child learns to eat that food in a variety of different ways, not just in *that* cup, or cut in *that* way, or dipped in *that* dip.

    Since our anxious eaters tend to eat familiar foods in the same ways, they often do not get this expanded practice on their own so we build in confidence experiences into our sequences.

Confidence S-t-r-e-t-c-h-e-s

1. Find a new food to like
2. Eat that new food from a variety of different bowls and plates
3. Eat that new food off of a variety of different tools
4. Eat that food from a variety of different people

This is not *change happens*

Earlier in the book we discussed the importance of helping your child manage change, any change at mealtimes. These are the children who are rigid about the color of the cup, the feeder, the non-broken shape of the cracker and the specific formula out of the specific can opened in front of them. We said these children might need to experience some tiny changes at the edges of mealtime to just begin to experience some flexibility of the mealtime environment before any change is considered in *their* food. The *change happens* is a starting point for these very, very worried eaters, often needed before any new food trying is considered. For example, we have shared stories of children who like one container for their formula, and a well-meaning adult changed the cup and the child was so worried he stopped drinking that formula altogether. Children have stopped eating their peanut butter sandwiches when the shape is changed, their cheese sticks when a new color is introduced, and their yogurt when a new brand was presented too quickly.

These confidence s-t-r-e-t-c-h-e-s **are best for children who already understand and are good with some mealtime change,** not those terribly worried about ANY change. *Change happens* is usually closer to the outer layer of the circle of sensitivity, the starting place, the *here*, and confidence s-t-r-e-t-c-h-e-s are close to the center of the circle toward the *there*. I usually ask parents directly and they usually know how their child might react. What would happen if we changed your child's cup? The parent might say, I would never do that because my child would stop drinking it altogether. Or the parent might say, I really do not think my child would care at all. I am the one that just always serves it that way. Parents usually know! This is why we tiptoe. This is why was listen to parents. And this is why we watch and learn from each child reaction.

Establish the food

Once your child tries a new food that he likes, we will want to help him have enough opportunities to eat it that so it becomes a favorite and an established food. So, it gets added to the *List*. Try adding that food into the family foods rotation so your child can get comfortable with it. When just learning new foods, our anxious eaters can try something one day and then forget about it the next. Offer more tastes and experiences with that food to help establish it as a food you are confident will be enjoyed and your child is confident that he knows and trusts it. We like to offer confidence s-t-r-e-t-c-h-e-s.

What is a confidence s-t-r-e-t-c-h?

A confidence s-t-r-e-t-c-h provides your child practice with the new food (or a familiar food) offered in a *new presentation*. The idea is that your child is offered the newly enjoyed food in as many new presentations as possible. Each new way gives her more tastes, more practice and helps to fully establish that new food into the daily eating routine. The confidence building opportunities add some novelty into the interactions and can help with diluting worry. **This should be fun and not pressure**. Of course, if your child is really worried about any utensil change, and this type of confidence activity is met with worry, you could accidentally push her away from the new food, so tread lightly, tiptoe toward these activities.

Change the bowls and cups

These are those changes around the edges we discussed earlier, but these changes are for the purpose of **establishing that food**. For example, you can change the bowls and cups in which the food is offered. By offering new bowls or cups you are saying, *you like that new food, great, can you eat it out of this bowl? How about that bowl? How about that new pudding out of this bowl or, maybe this short cup or this tall cup? What if we dipped the cup rim in the pudding and offered it as a tasting edge? What if you took a taste out of the bowl from your finger?*

Change the straws

You like this drink, Yum. Would you like some from this red straw? Or maybe this short straw? Maybe this Fourth of July straw or this crazy shaped one? We help the child generalize enjoyment of this new drink in a variety of these confidence building presentations. It helps her (and us) not to develop a ritual around the new drink (this drink must only be drunk from a red cup L) while adding some novelty and confidence in mealtime changes. It also gives her the opportunity to choose to drink a lot more tastes where the *ask* is, *which one do you want to drink from next* rather than, *it is my grownup idea that you drink two more ounces*. You got to a new food, it became established AND it was your child's internally motivated idea!

Change the "spoons"

So glad you like Grandma's soup, here is some with a new spoon. Would you like that new flavored yogurt off this picnic spoon or this truck spoon? Here is a fun spoon (a tall tea spoon) or how about using this straw as a spoon for your yogurt? OR, can you offer a bowl of spoons and your child can pick her favorite spoon each meal until you are comfortable that she is confident and that the new food is well established. Though the spoon changes may seem a bit trivial, my experience is that these confidence s-t-r-e-t-c-h-e-s can be a great way to build on *change happens*, that lifelong skill.

Let us consider "spoons" to mean utensils, implements to bring food or food tastes to your mouth. "Spoons" can also be fingers, forks, chopsticks, therapy texture tools, ladles, straws, spatulas and more! Be creative. These all have different shapes. This not only helps with *change happens* but also asks for a new motor plan, or way for the child to adapt his mouth in response to the new shape...another confidence builder. And by using textured toys, textured spoons or textured therapeutic tools, the child can have exposure to texture momentarily with the familiar food. These "spoons" can be a texture bridge.

Change the place and person

You can consciously change the place your child is offered the newly emerging food or drink. Some worried eaters only want to eat at their place setting at the table or with Mom. We know worried eaters can somehow rigidly connect a new food with a particular person. *I eat that only at Aunt Jane's house. I eat that food only with Dad. I drink that drink only with Mom or only in therapy or only at school.* By offering that newly added *List* food in different places and with different mealtime partners, you can help your child more firmly establish that food on his *List*.

Maybe you and your child can eat that new food in the park, at snack time in addition to meal time, at a play group or from the lunch box. Change it up as your child allows. Consider confidence s-t-r-e-t-c-h-e-s as a way to establish new foods and expand that *change happens* confidence.

Sample situation, be creative!

Here is a real story. Eva likes water from HER cup. She drinks HER iced cold water from HER green water bottle every day. As a confidence s-t-r-e-t-c-h we asked her:

Wait, wait, can you help me pour some water into this other cup for MOM? (This is a rehearsal that says, *Sweetheart, your water can be found in a different cup.*)

Can you hold this paper cup and I will pour water in it? You can have some. (We pour in a sip worth of water. She drank it.

Wait, wait, can you hold this again and we will pour more for Mom and more for you? Both drink it.

Wait, wait, can we find other cups around her to drink your water out of? Oh, here are two. Which one is for Mom?

Which one is for you? She picked one and gave Mom the other. Both drink more sips and we put more water in Eva's cup each time.

This activity continues with Eva drinking water sips out of seven different cups, a carved out apple and a carved out cucumber. She got to have rehearsals. She got to make choices. And she had fun! (And, by the way she learned about apple and cucumber smell and texture and a tiny bit of flavor!)

Another sample situation:

Tyrone tried a new pureed fruit from a pouch today. *Wait wait, which spoon shall we taste it with now?* (We gave him choices. He picked and we offered another spoon, a ladle a chopstick, a spatula, a cup rim, a yellow straw tip, a coffee stirrer, a fork, a therapeutic bumpy tool, a baby spoon, four regular spoons, and a large cooking spoon. We also asked him to taste off of her own fingers, one finger, two fingers, thumbs?

Tyrone had fun choosing and along the way had about 25 tastes of that new food with Mom and with therapist to fully establish it as a new *List* food, and also to confidently use his mouth in different motor plans as he adjusted to the shape of the many tools offered. The game was novel. It kept his attention. He was not strapped in. He was not required to participate. He was enjoying the activity, confidently practicing his motor mouth skills, and internally motivated to be there. This activity could be done in therapy time, or away from the family meal until Tyrone learns to interact with food comfortably in this way at home. Some families modify it by offering a bowl of tools at the child's place setting so he can try his foods in different ways.

Confidence is an important component or learning to eat. I think we adults have sometimes pushed too fast with new experiences. For example, once the child likes a texture such as smooth baby food purees, we are leaping off to more textured puree options or even mashed purees. We do not expect typically developing babies to taste purees one day and then eat a bowl of mashed food the next. We give them time to explore and let us know their readiness for next challenges. Some children just need more confidence building time at each step along the way.

I also think many different therapy treatments look the same day after day. *Sit* in the chair. Put your *seatbelt on*. I will feed you this food. You *WILL* take this number of bites or this volume! *I have chosen the food* and you *will* eat. Confidence s-t-r-e-t-c-h-e-s allow the child to be an active participant, make choices, and show internal motivation to participate. And, by the way, they are fun! Can't we aim for fun with internal motivation?

Dear Parent,

How might you help your child stretch confidence in a favored or new food or drink?

A new croissant

Sometimes eating away from home can provide an unexpected time to add new foods. We stopped for a snack after swim lessons and Teddy selected a croissant. I was a bit surprised because he'd never tried a croissant but ordered it to share. Little did I know that this would become a mini-ritual for him. Each time we finished a lesson he'd just expect our croissant date. Now croissants are one of his favorite, special breakfast foods. We had a very similar experience with bagels and cream cheese after dropping big brother off at school. For my son simplicity and routine are important. Having one food to think about also helps build his confidence. ~Laura Wesp

Bridging New Foods Home

"Parents' voices must MATTER above all else."
Shannon Goldwater

It is a partnership

As a therapist, I am sorry to say this, but your feeding therapist is not going to *fix* your worried eater! Not alone. It is absolutely a team effort. The one hour here or there that is spent in a clinic or at a feeding group can certainly help, but what happens at home the rest of the week will be key to your child's success. Helping your anxious eater *must* be a partnership between parents and clinicians and between parents and their children.

If you want your child to learn to like new foods, she needs to be around them. She cannot just try new foods at therapy. She needs to see others eating different foods than her *List*. She needs to find mealtimes inviting and learn from watching others. Her feeding team can help you find ways to incorporate food interactions into your day in a way that becomes a natural way of life.

When your child eats for others!?

Sometimes children try new foods for others and not you! This is common and may well be because of a change in the environment and the ritual expectations, maybe they are still re-learning trust with no pressure and healing from sensory surprises at home. It can be especially heartbreaking when you take your child to therapy week after week and she tries new foods there, but not at home, or actually eats that food regularly at the therapy clinic and not with you. This may be all confused with what your child expects and where she expects it and what food is associated with what feeder. But we need to re-think this.

When I was a therapy clinic owner, I saw this all the time. A clinician would say, *Sherry ate this or that new food this week*. The next question **must** be, will she eat it at home? Will she eat it with her parents? That <u>must</u> be our goal and we cannot settle for her to eat it only in clinic. However, these children have shown us time and again that transitioning a new skill to new places is challenging. We need to help transition new skills and new foods home. Once she likes a new food, we will want to help her build confidence around that food and establish it as a food she can eat anywhere and with any person.

Bridge the food home

We need to consciously focus on helping worried eaters learn to eat their new foods in a variety of places with a variety of people. That includes eating that new food at home. If your child learns to like a new food in a clinic or school setting, can you and the feeding therapist make a plan to transition that food home? Can you start by giving your child a number of experiences with that new food in that setting? *Really* establish that your child likes that food before making any changes in mealtime partner or environment. Build confidence.

Once your child likes that food consistently in the clinic setting, can you sit with your child and therapist or teacher and eat some of that food with them there? Maybe this happens once, or maybe a number of times. We want your child to understand that *I can eat this new food with my parent*. Can the therapist or teacher come to your house and eat that food with your child at your house with or without you? If not with you to start, add YOU in later. Can **you** offer your child and therapist the new food and eat with them? Mid-meal, can the therapist go to *take a phone call,* or *leave the table* for a few minutes so your child sees that he can eat that food with **you**, even if the therapist is not there. The sequence can have fewer or more steps as needed for your child's worry level.

When clinic sessions regularly occur in a therapy room without the parent, this challenge is compounded. Can you have a discussion with the team and let them know that you want to be in the feeding session? That you want to be included? You want to learn their strategies. You want to practice with the food interactions they are using and you want to take therapy successes home? If you try to help them like *that* therapy food at home and it is not working, let them know. Let them know that you need help bringing that food home. You may need a continuum of steps to get there.

And, remember the Circle of Sensitivity Hug. You are the food partner, the new food trying guide and you are letting your child know that YOU know this is hard. You are there as support. If you are always delegated to some different room, it is hard to be that emotional support. The goal must be YOUR involvement, your success and your child's success.

Clinic ◀——————————————————————▶ **Home**

Home visits

Some families have the option of home visits and others do not. Insurance and other funding sources may play a big role in where children are eligible to receive therapy. There are pros and cons to having therapy in your home. Many anxious eaters are much more comfortable learning to try new foods in the comfort of their homes. This is understandable. Home may well be more predictable with less worry. It can be more convenient for the whole family. It is the best place for therapy support for many children and families.

For some, home turns out not to be the best starting place. It is home where a child may have very specific requirements that things stay the same there. They may well already have figured out what is *supposed* to happen at home, what mealtimes are to look like at home, and sometimes when we feeding therapists go into the home it can be very, very stressful for a child because *we are not supposed to be there*. We are not part of their mealtime or eating expectation. We are making the environment different. We are the sensory surprise. We have known children that need that new environment of a clinic because for these kids, being in a new or novel place can reduce their expectations and allow them to make a change. Progress will be best in some type of partnership where in-home success is the end goal.

New food trying places and people

We have mentioned throughout this book that mealtimes should be peaceful. We absolutely want children to be exposed to new foods at the family meal in the passing and serving as non-pressured new food exposure, rehearsals. But, we therapists often suggest that *new food trying skills* be learned away from the mealtime for particularly worried eaters and brought back to the meal as the child gains skill and confidence. Any foods they learn to enjoy in new food trying can be added to a regular rotation in the family mealtimes.

We have also said that many anxious eaters have very particular requirements about how food should look and smell and feel and taste. Many anxious eaters also develop preferences regarding the person offering the food or the people they are comfortable eating with.

For example, Johnny eats yogurt at home with family but never at school. Johnny drinks apple juice at school with teacher and never at home. The food presenter is a part of the whole experience for Johnny. He has feeder expectations. *Mom is the one who gives me yogurt. Teacher is the one who gives me apple juice.* This is one of the factors that adds to the challenge of transition food experiences to home from other places. Children have expectations of us! This may be a reason to separate you and your child for some parts of some therapy settings but should not be the norm. In my experience, it should be a specific and prescriptive decision made by parent and therapist to get to a specific goal.

We have discovered that children will often try a new food in a new place when they had no preconceived idea of what eating in that place might be like. So, many parents will intentionally find a new-food-trying-place different from the mealtime table. One family had a little picnic table on the porch. When the siblings were playing there after school, Mom and Dad would put out a plate of familiar and new foods. They were amazed that their worried eater tried multiple new foods in that novel and stress-free place. He did not feel pressure at this picnic table and had no expectation that he should or shouldn't eat there. This little one was able to add a handful of new foods to his diet by trying them in that table.

Some parents take advantage of the different expectations of friends or relatives and focus on regular new food exposure with them. As you watch your child, you will notice the best places and environments for new food interactions. Parks, the back yard, on a snack sheet in the play room, when the cousins come over, or even at the mall or restaurant? Wherever the new food is tried and enjoyed, there will probably need to be a careful continuum of steps created to bring that new food skill home, just like the steps to bring therapy success home.

Groups

Many centers have feeding therapy groups. For many children this is a great way to dilute the worry. Children learn from watching others. The novelty of a group setting can be an inspiration for interaction with food in new ways as they interact with the other children in the group. Many parents say that their child has tried many different foods in their therapy group. But, be sure you have help in taking those new foods home and can establish them as comfortable *List* foods. Ideally parents will actively participate in groups so they learn about the creative ways to interact with foods. And, make sure you have input in the foods tried so groups success food make sense at your home.

Groups are not for everyone, though. For some, there is too much activity and stimulation and their focus is worse. Others are just not ready **yet** for group learning as their sensory sensitivities are currently too overwhelming to learn from imitation, turn taking and participation in the group in a focused way.

Two can be a group. Can you invite your child's friend over and have a play date? Ask the child's parent to send a favorite food. You all can try that food together while also offering one of your child's favorites.

Technology helps

In more recent years we have included technology into our therapy sessions. It used to be cameras, but now everyone comes to clinic with a cell phone equipped with a photo and video cameras with texting and sending possibilities. We use this technology in several ways.

The first way is to *dilute the worry*. As we are teaching new food trying, we use photos and videos as *rehearsals*. We take pictures of Mom kissing or licking the food. We take pictures of siblings or the therapist taking a *lip balm flavor or lipstick taste*. We take the photo of the other person to show the child what is coming next and give them a preview of the game we are playing. Rehearsals! We show the child the picture or they even help take the pictures. Taking pictures while interacting with and tasting new foods helps dilute the worry around new food trying. Taking pictures and videos also gives the grownups in the room time to gauge how the child is feeling about the food we are offering.

Secondly, we use the photos and videos to *celebrate* the child's participation in the activity. We can take that picture of Dad "trying" the food and then the child trying the food. We can take a picture or video of him doing his trying and text it home to celebrate his participation. The child can review these videos again when home with Mom. He can share his accomplishments with his grandparents who can help to celebrate his bravery.

We celebrate all the little tiny steps along the way. Parents will end up with a library of pictures and videos that documents their child's journey and shows their success. This documentation can also help a parent's perspective during those times of slower progress when they might just need a little boost! The picture library can be shown to the child regularly to celebrate his new food trying progress and his relationship with new foods.

The third way we use technology is to bring progress *back to clinic from home*. When a session ends, we ask if parent and child can take pictures of the child practicing these activities at home? The home videos are reviewed at the beginning of the next session in clinic and become another opportunity to celebrate the child! This keeps the conversation between clinic and home very active and shows parents we care about how things are going at home.

> Dear Parent,
>
> How can you bridge the transition of new foods from clinic to home and back?

Establish it

We encourage families to establish a new food. Once a child has found a new food he enjoys, we recommend putting that food in the regular rotation of mealtime foods so the child gets to practice it, to establish it as a predictable and enjoyable food. If you are having challenges establishing that new food at home, have a conversation with your specialist.

What works for you?

One of the techniques we use with families is to summarize each session. We ask, *of all the things we did today, what things are most reasonable for you to try at home? What things do you feel you and your child could have success doing at home?* A parent may say, *I can do this one thing, twice this week.* Great. What is important is that you feel you can be successful with a certain activity and are committing to a realistic amount of practice. Or another parent may say *I want to try these five things.* Each family is different. Professionals must to be sensitive when helping parents figure out how they can best work on tiny changes at home within the normal rhythm of their life. We are trying to help parents change their food habits little by little so the ideas need to be comfortably able to be incorporated into the family day.

Parents tell us they are most comfortable when *they* can pick what and how much to do at home rather than be given a list, a protocol or prescription of amount of time they should spend. When someone else decides for you, it can be distressing if you cannot meet their challenge or make the ideas work. Others do not understand your home, your reality and your energy. When **you** decide, it is more likely to happen, right?

When parents are continually given home programs that they were not a part of, when they are given assignments that they are not yet comfortable implementing, they tell us it is hard to continue with therapy. It is hard to comeback week after week. It is hard to understand where therapy is going when there is no identifiable progress and when ideas are not successful. Now your child might feel like he is disappointing you and you might feel you are disappointing the therapist. It is out of balance. Home ideas are so much more apt to be tried when they are created *with* parents and when they are easily implemented as a natural part of the day, rather than a specific hour of home therapy ideas. Help your child's team help you. Ask them, *how can I incorporate this activity naturally in my day?* Give them feedback. Work together, as a team.

> Dear Parent,
>   What food interaction activities do you feel would work in your home **this** week?

They are Listening

"Labeling a child creates a self-fulfilling prophecy. Telling children what they *can't* do, closes doors."
Jo Cormack

Our children are listening. Since they've been tiny, these children have been hearing that they have eating problems. They do **not** eat. They are picky. They are **not** eating what we think they should. They are **not** eating a balanced diet. They do **not** like to touch foods. They are **not** eating fruits. They do **not** like their food to touch. They do **not** feed themselves. They do **not** like to eat with friends. They do **not** meeting our mealtime expectations. We are **not** happy with how they interact with food. **Not. Not. Not. NOT!**

They are listening. First of all, when they are little we do not think it matters because they are too young to understand. That may well be true. But when these issues do not go away and all of a sudden our children are 2, 3, 4, or 8 years old, we find ourselves still having those conversations *in front of them*. As we tell the doctors about their eating, as we ask the dietitian questions, as we go to therapies and we describe the **NOTs**, they are there. We tell their friends' mothers at playdates and we tell their teachers. They hear us. They gradually GET the idea that they are eating differently. They are the ones who need therapy. They are the ones who are **not** right.

Some children are mildly picky eaters and when we continue to talk about them as *picky* eaters, we continue that story, we keep it going. We continue to narrate that they are *picky* and they continue to see themselves as *picky*. Children with milder challenges hear and can continue to believe, *Oh, yeah, I am a picky eater. I won't try that because I am a picky eater*. This can squash any bravery they might be mustering because, *I am a picky eater*.

Children with a significant level of worry can start to feel that the **NOTs** are a part of their identity. The **NOTs** may be interpreted as wrong, bad, abnormal, NOT good enough and disappointing. The **NOTs** of mealtime can turn into feeling sad, even more worried and can shape a self-image negatively. Instead of just worrying at each meal about the new foods that may lurk around the corner, the overwhelming sensory challenges of the mealtime, they may start worrying about how they are disappointing YOU, and how they are not good enough. I like to tell families, that *your child is doing the best he can, given his experiences and his wiring.* Can that be the starting point? Can that be the thought that helps you change your narrative?

They have ears!

We should proceed in complete awareness that they are listening. In combination with deciding to eliminate mealtime pressure, can you make a decision to **stop talking about these issues in front of your child?** Deciding to **not** talk about these issues in front of your child will take some coordination with family and friends, schools and medical professionals. Can you have a conversation with grandparents to let them know that from this day on, none of you are going to talk about this issue in front of the child as if they cannot hear? Can the conversations with specialists or friends be done separately? This is tricky when you are at an appointment and are asked lots of questions. Can you minimize this by writing out your concerns and getting them to the specialist ahead of time? Can you write out the diet (with the parentheses) and have that ready for the specialist? Can you bring another adult or responsible sibling who can wait with your child in the waiting room while this detailed conversation is going on? Some parents bring a special new computer game or coloring book as a great distraction. Some bring a toy the child has not seen before. Maybe borrow one from a friend so it is very new. OR Reserve a birthday gift that can be opened at a big appointment?

Some specialists do not **yet** think this way. Can you help them? Let them know your sensitivity on this matter. Specialists can learn and change too. In our clinic we would often interview the parent by phone first or ask them to have someone attend the appointment who can keep the child busy during that conversation. We try to gather information separately from the child then bring them together and be sure our conversations together are loving and careful without judgmental language.

As children get older we interview them separately if they are willing and able to separate from parents. This is especially important for children who are 8 or 9 and older depending on their communication skills and emotional maturity level. They often have had their parents talking about their eating and this is a respectful way of showing them that their opinion is very important in this story.

As children get older, they realize on their own that they eat and approach food differently from their friends. They absolutely deserve to have conversations with you about that, but could these conversations focus on information not labeling, on letting them know what great people they are, not how deficient. Their eating is different, unique, personal, but not deficient and not less. Can our words and our tone show we understand and support their worry? Can we acknowledge that this is hard for them and that we grownups want to be helpers? Can they center around loving who they are? Can we let them know we understand this is hard but we are going to help them gain skills to figure out food? As Brady said, "it's okay, help them."

Dear Parents,

What tiny changes can you make to have discussions about
your child's eating where they are not listening?

Acknowledge their worry

It can help children for them to know we *get it*. We understand. When your child says *No*, respect it. What needs to change? Can you give them words? Oh, that is a big smell? Or was that taste too big? Or tongue is not yet ready to try that? Once they have words they can use them next time to help us and them understand the challenge a bit more.

Give them words

Since they listen, let's give them words. Words of acceptance. Children need the words of acceptance. Our starting point is that each child knows she is great and wonderful and that food is something she might want to learn more about. It is not that SHE is wrong about the food. It is personal and she may believe that this food is not right for her. Remember we offer and children have the right to say *no* and that is our clue that this food, in this presentation, in this state, at this time, is not the right *ask*. We can adjust our *ask* so it does not elicit such worry. We can tell them that we can help them adjust the food to be okay for them. *You did not want to put that food on your tongue. Hmmm, how about trying to kiss it, or trying a finger taste? OR Oh, you did not want to use your fingers to touch that corn cob, how about I help you pass the corn with these tongs? OR If that is too big of a smell, next time if we can cover the cup with a lid. That might help? OR You did not like that applesauce. Is it too chunky? Next time we can make it smoother together in the blender.* We always want the child to know WE UNDERSTAND, and we can help…together. We are their food partner!

I often say to children, *your tongue is very careful (cautious, worried) about new foods and we need to think of ways to help your tongue learn to try new things.* I try to be careful that it is not that **they** are so different, (or less in any way) as a person. They are terrific, but their tongue or mouth needs some extra help learning about new.

Give them no *thank you* words. Not all foods we offer are the right ask. Not all foods will be enthusiastically tried this time or next time, or until many exposures later. Children will reject our offers but we can teach them words to navigate these situations. The skill of making a polite food rejection is an important one! *No thank you. Not today, thank you.* Your child can also learn to say *thank you* and place it on the side of the plate and then not eat it. These words will be their power and take the place of angry outbursts, crying, gagging, vomiting, pushing the food away or even tipping over the dish or running from the table. Words are much more socially appropriate! This is a lifelong skill to perfect! The challenge is that if we are giving children choices and giving them words. We, their caring grownups, need to listen to *their* words. We need to be trustworthy.

An adult anxious eater I know is still navigating these issues. He has learned a way to respond when colleagues invite his wife and him to dinner. Oh, can that be a terrifying situation when the two of you are going to someone's house where you are supposed to sit down and eat what is placed in front of you with others watching?! They figured out they can say, *it would be lovely to get together for dinner with you, but let's eat out to avoid all the work of cooking at home. Let's go out to a restaurant.* (Of course, in true anxious eater parenthesis style, he has three particular restaurants he likes in our town and orders the same familiar thing each time.) This is a polite *no thank you*, or, actually, a pivot. I know another anxious eater adult friend who just *owns* her eating issue. She says, *I would love to get together with you, but I am such a crazy picky eater that it works so much better if we can get together at this (particular) restaurant.*

And give them food words. We can help them identify that foods have looks, smells, textures and tastes. Can they learn to identify the sensory property that works for them and those that are hard for them? For example, by helping them identify that they like strawberry flavoring, we can let them know as a rehearsal (not a requirement) that this new food we are offering is also strawberry flavored. By helping them identify that we understand that they like crunchy foods we can help them know that this new food is also crunchy. The descriptors can help break down *worry walls* and help your child consider them. Words alone will not assure that your child is ready to try the new food but they give them the power to understand some of these variables and may reduce some of the surprise worry.

When a child lets us know *I do not want to touch that now* or *that smell is too big*, or *thank you, but may I have my spaghetti without the sauce?* It is great because they are beginning to identify some of the properties of foods that worry them. The touch, the smell, the look, texture or taste. When they can tell us the sensory properties that are challenging for them we can let them know there is a way to help them get more comfortable with that sensory property. We can let them know *if the smell of that drink is too big, you could try it sometime with a lid on the cup to take away some of that big smell. Or if you do not like the touch of that food on your fingers, (but you like the taste), you can use this fork, or these tongs.*

We can read the food package words and ingredients with children to use it as a time to talk about what is in the item, what things they can know about it before they try it. This is also where we can use the distant sensory properties to visually inspect the food, smell it, and touch it, break it, explore the texture, as a way to rehearse the new food. Also, when children cook with us, they begin to have routine experiences with particular ingredients that turn into food they like. For example, when they help make waffles with flour, and sugar and eggs and vanilla, they will find that there are the same ingredients in pancakes, or in cakes or muffin. Ingredient familiarity can help some worried eaters.

Give them words of partnership. We can help children *know*, *believe*, that we understand this is hard but we are here to help, to teach new food trying and that they are in our family and at our family meals. We understand *"it takes time to find new foods you like. We can find them together."* We will help them.

Give them words of hope. *Yet* is a hope word. *Your tongue does not like that strawberry*, **yet**, *but it might like strawberry flavor in a smoothie next time. Or your tongue did not like the taste (feel?) of broccoli* **yet***, but, don't worry, your tongue might like it another time. It might like broccoli in cheese soup instead of plain. Broccoli comes in all kinds of ways.* Yet is powerful for both parents AND children. Yet gives everyone hope

And give them words of celebration. We want to find the qualities in your child that can be celebrated and focus our words to convey that celebration. *You are a (brave) new food try-er. You found a new food to eat with Grandma. Your tongue likes grape juice now!*

These positive comments that support your child without value and judgement are encouraging as we find lots of tiny ways along each continuum to celebrate effort.

Dear Parents,

Can you think of words of celebration for your child?
(Words that have NOTHING to do with eating?)

Words help

Much as play therapists and child psychologists help children understand their emotions by teaching them a range of "feeling" words, teaching children a wider vocabulary to explain foods and their feelings about them can be very beneficial.

In rehearsing and exploring foods, can you help them expand their vocabulary from "good" or "yucky" to include more words that describe the physical properties of the foods? Foods give you a lot to talk about! You can talk about temperature (i.e. hot, cold, warm, just right, etc.), texture (smooth, lumpy, silky, grainy, soft, hard, etc.), appearance (color, size, shape, etc) and the list goes on. You get the idea! The more descriptive a child can be about a food, the more information you glean about how to adapt the ask. How much more informative for a child to say, "it's grainy" than to just say "yuck"!

To expand upon this theme, Teddy's wonderful occupational therapist, Rose Langston, routinely uses scented markers in her feeding therapy sessions. She and Teddy explore the scents of the markers and use a white board to make a sliding scale of how they smell. For example, the "Barnyard" marker is delineated as "disgusting" and the "Watermelon" marker is deemed "amazing." Right in the middle is "Fresh Air." This helps Teddy understand that scents (and by extension flavors) appear on a continuum. When Teddy rejects a food in a session, Rose will sometimes say, "Is it disgusting like a barnyard? Or, just "okay" like fresh air?" She'll sometimes hand Teddy a marker to put an "x" on the sliding scale to indicate where a food falls. These sessions have translated extremely well to home. They've helped us see which foods he thinks are amazing. (Who would've guessed Julia Child's vinaigrette recipe?!) Additionally, we've been able to tiptoe toward learning to accept and eat a small portion of foods that are just okay. We talk about how we all have favorites, but that not every food at every meal can be a favorite. It's still a good idea to eat a range, and sometimes we find a favorite the more we give it a try. ~Laura Wesp

Nutritional Health

Children who are anxious eaters, by the definition described in this book, have narrow diets. They often eat few, or no, fruits or vegetables and very limited meats. Some drink lots of milk and eat lots of yogurt so the dairy food group dominates their *List*. Others consume no dairy, or even protein, at all. Many have a parentheses diet primarily comprised of brown, crunchy, familiar, and specific processed foods. They may consume mostly carbohydrates and often lots of sugar and salt. You, understandably, worry about their nutrition when your child will not try new things!

> Dear Parent,
>
> Have "food amnesia". One of the biggest changes I encourage parents to make is to keep offering foods to their child, even and especially, if you know they won't eat it. Have amnesia about what they ate or didn't eat the last time you served that particular food. So often, concern about a child not eating enough food or a particular type of food, can lead to catering to their preferences. For example, if a child eats broccoli, but not carrots, a parent may not make carrots and only offer broccoli so the child "gets in her vegetables." The problem with this is that the child will never learn to eat carrots if she isn't offered them. You may need to offer the carrots for years before she eats them, but she will never wat them if they are not offered. ~Anna M. Lutz, MPH, RD/LDN, CEDRD-S

Ask a professional

You tell us you do not need a professional to tell you your child's diet is incomplete. It is obvious to you. With no fruits or vegetables in sight, hardly any meats, and an abundance of brown crunchies and such limitations, the just diet cannot be good! The question is not whether the diet needs improvement, it does, but how to get those more nutritional foods **in your child** without creating a battleground. This is where you and the professionals need to work closely together.

Many parents tell us their child's pediatrician has zero concern about the diet if the weight is okay. Maybe there will be a statement to have him "eat a rainbow". But you are seriously concerned about the narrowness of your child's *List*. You will need to be the advocate for your child. Consider writing down your child's diet for a week or so. Document the foods eaten that the volume of drinks. Tell the pediatrician you really do want help, a referral, some support. When pediatricians realize how concerned you are about the sustainability of such a *List* diet, maybe you will be heard. When you ask directly for help and support, SOMETHING to make you feel better about mealtime, and you cannot get it, it may be time to get a second opinion. YOU DO NEED SUPPORT.

We encourage you to schedule routine health checks with your child's pediatrician. The pediatrician can follow height and weight data and look at how your child is growing over time. Is he trending toward underweight or overweight? The pediatrician can also check blood levels to look at overall health. Registered dietitians can provide you with specific nutritional analyses that can help you pinpoint areas of specific macro and micro nutrient deficiencies and guide you in prioritizing food, food groups or supplements to work toward. Each child's health and nutritional needs will vary, but it is important to look at the big picture of your child's nutritional health. Some children will need extra nutritional supplementation, formulas, vitamins. Working with your medical team can help you prioritize nutritional strategies.

Role model

Throughout this book we discuss the importance of role modeling the mealtime manners and food exploration you want your child to experience. Observing you eating *your* varied and nutritional diverse foods provides rehearsals for *new food trying* for your child. Including your child in food interactions and preparations provides sensory rehearsals to tiptoe toward more sensory comfort for your child. Specifically, teach new food trying skills and carefully give confidence s-t-r-e-t-c-h-e-s so a new food joins the preferred *List* foods.

Add a vitamin or medication, how?

Each family may have their own strategy for helping their children take vitamins and medications. Once you have a vitamin or medication recommendation the challenges is figuring out how to help your child take it. (Check out the Vitamin/Medication S-t-r-e-t-c-h chapter.)

Special formula

Sometimes the pediatrician or registered dietitian suggests offering a special formula drink that provides a balanced liquid nutrition. Some are ready-to-serve liquid drinks and others are powdered drinks to be added to other foods or liquids. These can be introduced in a continuum of diluted steps as needed for your child or may be accepted all at once.

Some cautions here! We often suggest if one container of formula supplement is needed, can it be given at the end of the day, after dinner as their *Power Drink*? This way, it will not be as apt to interfere with the appetite for oral foods for the day. If it needs to be offered during the day, or if more than one is suggested, can your child sit at the table and drink it as a meal rather than sip at it over hours? The sipping approach can mess with appetite for the next time meals are offered. Also, can it be offered some days from the original container, sometimes from a glass or cup, or sometimes with a straw? We see many situations where the child learns to only drink this supplement from the original packaging, opened in front of the child in a ritualized way, at a certain temperature. (Note: manufacturers change packaging from time to time and children who learn to trust only one label design or container may panic when it suddenly changes.

To avoid those *parentheses challenges* later, can you change it up from the beginning? Also, can you offer the drink at a meal or while sitting so your child does not wander around the house sipping that high calorie drink? We have already discussed how meals need a "where". Meals should be in a *place*, when possible, and drinking this high calorie drink over a longer period of time takes the edge off appetite and can affect the next mealtime interest. There are situations where the medical team suggests three, four or five cans of this drink in a day to more completely enrich nutrition. When this is necessary, can the drinks, again, be regularly offered in and out of the container, with and without straws and always at a mealtime rather that while wandering? These will help you prevent the rigid challenges that can occur. Can oral foods always be offered first before the drink so you do not end up with a situation where your child only sees the nutrition drink as food and eliminates all else?

Fruits and vegetables

Since fruits and vegetables are often scarce in the parentheses diet, they are often a priority in helping anxious eaters in trying new foods. We have discussed crumbing freeze-dried fruits and vegetables and a continuum of smoothie s-t-r-e-t-c-h options in other chapters. Most anxious eaters we know have some type of goals to support adding fruits and vegetables in one of these options. (Check out the S-t-r-e-t-c-h-e-s sections for more ideas.)

> Dear Parent,
>
> How can you help your child find some enjoyable fruits and veggies for his diet?

Hydration

I live in the desert so we constantly think about hydration. But, all children need fluids. When children have limited diets and parentheses lists for liquids, helping your child take in enough fluids can be quite a challenge. We need fluids for plenty of bodily functions, not the least of which is good digestive health. Constipation can be quite a challenge for children who have limited diets, limited fiber, limited exercise and lots of carbohydrates. It is worth the effort to figure out how to help your child take in more water or other fluid during the day.

We have discussed when children like their water from a certain container. That is your starting point. Use their love of water *in that container* to offer fluid plenty of times a day. Your child usually drinks less liquid than you think and needs more liquid than you think. (Check in with the pediatrician or registered dietitian to estimate your child's daily fluid needs.)

Some families work out predictable, *routine* times each day to drink water together. Routines help. Children, then, *expect* them. Since worried eaters often like rituals and routines, can you offer a drink before getting in the car or before taking a walk to the mailbox? Perhaps every meal ends with a bit of water? What would work in *your* family? Remember this cannot be a battle so your first offers of water need to be small amounts, a tiptoe on a continuum toward a full glass! Can your child chug an ounce of water then you go to the mailbox? (Be sure everyone going to the mailbox is also chugging their ounce of water.) Gradually the amount consumed increases as your child learns and adapts comfortably to the routine.

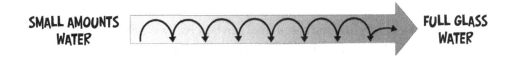

SMALL AMOUNTS WATER → FULL GLASS WATER

Exercise

All children need exercise and your worried eater is no exception. Establishing a good routine of exercise is important for good health, balancing caloric intake to prevent obesity, and for helping reduce constipation. Is there an exercise routine that works for your child, even if it is a walk to the mailbox, or around the block? Helping your child get exercise can be good for you too! It gives you two something to enjoy together that has nothing to do with "take another bite"!

Diets

There are many diets out there. And diets, as in food preferences, are often very family specific. When anxious eaters, for example, have specific diagnoses of autism spectrum disorder, families will be bombarded with diet choices. There are many theories about diets, sugars, dairy, gluten, probiotics, omega three fatty acids, vitamins and more. I leave discussions about those diet variations to pediatricians, dietitians and families. As a feeding therapist, I will try hard to help you help your child eat whatever foods are recommended for her diet.

However, I do have an opinion about diets that are big changes and highly restrictive. For example, many families decide to change the diet to gluten free and casein (essentially dairy) free. This diet may or may not be a great idea for your child. Some families swear by it and other see no difference. Please discuss with your child's pediatrician. As with many diets these days, we need more information and good research to know their full value. BUT, I do recommend caution as you make decisions. If a child's main diet is yogurt, milk, cheese, crackers, cereal, nuggets with breading, and waffles, going gluten free and casein free can be a really big challenge for a really anxious eater. If you take away all their favored, *List* foods what do they have left?

I have a friend who took all the gluten and casein out of her child's diet all at once. Mom and Dad were worried about how these foods affected their child and hoped that the new diet would help in important ways. However, their very anxious eater then was only able to eat what he *knew*. So, for the next two years he ate ONLY potatoes. Potatoes in the form of potato chips (ONLY a particular brand of potato chips in certain shapes) and French fries (ONLY hot from one particular fast food restaurant). *Hot* meant three or four trips to that fast food chain restaurant *every single day*. The child was eventually given a feeding tube as they found their way back to other foods. My caution here is **not** that the diet idea was bad. It is that we have to be very careful when we change diets for worried eaters all at once.

When change is the biggest worry for the child, SLOW and careful tiptoeing is usually better. We suggest that if a family has decided, for example, to eliminate gluten, can we FIRST help the child establish some non-gluten food options first? If all their browns, their cereals, their crackers are gluten based, can there be a concerted effort to help them learn to like rice-based crackers or cereals? You are still offering the brown and crunchiness that is appealing to them, but can you help them add the rice food group so that gradually you can replace the wheat-based brown foods with rice-based foods? Or if you are going to eliminate milk-based foods, can you help your child like a different drink substitute such as a soy, rice, coconut, pea, oat or hemp-based drink? (Check out choices with your dietitian). Can you help them like this new drink BEFORE eliminating all dairy? If cheese or yogurt is a staple of the diet, can you find non-dairy substitutes for them to enjoy and establish FIRST? Add the new food first before eliminating the *List* food. Your child's dietitian can help you find the best substitutes for your child.

Dear Parent,

Where are the nutritional gaps that need support?

Mealtime for Siblings, too

"Food in my house is all about my brother!"
Loving sibling

When a child is an anxious eater, mealtimes can lose their balance. It is no wonder that a loving sibling can become a bit frustrated that mealtimes are all about the challenging mealtime needs of the anxious eater sibling. *Even choices of where to celebrate **my** birthday are influenced by my brother's issues!*

Brothers and sisters notice the worry surrounding mealtimes when they have siblings who are anxious eaters. Maybe they are quietly observing the interactions and seeing how hard parents are working to help their sibling. Maybe they notice when there is heightened worry, pressure, anger and frustration. Maybe the sibling realizes the anxious eaters gets a lot of attention when they do not want a food. Maybe he wonders why he cannot have a *snack food* dinner and why he is offered different foods. Maybe the sibling wonders why he is supposed to stay at the table until everyone is finished when the anxious eater does not have to. Maybe he wonders why the anxious eater can sit at a different table. Maybe the sibling wonders why he can't have his own computer at the table when he is eating. It can be confusing.

Mealtime peace

We have discussed that *mealtime peace* is an important starting point for your anxious eater. But, it is also important for siblings. Turning the pressure off and re-finding that peaceful starting point helps everyone.

Siblings need information

Sometimes parents do not want to bother the sibling with too much information, but they notice our reactions. Can you have ongoing conversations to let them know what is going on with your worried eater? Can you help them understand that your anxious eater is doing the best he can and that you, as a family, are trying to help him become more comfortable with foods and mealtimes? Can they be included so they feel like a part of the solution?

Siblings need to be heard

We know siblings of children with special needs can become more empathic, more resilient, more responsible than some of their peers. They often want to help and absolutely do not want to make things harder for parents. They can be more compassionate, helpful, loyal and patient. They can see our stress and do not want to add to it. Some try really hard to never disappoint us, never be a burden, and, in essence, to be perfect. That is a tough goal!

We also know some siblings can become just plain angry, frustrated or sad. Some can turn resentful, jealous, angry, worried, and then guilty for feelings those feelings! The emotions are complicated. They may not get the one on one time with parents. We need to listen and give them the opportunity to share feelings.

Siblings may find themselves in situation where they need to find words to explain their worried eater sibling to friends. They may feel isolated and even embarrassed. They may feel stressed if others make fun of their sibling and need words to make sense of it all. Can we talk about this with them and help them find the words they need?

Perspective in helping

It is common for siblings to want to be the helper. But, can you keep a perspective on this? Being a helper and being a part of the positive mealtime environment will be important, but the sibling also needs to not feel as though there is too much pressure on her. Pressure does not work for anyone. Helping is important, but too much responsibility can also be overwhelming.

Siblings could be a part of the family multiple exposures and rehearsals. Can you explain why you will be incorporating more conscious food interactions into your mealtimes from here on? They can participate in the new mealtime interactions. They can learn about the new family definition of re-defining TRY IT. They can model mealtime jobs, food preparation and making smoothies or crumbs. They can help with grocery shopping and putting food away. They can help with the garden. They can use food in their food academics and food math too. They can practice spelling words by drawing them in crumbs, too. They can be included in so many of the strategies shared in this book.

The sibling actually can be a *worry diluter* by role modeling the steps of new food trying, touching, passing, smelling, kissing and licking new foods. Perhaps they can participate by taking pictures of their sibling or parent trying food in new ways. Perhaps they can be the picture taker in the celebration of the worried eater's new food trying?

Sibling influence

Though siblings can be a great help at mealtimes in a positive way, anxious eaters can also be poor role models for the other children at the table. This can be quite challenge in any home, especially for families where the anxious eater is older, subsequent eaters can watch the picky eater refusing many food offers and learn that that is the norm at mealtimes. Creating more peaceful mealtimes will help everyone.

Siblings need their own time with parents

It is easy to get into a situation where the worried eaters take up a disproportionate amount of time as worried parents try and try and try to *get them* to eat new foods or more foods. And then, there are all those appointments! Maybe the sibling has to stay home, left alone. Or, maybe the sibling needs to come to many appointments that are not theirs. Either way, it can be a challenge if it happens a lot.

Maybe family activities are restricted due to the worried eater's relationship with food. Perhaps the family can only go to one pizza place or can only bring pizza home and avoid restaurants altogether. Perhaps family events such a birthday parties or school events take on a whole different feel because of the eating restriction of the worried eater. Siblings will need their own time with parents as well as their own restaurant experiences.

Can parents set up special meals with the sibs? Perhaps they can go out to eat with each parent once a month to just have fun, try a new restaurant that otherwise would not have been a family choice, and to just have conversations that have nothing to do with the worried eaters issues?

Siblings need their own interests

Some siblings are worried because they feel their whole day is about the sibling who has special issues. Siblings not only need their own time with parents, they need to have their own interests. They need to be able find their own interests to be celebrated.

> **Dear Parent,**
>
> **How can you celebrate the siblings?**

Anxious Eaters at School

Anxious eaters can be particularly challenged eating at school. Mealtimes tend to be loud and very exciting, maybe too exciting, as lots of schoolmates eat enthusiastically. There is lots of sensory going on. Sounds of chairs scraping the floor as children pull up to and away from the table. Sounds of forks tapping on plates. Sounds of others talking and chewing. Sounds of plates dropping to the floor. Smells of cafeteria foods. Smells of your neighbor's pickles and tuna fish sandwich. Smells of the cleaning fluid the janitor uses to clean up. Smells! There are food textures, new and familiar. There is lots to see. There are the food differences, the many schoolmates, their foods, your child's foods, the view of friends mouths as they talk, giggle, and chew with open mouths. There is the school pizza that looks different today than it did last time. There is the school milk box that is a new brand and not the same box as last week. There is the texture of the milk spilling nearby, the texture of the pizza that changed because it is cooler today than it was last time it was served…and on and on and on. Sensory and sensory and more sensory.

And the time allowed for school meals is limited and requires very focused attention. With all the sensory distractions and eating challenges, many worried eaters run out of time to finish and end up hungry. If they only drink apple juice, but only water is allowed in classrooms, they then add thirst to the day. Hunger complicates mood. It complicates learning. Disruptions in both do not help them get the maximum benefit from their school experience. Some children may even be labeled behaviorally challenged when, in actuality, they just are not eating enough in the challenging environment of school.

It is no wonder many anxious eaters choose to eat alone as they get older and avoid the sensory chaos altogether. It is no wonder that teams often support anxious eaters by allowing them to eat separately at a different time or place or with a smaller group of classmates. It is no wonder that many anxious eaters prefer to bring their own lunch, the same foods, same brands, same packaging in the same lunch box. Their own lunch box can provide the only really predictable part of the school lunch time for them.

Your child's lunchbox

When your child is making a transition to a new school, there is lots to figure out. Consider how much is new for him. Because of the unpredictability of school mealtimes, worried eaters may cling to the routine or predictability of their own lunch. They may well need the same lunches (predictably packed) to come to school repeatedly until they *get* the school lunch routine, until they find their eating rhythm at school.

But remember, it is very easy to get in a rut of the exact same lunchbox foods offered in the exact same way. Once you have found that lunch box mealtime peace, can you gradually make some little changes so your child knows *change happens* in lunch boxes too? Could the plastic wrap be a color? Could the size of the zipper bags change from full size to snack so change is occurring around the food but initially not to the food? Could you have a conversation with your child that a new food will come to lunch each day and it can be tried when he is ready, or not. Can you child help pack his lunch so he has a rehearsal about what is in it?

Some parents decide to add a *new food trying container*, or a zipper-bagged-new-food to the child's lunch box, warning them in advance and reminding them they can try the food if they want, or not. *What try food can we put in your lunch box today? You can eat it only if you want.* When faced with new foods in this manner, sometimes children will choose to try them after they have had enough exposures to the new food in a non-pressured opportunity. The rehearsals that the food is coming, or that the child helped pack his own lunch will be very important to minimize the surprise of the new food presence.

Grocery store excursions

Sometimes we take a trip to the grocery store solely from Teddy's perspective. This visit is not when I stock up on family basics, but rather a time when I offer Teddy the opportunity to make food selections for his snacks or lunchbox. Often, when Teddy sees the packaging or items that he recognizes from his classmates' lunches he wants to buy them. He sees friends enjoying them and wants to try, too. Sometimes he may have a memory of having tried a food in the past and wants to have it again. It may not be on my radar at all! We also just walk through the colorful produce selection and often end up adding a few foods that I am simply not in the habit of purchasing. I may default to apples, bananas, and berries, but we may leave that day what a pomegranate and star fruit. Not everything that makes it into our cart

Create rehearsals

In order to help your child with change in his lunch box, you may need to create rehearsals at home first. Can he learn about new foods for school at home and when he is comfortable with them at home, can he help add them to his lunch box? Can he help put his food in different zipper bags or different sections of the box so he will know they are there? Can you make a lunch box with a surprise new food in it and open it together at home to practice his reaction? Can you and he practice touching it through the zipper bags and smelling or even trying it with finger or lip tastes? Help him apply his new food trying skills to his lunch box exploration.

Dear Parent,

How can you create *new food* rehearsals in your child's lunch box?

Peer modeling

School snacks or lunches can also be a great opportunity for your child to see others eating their foods nearby. He can see kids eating and enjoying different foods, that are not in their own usual routine. Many worried eaters find new foods they like when they have tried them in this setting. The novelty, the role modeling from peers, and the reduced pressure to try the foods can be an advantage. Your child will let you know if he is ready to learn from eating with school mates, or if they are not yet ready.

School parties

Many schools have food as a part of the curriculum or part of the many rewards and celebrations that occur. And these foods may or may not, often NOT, be familiar for your child. You may need to have a conversation with the teacher about your child's food worries. One option is to send in a package of a snack food your child does like, so he has options if there is no option available that day that is on his *List*. Another option is to find out some of the usual treat foods offered at school, and work on exposure to them at home. Yet another option is to become one of the classroom parents who provides these snacks and be sure to provide ones your child enjoys. And, many children will surprise you by just trying classroom treat foods because their friends are eating them. Give them the opportunity to be around those foods.

Teaching moments

Many parents tell us their frustrations when school personnel just do not understand. They can say things like *why do you send just junk food to school for your child? Or your child's lunch is not healthy OR we recommend every child's lunch has a fruit and /or vegetable.* As if it is YOUR WISH to send this brand of crackers, and this brand of chips and this exact box of juice every day!? Many parents say they would love to send ANYTHING else, but the change is just too much for their child. Parents feel judged and shamed when school professionals who do not understand your child's relationship with food offer advice. Unhelpful advice.

But, remember this. Until your child had these issues, you probably did not even know picky eaters, or anxious eaters existed. Right? Many well-meaning school personnel clearly do not understand your child's eating. Their comments, intended to nudge you into offering different foods, can feel very hurtful and shaming, but most likely they have no experience with a child who is a sensitive and worried eater. When you get over your hurt and anger, can you think of this as a teachable moment? Can you make an appointment with the school personnel and have a conversation about your child's eating, his challenges and what you are doing to support him? Can you let the teacher know that you could use her help in this effort and work out details that will improve your child's school mealtimes? Your child's feeding therapist or other supportive professionals can support families as they interface with schools. Ask them to help.

School lunches

No parent relishes packing lunch every day, and for parents of kiddos with restrictive eating it can feel especially burdensome. I have found that using the YumBox™ greatly helps me. I LOVE it! There's a bento-style tray, and each food group is labeled with a cute, friendly graphic. For the most part, I try to pack according to the food group labels, and that has definitely helped drive variety. For the less-preferred categories, I keep things super manageable and may only put one or two bites in those compartments. Think two blueberries or one small curl from a fresh carrot. On days when we have time, I pack most of the lunch and then show it to Teddy. "What do you think about your lunch?" That gives him the opportunity to suggest a food to fill one or two of the empty compartments, or if he really objects to something I have time to ditch it! ~Laura Wesp

Advocating for Your child

Feeding team specialists have experience and knowledge that is very important in getting to the bottom of the issues. They understand the medical and social complexities of eating. They know other families who struggle with these issues. They have ideas. But, the answer for your child lies in a cooperative partnership between you both. You know your child. You know the challenges your child is having with eating. You know mealtimes at your house. You are the advocate that will help your family navigate the system of support.

Perspective

This is a big issue for you. Eating well is an important issue for your child. Of course, you need to deal with the immediate medical and health challenges as they come up. But, for chronic anxious eaters with *List* foods, we want to also keep perspective. Your child may well be doing the best she can, given her life experiences, her wiring, and her skills. Your interactions need to go way beyond the daily mealtime struggles. Can you be your child's guide not her adversary along this journey of mealtime struggles?

Communication

Children generally want to eat, so when they do not eat well, or when change is the strongest influencing factor in eating, children will find whatever way they can to communicate that to us. They will let us know what is working and what is not, and it will be our adult collective job to listen and try to help. We want to find ways to celebrate and communicate our joy for who they are as a person not inadvertently communicate disappointment meal after meal.

Advocate with well-meaning relatives

Advocacy for your child can feel like a full-time job. Well-meaning relatives and friends who want to help but do not *get it* can be a source of sadness, frustration and anger. Their suggestions of *just make them hungry,* OR *if you did not just feed them junk food... OR in my day... OR stop spoiling your child* may not only **not** help but can put a wedge in your relationship. And, sadly these are the very people you would usually go to for support.

Remember that these well-meaning comments often come from a place of caring without a clear understanding of what you are going through. Others who have not been in your shoes, who have not tried to feed an anxious eater who has a *List* of specific favored foods can find it very hard to understand. Actually, YOU probably find it hard to understand when your child's choices are so personal and defy your usual logic. Can you advocate for your child and yourself by giving feedback to this person? Can you tell them more about the struggle and let them know you need their support, but not their judgment and that you and your child are doing the best you can? Do you need outside counseling support to strategize your responses to find ways your friends and relatives CAN better understand your situation? And there are many situations where that relative or friend just cannot *get it* and you need to find your support in other places as you advocate for your child.

Advocate with the pediatrician

The pediatrician is often the first medical professional to hear your concerns about your child's eating. This is a great starting point for many concerned parents. However, too many families have described feeling dismissed as they have related their worries about their anxious eaters. Pediatricians deal with parent concerns daily. So many parents of toddlers come in describing the typical toddler picky stages of eating and the usual pediatrician response is that the toddlers will outgrow this stage. And most do. (But not your child).

Pediatricians monitoring growth will often not have concerns about your child because so many anxious eaters are actually growing quite well with no major alarm bells going off on their growth charts. **But you know your child**. You know eating five or ten *List* foods in your child's *parentheses diet* is not normal, and not a healthy diet. If your pediatrician gives you advice that does not fit for what you see, give feedback. Explain your concerns further. Let them know you want help. You are the advocate who knows your level of worry about your child. If the pediatrician still does not hear your level of concern, consider a second opinion.

Advocate with the extended medical team

Many anxious eaters are referred to specialists, from feeding specialists to sensory specialists, gastroenterologists to allergists, dietitians to developmental specialists, psychologists to psychiatrists to rule out contributing factors in their eating limitations. Though they do not want to over diagnose eating challenges or create more worry than necessary, they also need to listen to you and your worry and not minimize the challenges you see in your children.

The team will help to rule out or treat any underlying medical difficulties that influenced your child's enjoyment of foods. Teams will make recommendations. They make the best recommendations they know based on their experience. Most times these recommendations will be the absolute best recommendations for your child. But sometimes the recommendations just **do not fit** for you and your family. Sometimes you just cannot make the ideas work at your home, or they just do not fit with your parenting style. Again, give feedback. The more the team can learn specifically about you, your beliefs, your parenting style for family mealtimes, the better they will be able to help you.

But remember, just because the underlying medical issue is being treated, does not mean that your child will all of a sudden start eating. Remember, the unique children we are discussing in this book have worries; they worry about change. In order NOT to push into their worry, we need to start from a place of calm and help them tiptoe toward change. It takes time for worried eaters to trust the mealtime peace that is presented. Just because a specialist says your child needs an expanded diet, or that you should add fruits and veggies, does not mean you are successful at *getting those in your child*. You need to partner with your team for the ideas and the strategies to make them successful for you and your child.

Your child's eating issues may require further testing and further discussions. Remember throughout that your child is listening, (See They are Listening chapter), and advocate for discussions about your child's eating to take place, as much as possible, without you child having to repeatedly hear, yet again, about what they are NOT doing.

Partner with the team

Probably no particular specialist is going to fix your child's eating. It will be your partnered effort with their input and your input, and you both finding ways to make successful, tiny steps of change at home.

Specific feeding therapy can help. Feeding specialists and teams can help determine the issues influencing your child's eating and help you break down the issues into tiny achievable steps. They can offer individual therapy as well as feeding group settings. They can offer ideas you can try at home. But this support needs to empower YOU also.

Here are some considerations when picking a feeding therapist or team members:

1. **Do they listen to YOUR concerns?**

   When you go to the team with your concerns, are they listening? Parents can feel that their worries are minimized and sometimes even feel blame from team members. This is probably not helpful! Give them feedback. You need to feel you are being heard.

2. **Is the support timely?**

   No parent wants to be put on a four-month waiting list when their child is not eating. That is not okay! Mealtimes happen every day, multiple times. You need support **now**. Your worry grows and the problems can actually get worse as your child is continuing to practice anxious meals with anxious interactions. Find the support that understands that these are powerful worries and that support needs to be timely.

3. **Do they seem to understand YOUR child?**

   Does the team seem knowledgeable? Do they seem to *get* what is going on with your child? Do you feel they are taking an individual approach or fitting your child into a mold? You can provide the specialist with more information, take videos of what you see at home, and have conversations. If they still do not seem to understand your child in the sensitive way you prefer, you might consider a second opinion.

4. **Does your child enjoy interactions with the team, individual or group activity?**

   Does your child enjoy going to feeding therapy? Is he happy to be there or does he actually have an increase in his worry? Many parents tell us their child cries when he sees the parking lot of the clinic. Or fights and gags or vomits regularly in therapy sessions? We absolutely do not want to create therapy situations where your child is increasing his worry. We do not want therapy to be experienced as another pressure? We do not want the situations we choose to help children to be causing increased trauma and adding to their memory bank of negative experiences. If your child is not enjoying the therapy, can you discuss this with the specialist and find ways to grade the asks and tiptoe from the starting point of success? Can you and the team make the changes that must be made to reduce pressure and worry?

5. **Are their ideas realistic in YOUR home?**

Is the team making suggestions that fit for you in your home? Are they giving you enough suggestions that work or are they overwhelming you with too many suggestions that are just not achievable in your home? Many therapy suggestions work well. That is why feeding teams make those suggestions. However, they may not work in your home. You may have triplets and need to balance the suggestions with your reality. Maybe you do not have the funds to purchase sixteen new therapeutic foods. Maybe your family does not eat cheese? Maybe you do not like food play at your house and just cannot *do messy*. The ideas must be able to work in the context of your day-to-day life.

Have a conversation with the specialist to help her understand how you are feeling about the suggestions and ask for help in adapting them to your situation. Discuss your family food choices and eating preferences. Provide a video so the clinician can see your family mealtime scenario and better help you adjust your *asks* in your home.

6. **Are their suggestions helping you and your child make change or are you working on the same goals forever?**

Many families describe working on the same goals for months and months. You do not see progress when the same goal lingers for months and months, but also you are losing valuable time that your child could be experiencing mealtimes in a new way. Is the team starting from familiar, safe and mealtime peace? Are they grading the *asks* small enough that your child can be comfortable with the stretch toward new mealtime interactions, new trying and new foods?

7. **Does the team empower YOU to be successful?**

Are you being successful at home? Are you able to transition clinic success to home success? Are you given ideas on what you can do daily to see success at home? To be successful at home, you need to be included in the therapy settings so you can participate and see what ideas would be comfortable at home. Too many times clinicians give a standard list of ideas that they have not specifically tried with your child. Ask the clinician if you can try them together in the therapeutic situation so that you can try them at home. (See Bridging New Foods at Home chapter.)

Advocacy Checklist

☐ Do they listen to YOUR concerns?
☐ Is the support timely?
☐ Do they understand YOUR child?
☐ Does your child enjoy interactions with the team, individual or group activity?
☐ Are their ideas realistic in YOUR home?
☐ Are their suggestions helping you and your child make change or are you working on the same goals forever?
☐ Does the team empower YOU to be successful?

Advocate with school

Your child's eating issues affect his eating at school. You will need to be his voice at school to advocate for the optimum environment for your child to eat meals at school. (See Anxious Eaters at School chapter.)

Advocate for yourself

And, in order to take care of y our child and your family, you will need to take care of yourself. (See Taking Care of Yourself chapter.)

The constant stream of advice from well-meaning observers can become tiresome. It seems as if everyone believes he or she has the one idea that will unlock my son's restrictive eating. When you are in the trenches doing everything you can, I know that unsolicited advice can be annoying at best and hurtful at worst. It's helped me to categorize these comments in two ways: 1) "He looks fine to me," or, 2) "Have you tried this..." On the surface, the first type of comment can feel like marginalizing the issue and the second seems like judgment. By looking a little deeper, I've learned to reframe those two phrases into something more helpful.

Rather than feeling misunderstood by the "can't see it/don't acknowledge it" comments, I try to take them as a compliment that Teddy looks healthy and vibrant. With his medical condition it's very hard for him to maintain a healthy weight. I know what has gone into getting him to that point, and it's a lot of work!! So, when told that he looks "fine," I've learned to reply with, "Thank you, he has an excellent medical team and I'm very grateful."

When confronted with the "have you tried?" type of advice, I try to see this through the eyes of compassion. Whoever is offering advice is really saying, "I wish this were different for you." I have dubbed this type of advice the "chicken nugget" comment, because it reminds me of a time when I was serving Teddy grilled chicken and he was being pretty adamant in his refusal. A well-intended observer looked at me and, in all seriousness, asked, "Have you tried chicken nuggets?" I had to muster a lot of patience in that moment to maintain a kind smile as I replied that yes, I had indeed tried chicken nuggets.

Inside my head I was screaming, "YES, about 1,000 times!" I've found it a lot easier to brush off the never-ending suggestions about what works for someone else by just saying in my head, "Oh, that's a chicken nugget comment." While thinking that, I find the grace to say, "Thanks; I'll give it a try." ~Laura Wesp

Taking Care of Yourself

When your child is an anxious eater you invest a lot of energy (and emotion) to improve the situation, *get your child to eat*, balance his diet, get to appointments and *fix things*. But you need also to find time, to make time, to take care of yourself. I remember a psychologist friend who once described our energy level as a basket of apples. She had us consider that when we do for others, help others, it is like giving them an apple from our basket each time. We give out apples over and over again. Apples in our basket diminish. We need to find ways to fill our apple basket back up before we run completely out. We need to give back to ourselves to refill that basket. If you run out of apples, it is hard to help your anxious eater! Let's think of ways you can replenish your apple basket.

Nourish your relationship with your child

Are you nourishing your relationship with your child in ways that have nothing to do with eating more or eating differently? Pull that video camera on your life back to see the bigger picture. Is your main interaction with your child 4-5 times a day all about coming to the meal, eating the food, the bites, staying at the table, and trying new things? If it is a struggle, and is hard on you and hard on him, you are using up a lot of apples. Can you replenish the apple basket by finding other special things to do with your child? Read a book, take a walk, play with the puppy, listen to music, do homework, do something, anything, that has nothing to do with *take a bite* and everything to do with enjoying your time together?

Nourish YOU

You are worth it, too! What do you need to do to nourish YOU? Are you finding any time during the day, or week, for celebrating YOU? Maybe it is a bubble bath, reading a book, feeding YOURSELF good food, taking a walk, talking with a friend, having a date with your partner? Are you nurturing YOUR interests? And *yourself*?

Remember to feed yourself good foods that make YOU feel healthy. Can you sometimes grocery shop for those special ingredients that could go into a gourmet sandwich or scallop dinner that are YOUR favorites? (Someone else in the family might just try them!) Exercise regularly to feel your best. Start at your starting point of exercise and tip toe toward more healthful and varied exercise. Keep hydrated and, while keeping yourself hydrated, offer your child a drink to keep her hydrated. ☺

Sometimes you need a break

Sometimes nurturers just need to take some time off. Parents need a break. Sometimes that could be a date that allows the baby sitter or grandparents to take over for an evening. Sometimes is it other parent's turn to do the cooking? Sometimes could you order out take-out food? Sometimes is it scheduling a babysitter so you can have a nap? Even though we recommend eating with your child as great opportunities for multiple positive exposures to food, can you declare a night where grownups-eat-alone-with-candles-night where you just feed the kids and then have your own grown up meal later?

Nourish your relationship with food

When there are anxious eaters in the house, mealtimes and food prep can become highly stressful. You create a new dish and no one wants it? Do find yourself eating the same foods every night and they are *kids foods* not *your taste* in foods? Have you become a short order cook making a different meal for each family member? Did you used to love to cook and now you hate it? What can you do to nourish *your* relationship with food?

Can you get away for a meal by yourself with partner or friends where you can order ANYTHING you want and *someone else* fixes it? Can you create a few new recipes that you enjoy, knowing that if no one else likes them, YOU will have delicious leftovers?

Let others help you

Can you let others help you? It has been said that it takes a village to raise a child. It takes a committee of loving grownups to nurture and nourish your whole child, and I do not just mean his diet. Can you cultivate and celebrate the support systems in your life? Can you let grandparents help when they ask? Maybe they are able to babysit so you can have a break, or maybe prepare a dinner once a week? Maybe they do not fully understand your child's eating issues, but they certainly can make some food you like! Can you include them in your anxious eater's life in other ways that celebrate who he is, rather than the foods that he does not eat? We love it when children can be celebrated by multiple grownups!

You may need to cultivate those babysitter options so that you will have the option of breaks. You will not always find the perfect babysitter the first time but try and try again because in the long run, it will be worth it to have a sitter you trust with your children so you can have breaks. Once we found the best baby sitter for my children, I remember telling them *you boys get to spend the evening with* (babysitter) *Mandy on Friday* and they would shout *hooray* in celebration and look forward to it. It took away any guilt I may have had about leaving them for the evening while my husband and I re-charged our own parenting batteries. And once you have a babysitter who really understands your child's eating worries, babysitting time can include multiple exposures to new foods. Perhaps you and the babysitter can plan some playful and fun food preparation interactions to have together with your child during their time together. Maybe together they can make some part of the dinner meal so your child's participation gets to be celebrated.

Growing an anxious eater is hard work. I realized friends and family wanted to help but had no idea how. I kept isolating myself. I had an idea that has made all the difference. When my daughter was at school one day I had a few friends over for lunch. I described the worries, mine and my child's, in detail. I told them I knew they wanted to help and understood that they just did not know how. They asked how they could help.

I asked if they could help me take some of the mealtime pressure off if they could each make an evening meal for our family once a month. They were thrilled to help. It was unbelievable how that helped us! I would look forward to those nights when I knew, I did not have to make the meal. (Of course, I still usually needed to figure out my anxious eater's food, but it was such a treat for ME that food was being created for ME). Truthfully, I had not realized how I was hating cooking, eating and mealtimes in general. Now I actually looked forward to these nights. And several friends have brought meals over a couple times a month! My friends are happy helping in the way they can and I am happy with their gift of love. ~Appreciative Parent

Support

Sometimes the best gift you can give yourself is the gift of some counseling to help you put all the worries of mealtime and parenting in perspective. Individual counseling can help you understand your emotions in this situation and help make the changes you want to make. Many clinics have feeding support group options for parents of anxious eaters to discuss the common challenges in feeding these children. If your child's feeding clinic does not have a group, ask them to start one!

Give yourself permission to be human

As an overachiever, I fully understand those who want to do it all and be a perfect parent. As you read this book, maybe you are not starting at mealtime peace. Maybe your family meals are currently out of balance. It is okay. You meant well. You were trying to help. Give yourself permission to consider this your starting point. You are human!! You know now how to tiptoe toward more success with tiny steps for your child, and for yourself.

Find a balance

Every consultant you ask has suggestions for how you can help your child. This one has three. This one has six. This one has thirteen. You can be enthusiastic about the suggestions when you are face to face with them at the consultations, but three plus six plus thirteen is twenty-two suggestions! These suggestions add up and where is the time in the day to carry out twenty-two suggestions going to come from? Chances are the time comes out of YOU time, family time, sibling time, daily *life* time! The time you spend on each suggestion is time you are not spending on something else. To find a balance, you will probably need to figure out which suggestions make the most sense for you and your family and think about how can they become a part of your day? How can these ideas be incorporated into your natural routine and without the need to do a three-hour prescriptive therapy routine every single day? Ask your team members for help in finding this balance if you need to. How can these ideas be naturally included in your day or week? Talking with other parents can help, too.

Dealing with Frustration

I am writing this after making pancakes with Teddy and building fruit kebabs. I also presented a yogurt squeezer, feeling proud of the balanced breakfast I'd made. After all that effort, my son tried one bite of the pancakes and declared them yucky. He did eat three small bites of fruit, but then requested something "crunchy." He ended up eating half of a Ritz cracker. It can be extremely frustrating to plan and make meal after meal and have them so frequently rejected.

I have heard the suggestions to involve Teddy with as much of the food prep as possible. I take him shopping with me and do my best to engage him in the kitchen. Even so, we still deal with frequent refusals. The urge to give up can be tempting. One sanity-saving strategy is to have a few meals off. I try to find one or two meals each week when I can eat somewhere other than home and just enjoy a meal that someone else prepared for _me._ Daily exercise also really helps me deal with the constant stress. Carving out time for myself is as much a benefit for my family as it is for me. I reach that point of discouragement or frustration a lot sooner when I haven't built in mini breaks for myself! Give yourself permission to take care of yourself! ~Laura Wesp

Summary Hugs

I have described this journey in words, in pictures, in my voice and the voices of parents. It is my hope that each reader has found some answers, or at least some more good questions to ask. It is my hope that parents and medical professionals both have some new ideas or a new perspective, or some glimmers of strategies to add to what is already working in their feeding journeys with anxious eaters. My heartfelt wish is that you are able to find ways to celebrate your child and yourself.

There are many words and phrases unique to this book. Mealtime peace, *change happens*, here to there, rehearsals and Re-define TRY IT and s-t-r-e-t-c-he-s are some. For those interested, I have included a glossary to follow that can help you think about the ideas in this book in a kind of summary list. If it helps, use it and share it. The pictures in the book are meant to provide a visual for the ideas shared. If some are meaningful to you at the place you are in the journey, I encourage you to photocopy them and put them up on your refrigerator as a small reminder. Particularly popular ones are Yet, Celebrate, Mealtime Peace, and the Circle of Sensitivity Hugs, but you may have your own favorite.

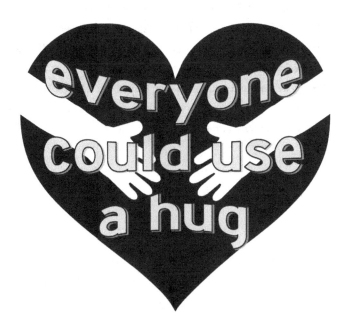

It is a journey.

Maybe because cars are often top-of-mind as the mom to two boys — we watch car movies, race toy cars, build Lego cars, and practically live in our car — these road trip analogies come to mind as I reflect on our story with eating challenges.

1. **This is not a one-lap race.** This is a cross-country journey with detours and road-blocks. It is not for the faint at heart, and you will not be the same because of it.

2. **You will need to stop and refuel.** Use the rest stops! For me this means exercise and stepping away. For my son, it means trips to the park and just getting breaks from meals and food. ~~work.~~ For our family it may also mean take out. Do what you can to care for yourself.

3. **Know when to change lanes.** I desperately wanted to drive in the fast lane, but we were burning out. For our family, we needed to find a pace and an approach that was sustainable and pleasant. Now that we've chosen the slow lane, we find that we enjoy the journey a lot more.

4. **Road trips are better with friends.** Reach out to other parents facing similar challenges, even if they are hundreds of miles away.

5. **When you are broken down, let others help.** (Advice more easily spoken than taken!)

6. **Don't fight with the other passengers.** Remember they are on this journey, too. Think about it like riding down the road. The view from the windshield is not the same as the view out the side window. My husband and I do not approach feeding in the same way. He doesn't attend therapy sessions, read books, or watch video tutorials about feeding! Sometimes it's easy for me to lose patience with him, but our family runs best when I realize that different can be a very positive thing.

7. **There is no map** and your destination may be unclear. There is no guarantee that your child will ever become an "adventurous" eater. Enjoy the now! Try your best to enjoy your journey and your child. ~Laura Wesp

Anxious Eater Anxious Mealtime Glossary

Active Encouragement: Active encouragement is a sensitive and responsive way to encourage children to learn something new. It is an *ask* with a choice. It is a way to creatively invite or encourage a child to interact with a new food, or mealtime experience without pushing into their worry. It may use words, interesting plates and utensils, and interesting interactions or choices to help the child WANT to interact. It is not a requirement or demand. The child is making the choice to participate. It is a strategy to help them develop internal motivation to eat. There can be no pressure.

Anxious Eaters: For the purpose of this book, we are describing children who are worried about mealtime change as anxious eaters. Anxious is used colloquially as a descriptor of these eaters. The word worry is often used interchangeably in description of these children.

ARFID: Avoidant restrictive food intake disorder, an eating disorder diagnosis found in the Diagnostic and Statistics Manual of Mental Disorders, Fifth Edition.

Ask: This is the offer. This is what we *ask* children to do. We will be careful that our *ask* is the right safety *ask*, developmental *ask,* sensory *ask*, motor *ask*, emotional *ask* and independence *ask*.

Beginning and an End: When there is worry, it helps to have information. When there is a beginning and an end to the activity, children are more able to take themselves out of their immediate comfort zone to try something new, briefly. For example, when ask a child to hand something to someone else he may be more willing to touch that new food because he can see the end of the activity.

Binder Foods: These are foods that stick together in your mouth like mashed potatoes or refried beans. They can be mashed with the tongue and swallowed whole or with minimal chewing.

Bouquet of Straws: The child is offered several straws in a cup, like a bouquet, when drinking a drink and can choose *which straw is next? And now which straw?* It can be a strategy that dilutes the worry as children make the choice to take in more volume.

Brand S-t-r-e-t-c-h: This is a s-t-r-e-t-c-h from one brand of a particular food to another brand starting with familiar.

Change Happens: This is a strategy in support of anxious eaters. We want to help them be comfortable with *change happens* at mealtimes. This is very important for worried eaters who require every part of the meal to be the *same*. We begin *change happens* at the edges of worry, rather than pushing right into it.

Circle of Sensitivity: This is a visual with a heart in the center and layers around that heart. The heart represents the child's new food trying, eating and enjoyment in the center. The layers around that heart represent the layers of protection that the child creates to protect him from worry. To help the child try new foods, we tiptoe toward the center of this circle of sensitivity toward his worry one tiny step at a time, one layer at a time, so he can enjoy the process and so we do not push directly into their worry. We move toward that heart in a continuum of tiny steps here to there.

Circle of Sensitivity Hug: This is the concept that we can become a child's new food trying guide and embrace their efforts to try new foods, not push into their worry. We want worried eaters to feel our arms around them physically or emotionally in encouragement as they bravely try new foods.

Complimentary S-t-r-e-t-c-h: This is a s-t-r-e-t-c-h from one food to another in the same flavor category, for example, one berry yogurt to another, starting with familiar.

Confidence: We aim for confidence with food when children find new foods they like. Can they confidently eat that food in new ways (motor asks) and with different people, in different places, different utensils? This helps establish that food more securely into the routine.

Confidence S-t-r-e-t-c-h: These are s-t-r-e-t-c-h-e-s accomplished by giving practice opportunities with a new food by offering the familiar new foods in different presentations. For example, you can offer the new food off of different spoons, bowls, cups or straws to build motor and emotional confidence in that newly presented foods.

Continuum: A continuum is continuous sequence in which adjacent elements are not perceptibly different from each other, although the extremes are quite distinct. These are the tiny steps from here to there.

Crumb Kisses: These are crumbs left on the lips from kissing a pile of crumbs. This is a way to get friendly with crumbs without worrying about them on the tongue (YET)

Demand: To ask brusquely or in an authoritarian fashion. Synonyms include order, command, urge. It is the opposite of an offer.

Dilute the *Ask*: We want to dilute the worry when trying new foods if the worry is great. We can do this by masking some of the sensory variables such as putting a lid on a new drink to mask (dilute) the new smell or by offering a new food in the tiniest amount paired with a familiar food such as offering the grasshoppers with tortilla and guacamole! We can also dilute the ask with a distraction that reduces the worry such as focusing on the mouth math or touching a new food by handing it off quickly to another person. A Sandwich TRY dilutes the *ask*. A s-t-r-e-t-c-h dilutes the *ask*. Re-Define TRY IT dilutes the *ask*.

Dip and Stir: This is a strategy for offering the tiniest flavor (or color) change in a drink by dipping a straw, stirrer or spoon in a juice, nectar or puree and stirring it in the drink making the slightest change.

Distant Sensory: These are the sensory variables of looking, smelling and touching foods with fingers, that give a rehearsal or preview of the new food without it needing to go into the mouth yet.

Division of Responsibility: This is a theory which Ellyn Satter[21,22] uses to describe the division of child and adult responsibilities during mealtime. She tells us it is the adult responsibility to decide the menu, the where and the when of mealtimes and the child responsibility to decide how much to eat, and if they want to eat the food offered.

Dry Meltables: These are dry foods that melt easily or mix easily in saliva, requiring minimal grinding chews.

Enjoyment: Enjoyment is one of our goals for children in search of new foods to like. The sensory aspects of the foods have a lot to do with the enjoyment of the food. The tastes, textures, smells, sounds, and sights of foods contribute to the enjoyment. We are looking for what foods does your child love.

Established Foods: These are foods well established in the child's diet that the child will comfortably eat most of the time when offered. We try to *establish* new foods with multiple tastes and practice and confidence s-t-r-e-t-c-h-e-s after the child shows she likes them.

Externally Motivated Eating: The child is eating because of external factors such as pressure, the adult said so; the adult decides what and how much he is to eat; the adults continue the meal until the adult determines it is the end of the meal; the adult gives reinforcers, treats, praise for the child to eat. This is not internally motivated, child directed eating.

Familiar: Familiar is the starting point for new food trying. What foods does the child love? Since new food trying can be worrisome for our anxious eaters, we always start with a familiar food, or familiar routine or familiar activity so the child starts from a comfortable place. We tiptoe from there!

Favored Foods: These are preferred foods, comfortable foods, foods on the *List*.

Feed the Birds: In this activity we ask a child to put a food in her mouth (or between her lips) and spit it out (maybe outside near a bush) to feed the birds. This is spitting out practice and it has a beginning and an end. It can be a limited sensory exposure to that food. It is a way to refine oral motor planning skills as well as be introduced to new food flavors, or textures in the mouth, briefly.

Finger Taste: The act of tasting foods by rubbing the finger on or in the food then tasting it. This is often done first with flavor only and then with taste that also includes texture.

Flavor: Flavor, for the purpose of this book, is defined as the taste of the food without the texture, as in rubbing a finger on an apple and then tasting it.

Flavor S-t-r-e-t-c-h: This is a s-t-r-e-t-c-h from a familiar flavor to a new flavor with tiny steps along the way. The flavor does include texture, just flavor.

Food Academics: The use of foods in pre-academic activities such as color, size alphabet, math and shape sorting as a way to provide a multiple food exposure interaction.

Food Rehearsals: Interactions with foods in a variety of ways that allow the child to learn about the food without the requirement to try or taste it.

Garnish: This is a piece of food put on a plate to decorate the plate. Teaching about garnishing is a way to have a child understand this is an extra food on everyone's plate that can just be there and is not required to be eaten. It can be an activity that bridges to acceptance of new and unfamiliar foods on the plate. We encourage children to participate in garnishing, or that garnishing become a mealtime routine.

Goal Foods: These are foods or food groups parents would really like their child to be able to eat.

Grade the *Ask*: Grading the *ask* is the strategy of offering the child a new food to try that has a careful *ask*. In other words, are we offering the new foods in a sensitive, calibrated way that takes into consideration the child's skills and experiences as well as the specific sensory properties of the new foods. We can grade the safety *ask*, the developmental *ask*, the sensory *ask*, the motor *ask*, emotional *ask* and independence *ask*.

Hard Chewables: These are foods (or mouthing toys) that are hard, that can be mouthed and explored to help the child learn more about her mouth, tongue, jaw, chewing and food exploration. They need to be safe and not easily broken off as a choking hazard. They are used with care and supervision.

Here: The starting place of what works for the child. What works today, *here* and now? This could be a feeder, a food, a texture, flavor or sensory property, utensil, a particular environment or presentation.

Internally Motivated Eating: We are looking for eating to be internally motivated, where the child determines the *amount* and the *what* of eating. The child makes those decisions. This is in contrast with externally motivated eating where the parents decide how much the child will eat or provides external motivators such as pressure, toys and rewards or "I am proud of you" praise for eating.

Ice Cube Meltables: An ice cube meltable is a strategy of adding a flavored ice cube to a familiar drink to change the flavor, smell, color or temperature in a very gradual way.

Lip Balm (or Lipstick) Flavor: This is a flavor put on the lips with a finger, or put on with the actual food, that is similar to putting on lip balm or lipstick. Because this is a flavor, it has taste, but not residual texture. The flavor is not required to go in the mouth, but on the lips. It is a way to help the child get the food near the nose for smelling, and in the vicinity of the tongue if he wants to lick lips. There is not residual texture. This might be achieved by rubbing a finger on a cucumber and then putting that flavor on the lips, or rubbing an actual cucumber pieces on lips.

Lip Balm (or Lipstick) Taste: This is a lip taste that is flavor with texture put on with a finger or utensils similar to putting on lip balm or lipstick. This taste is not required to go in the mouth. It is a way to help the child get the food near the nose for smelling, and in the vicinity of the tongue if he wants to lick lips. There is residual texture. Dipping a finger in a new sauce and rubbing it on the lips could be a lip balm or lipstick taste, as it leaves the sauce on the lips.

Lip Taste: This is the strategy of tasting a new food at the lips and not yet at the tongue. This taste would be a lip flavor if it was taste alone without texture and a lip taste would be the flavor with texture (as in puree or crumbs).

List **Foods**: These are the favored foods the child eats daily. This is the narrow diet that includes qualifiers, descriptors, parentheses. This is the *List* the child will eat, must eat, no deviations.

Look S-t-r-e-t-c-h: This is a s-t-r-e-t-c-h that changes the look of a food or drink, starting from familiar.

Mealtime Peace: Mealtime peace is the starting point for this journey of mealtime change. It is that peaceful place that no longer causes the mealtime to be a battlefield of stress and worry for everyone. No pressure.

Meltables: These are dry foods that dissolve easily in saliva and require minimal or only beginning chewing before swallowing.

Mouth Math: This is the activity of doing math with the mouth, such as figuring out how many frozen peas are in the mouth or subtracting (spitting out) one pea and how many are left or counting the cereal pieces in the mouth with the tongue. The math as part of the activity can dilute the worry focus of trying a new food.

Multiple Exposure Rehearsals: Multiple exposures are those food interactions that included watching others eat and prepare foods and interact with foods without the *requirement* to taste or try them. These include inviting the child to the table, modeling mealtime interactions and routines, including the child in family food related activities. They are one of the important types of rehearsals.

New Food Try-er: We call children who are learning to try new foods new food try-ers.

New Food Trying: We describe a continuum of ways to try new foods. Some children like the Sandwich TRY where the new food is paired with a familiar food, such as a tiny taste put between two pieces of bread to dilute the look, flavor, texture and smell of the new food. Some learn finger tastes. Some learn new foods through s-t-r-e-t-c-h-e-s and others need to completely Re-define TRY IT.

Negative Tilt: The negative tilt occurs when the adult offers the food and the child adamantly leans away from the adult and the food. This is not part of the normal pacing of the meal. It is a strong response that comes from a history of multiple negative experiences with the mealtime.

Offer: The offer is the food (or activity) the adult invites the child to try with no demand that they MUST try it.

Pair it with Familiar: Offer a new food with a familiar food to dilute the flavor, smell, and texture *ask*. This type of new food try could also be called a s-t-r-e-t-c-h.

Parentheses Diet: The parentheses diet is what we are calling the restricted diet of favored foods for an anxious eater that includes the specific qualifiers of each that specify particular qualities in that food, the need for same brand, flavor, presentation, taste, or texture. The *List*.

Positive Tilt: The positive tilt of mealtime occurs when the adult offers the foods and the child leans toward the adult or food, physically or emotionally, to indicate a readiness to accept or try that food.

Pressure: The use of persuasion, influence, or intimidation to make someone do something. This is what we are trying to avoid at mealtimes!

Pressure Free Zone: This is what we call the mealtime where there is no pressure. No conversation about trying to eat, or eat more, or take a bite. We encourage the family to get back to a pleasant, no pressure mealtime environment.

Puree to Puree: This is the concept that purees vary widely in their texture and that we need to consciously give opportunities of children worried about new and worried about sensory change to systematically try new and expanded puree textures. We want to help a child s-t-r-e-t-c-h from one puree to another with careful asks.

Pushing into Worry: This is an offer that is too great an *ask*. The child pulls away, worried, and instead of a careful pivot to a new lesser, successful ask, the grownup pushes the child more into their worry, creating more pressure, worry and more resistance.

Re-Define TRY IT: We have re-defined what we mean by the expression *TRY IT* by breaking new food trying into tiny less worrisome steps for worried eaters that tiptoe through a Circle of Sensitivity.

Rehearsals: Experiences that provide children with information, a preview, about what to expect in upcoming food interactions. Multiple food exposures are rehearsals. There are also two types of sensory rehearsals, distant sensory rehearsals and up-close sensory rehearsals. Rehearsals help reduce the worry.

Sandwich TRY: This is a new food trying method where the new food is paired with a familiar food to dilute the *ask*. It is a way to pair the new food with a familiar food. An example would be sandwiching a new taste of cheese between two tiny pieces of read or two crackers. The bread and crackers dilute the smell, flavor and texture *ask*.

Scatter foods: These are foods that separate or scatter in your mouth like peas or crackers, white rice. Due to their scatter properties they require more oral organization to get them in the bolus form of readiness to swallow.

Sensory Rehearsals: These are food interactions that bring the child close to the distant and near sensory properties of the food as a preview to trying or eating it.

Sensory Step Down: This is the concept that there is a hierarchy of difficulty along a continuum in new food trying and sometimes we ask too much of a child and need to step down the sensory *ask*. For example, if a child is asked to taste a food and is uncomfortable with that he could be asked to lick it, kiss it, or even just touch it to hand it to someone. If even that is too much, he could touch your hand while YOU hand it to someone. The goal is to make the *ask* achievable and step down slightly going from your original ask, quickly to success without having the child spend much time in a state of worry.

Sensory Surprises: A sensory surprise occurs when your mouth expects one particular food texture or flavor and unexpectedly gets another. Avoid these!

Sometimes Foods: These are foods that, when offered, will sometimes be eaten and sometimes not. Parents often describe these foods as unsure foods, foods that they cannot count on, but foods that may be eaten now and then.

S-t-r-e-t-c-h: A s-t-r-e-t-c-h is new food trying technique that helps a child learn to like a new food or food property in tiny steps starting from a familiar food or food property. You s-t-r-e-t-c-h from familiar.

Success: Important for both parent and child. ☺

Systematic Desensitization: A process of that uses principles of classical conditioning to replace a person's phobia, or fear response, with a new response in a systematic way.

Taste: The taste includes the flavor and texture of the food.

Texture S-t-r-e-t-c-h: A s-t-r-e-t-c-h from one textured food to another in tiny steps.

There: Our goal, where we want to end up. (Enjoyment, confidence and internal motivation) *Here* was the starting point, *there* is the end point

The *List*: This is the list of the favored food or preferred foods comfortably eaten by an anxious eater. It includes parentheses qualifiers.

The NOW of Eating: This is a way to describe what the child **currently** does at mealtime, what the current mealtime is like, what works and does not work about the current mealtime. The NOW.

The THEN of Eating: This is the collective eating experience until now, the eating history, the eating memories and eating experiences that have led to the NOW meal-time interactions. Children and parents bring the memories of the THEN mealtime experiences to the table.

The YET of Eating: This is the hope for future change at mealtimes, the **not quite yet** of skills and food interactions. For example, instead of saying Nancy cannot chew, we would say Nancy is not yet able to chew. OR Barb likes very smooth baby food textures and is **not yet** comfortable with more textured purees. **Yet** gives hope.

Tongue Taste: This is a taste on the tongue. It can be flavor only or a taste that includes texture.

Touch Sequence: This is a sequence of handing the food to someone else and then getting comfortable with the texture of the food in the palm as a rehearsal to new food trying.

Up-Close Sensory Rehearsals: These are sensory rehearsals where the child is interacting with the foods in a way that provide her with near sensory variables of close smell, vision, sound and taste and mouth texture.

Used to Foods: These are foods that used to be on the *List* and are no longer accepted or eaten.

Vitamin Crumb S-t-r-e-t-c-h: This is a s-t-r-e-t-c-h to help the child eat a vitamin using the crumb stretch principles.

Wait Wait, Pivot: This is the stated or unstated moment of "wait, wait", where the grownup pauses after a child's "no" and then pivots to a lesser sensory or emotional *ask*, a sensory step down. The grownup might offer a piece of banana for the child to smell and the child seems disgusted, worried. Instead of pushing into the worry or ending the activity right then, the grownup says something like, "Wait, wait, can you help me put this food away?"

Worry Diluter: Using a worry diluter is a way to reduce the worry of new food interactions for an anxious eater. Sometimes it dilutes the worry to mask the sensory properties of that new foods by pairing it with another familiar food as in a Sandwich TRY. (Ex. Grasshoppers with guacamole!) Sometimes the diluter is a conversation, a distraction, or the novelty of the presentation.

Yet: Gives hope. Not now, but later.

References

1   Dweck, C. S. (2008). *Mindset: The new psychology of success*. Random House Digital, Inc.

2   Dweck, Carol S. "The Power of Yet." *TED*. https://youtu.be/J-swZaKN2Ic, 12 Sept. 2014.

3   Oxford Online Dictionary. Retrieved 19 April 2019 from https://en.oxforddictionaries.com/

4   Bailey, R. A. (2015). *Conscious discipline: Building resilient classrooms*. Loving Guidance.

5   Birch, L. L. (1999). Development of food preferences. *Annual review of nutrition, 19*(1), 41-62.

6   Galloway, A. T., Fiorito, L. M., Francis, L. A., & Birch, L. L. (2006). Finish your soup: counter-productive effects of pressuring children to eat on intake and affect. *Appetite, 46*(3), 318-323.

7   Star Institute. https://www.spdstar.org

8   Zickgraf, H. & Mayes, S. D. (2018). Psychological, Health, and Demographic Correlates of Atypical Eating Behaviors in Children with Autism. *Journal of Developmental and Physical Disabilities*, 1-20.

9   American Psychiatric Association (2013). Autism Spectrum Disorders. In *Diagnostic and statistical manual of mental disorders*. 5th ed. Arlington, VA: American Psychiatric Association.

10   Cormack, J. (2018, October 10). How to Help a Child with Autism Feel Good About Food. In *Issue 75 – Helping Your Child with Autism Thrive. Autism Parenting Magazine*. Retrieved from https://www.autismparentingmagazine.com/autism-feel-good-about-food/

11   Fisher, M.M., Rosen, D.S., Ornstein, R.M., Mammel, K.A., Katzman, D.K., Rome, E.S., Callahan, S.T., Malizio, J., Kearney, S. and Walsh, B.T. (2014). Characteristics of avoidant/restrictive food intake disorder in children and adolescents: a "new disorder" in DSM-5. *Journal of Adolescent Health, 55*(1), pp.49-52.

12   Goday, P.S., Huh, S.Y., Silverman, A., Lukens, C.T., Dodrill, P., Cohen, S.S., Delaney, A.L., Feuling, M.B., Noel, R.J., Gisel, E. and Kenzer, A. (2019). Pediatric feeding disorder: Consensus definition and conceptual framework. *Journal of pediatric gastroenterology and nutrition, 68*(1), p.124.

13   Feeding Matters. https://www.feedingmatters.org

14   Just, M. A., Cherkassky, V. L., Keller, T. A., & Minshew, N. J. (2004). Cortical activation and synchronization during sentence comprehension in high-functioning autism: evidence of underconnectivity. *Brain, 127*(8), 1811-1821.

15   Pliner,P. & Loewen, E. R. (1997). Temperament and food neophobia in children and their mothers. *Appetite, 28*(3), 239-254.

16   Green, S. A. & Ben-Sasson, A. (2010). Anxiety disorders and sensory over-responsivity in children with autism spectrum disorders: is there a causal relationship? *Journal of autism and developmental disorders, 40*(12), 1495-1504.

17   Merriam-Webster Online Dictionary. Retrieved 19 April 2019, from https://www.merriam-webster.com/dictionary/

18 Collins Online Dictionary. Retrieved 19 April 2019, from https://www.collinsdictionary.com/us/

19 The Free Online Dictionary. Retrieved 19 April 2019, from https://www.thefreedictionary.com/

20 Morris, S. E. & Klein, M. D. (2000). *Pre-feeding skills: A comprehensive resource for mealtime development.* Austin, Texas. ProEd.

21 Satter, E. (2012). *Child of mine: Feeding with love and good sense.* Boulder, CO: Bull Publishing Company.

22 Ellyn Satter, MS, RD. https://www.ellynsatterinstitute.com/

23 dictionary.com. Retrieved 19 April 2019, from https://www.dictionary.com/

24 Klein, M. D. (2018). Get Permission Approach to Pediatric Feeding Challenges Workhops.

25 Lumeng, J. C., Miller, A. L., Appugliese, D., Rosenblum, K., & Kaciroti, N. (2018). Picky eating, pressuring feeding, and growth in toddlers. *Appetite, 123,* 299-305.

26 Birch, L., Savage, J. S., & Ventura, A. (2007). Influences on the development of children's eating behaviours: from infancy to adolescence. *Canadian journal of dietetic practice and research: a publication of Dietitians of Canada, 68*(1), s1.

27 DeCosta, P., Møller, P., Frøst, M. B., & Olsen, A. (2017). Changing children's eating behaviour-A review of experimental research. *Appetite, 113,* 327-357.

28 Cambridge Online Dictionary. Retrieved 19 April 2019, from https://dictionary.cambridge.org/us/

29 Skye, L. (2018, June 1). Autism and controlled eating. Network Autism, National Autistic Society. Retrieved from https://network.autism.org.uk/knowledge/insight-opinion/autism-and-controlled-eating

30 Rowell, K. & McGlothlin, J. (2015). *Helping Your Child with Extreme Picky Eating: A Step-by-step Guide for Overcoming Selective Eating, Food Aversion, and Feeding Disorders.* Oakland, CA: New Harbinger Publications.

31 Zucker, N., Copeland, W., Franz, L., Carpenter, K., Keeling, L., Angold, A., & Egger, H. (2015). Psychological and psychosocial impairment in preschoolers with selective eating. *Pediatrics, 136*(3), e582.

32 Mascola, A. J., Bryson, S. W., & Agras, W. S. (2010). Picky eating during childhood: a longitudinal study to age 11 years. *Eating behaviors, 11*(4), 253-257.

33 Thomas, J. J., Lawson, E. A., Micali, N., Misra, M., Deckersbach, T., & Eddy, K. T. (2017). Avoidant/restrictive food intake disorder: a three-dimensional model of neurobiology with implications for etiology and treatment. *Current psychiatry reports, 19*(8), 54.

34 Minshew, N. J., & Williams, D. L. (2007). The new neurobiology of autism: cortex, connectivity, and neuronal organization. *Archives of neurology, 64*(7), 945-950.

35 Farrow, C. V. & Coulthard, H. (2012). Relationships between sensory sensitivity, anxiety and selective eating in children. *Appetite, 58*(3), 842-846.

36 Zickgraf, H. F. & Elkins, A. (2018). Sensory sensitivity mediates the relationship between anxiety and picky eating in children/adolescents ages 8–17, and in college undergraduates: A replication and age-upward extension. *Appetite, 128,* 333-339.

37 Taylor, C. M. & Emmett, P. M. (2018). Picky eating in children: causes and consequences. *Proceedings of the Nutrition Society*, 1-9.

38 Mayer, E. A. & Burns, T. (2016). *The mind-gut connection: how the hidden conversation within our bodies impacts our mood, our choices, and our overall health.* New York, NY: Harper Wave.

39 Koloski, N. A., Jones, M., Kalantar, J., Weltman, M., Zaguirre, J., & Talley, N. J. (2012). The brain–gut pathway in functional gastrointestinal disorders is bidirectional: a 12-year prospective population-based study. *Gut, 61*(9), 1284-1290.

40 Shields, G. S. & Slavich, G. M. (2017). Lifetime stress exposure and health: a review of contemporary assessment methods and biological mechanisms. *Social and personality psychology compass, 11*(8), e12335.

41 Shonkoff, J.P., Garner, A.S., Siegel, B.S., Dobbins, M.I., Earls, M.F., McGuinn, L., Pascoe, J., Wood, D.L., Committee on Psychosocial Aspects of Child and Family Health and Committee on Early Childhood, Adoption, and Dependent Care. (2012). The lifelong effects of early childhood adversity and toxic stress. *Pediatrics, 129*(1), pp. e232-e246.

42 Sanders, M. R. & Hall, S. L. (2018). Trauma-informed care in the newborn intensive care unit: promoting safety, security and connectedness. *Journal of Perinatology, 38*(1), 3.

43 Van der Kolk, B. (2000). Posttraumatic stress disorder and the nature of trauma. *Dialogues in clinical neuroscience, 2*(1), 7.

44 Perry, B. D., Pollard, R. A., Blakley, T. L., Baker, W. L., & Vigilante, D. (1995). Childhood trauma, the neurobiology of adaptation, and "use-dependent" development of the brain: How "states" become "traits". *Infant mental health journal, 16*(4), 271-291.

45 De Bellis, M. D. & Zisk, A. (2014). The biological effects of childhood trauma. *Child and Adolescent Psychiatric Clinics, 23*(2), 185-222.

46 Irene, Chatoor, MD. Director Mental Health Infant and Toddler Mental Health Program. https://childrensnational.org/choose-childrens/find-a-provider/irene-chatoor

47 Rowell, K. (2015, December 15). Avoiding Trauma in the Therapeutic Setting: Considerations for Pediatric Feeding Therapies. MN Trauma Project. Retrieved from https://www.mn-traumaproject.org/single-post/2015/12/19/Avoiding-Trauma-in-the-Therapeutic-Setting-Considerations-for-Pediatric-Feeding-Therapies

48 Powell, F. C., Farrow, C. V., & Meyer, C. (2011). Food avoidance in children. The influence of maternal feeding practices and behaviours. *Appetite, 57*(3), 683-692.

49 Tan, C. C. & Holub, S. C. (2012). Maternal feeding practices associated with food neophobia. *Appetite, 59*(2), 483-487.

50 Levine, A., Bachar, L., Tsangen, Z., Mizrachi, A., Levy, A., Dalal, I., Kornfeld, L., Levy, Y., Zadik, Z., Turner, D. and Boaz, M. (2011). Screening criteria for diagnosis of infantile feeding disorders as a cause of poor feeding or food refusal. *Journal of pediatric gastroenterology and nutrition, 52*(5), pp.563-568.

51 Nourish AZ. (2019, January 07). *Grasshopper Story.* Retrieved from https://youtu.be/V675_yjFQRE

52 Ziemba, Brady. (2018, October 9). Brady's Tasting Tips for exploring new foods. From Franken Brady. Retrieved from https://youtu.be/xWiP_MU7frk

53 Jennifer McGlothlin MS-CCC-SLP. Coauthor of Rowell, K. & McGlothlin, J. (2015). *Helping Your Child with Extreme Picky Eating: A Step-by-step Guide for Overcoming Selective Eating, Food Aversion, and Feeding Disorders*. Oakland, CA: New Harbinger Publications.

54 Kay Toomey, PhD. SOS Sensory Oral Sensory Approach. https://sosapproach-conferences.com/

55 Macmillan Online Dictionary. Retrieved 19 April 2019 from https://www.macmillandictionary.com/us/

56 Heidi Liefer Moreland, MS, CCC-SLP, BCS-S, CLC. Clinical coordinator and feeding therapist at Thrive with Spectrum Pediatrics. http://www.thrivewithspectrum.com/

57 Jo Cormack, MS. Emotionally Aware Feeding. https://www.jocormack.com/

58 Addessi, E., Galloway, A. T., Visalberghi, E., & Birch, L. L. (2005). Specific social influences on the acceptance of novel foods in 2–5-year-old children. *Appetite, 45*(3), 264-271.

59 Dovey, T. M., Staples, P. A., Gibson, E. L., & Halford, J. C. (2008). Food neophobia and 'picky/fussy' eating in children: a review. *Appetite, 50*(2-3), 181-193.

60 Online Google Dictionary. Retrieved 19 April 2019 from http://googledictionary.freecollocation.com/

61 Clear, J. (2018). *Atomic habits: An easy & proven way to build good habits & break bad ones*. New York, New York: Penguin.

62 Kill, K. Hope With Feathers Blog. Retrieved from http://www.thenewyorkperch.com/journal

63 Shepherd, G. M. (2011). *Neurogastronomy: how the brain creates flavor and why it matters*. New York, NY: Columbia University Press.

64 Coulthard, H. Harris, G., & Fogel, A. (2016). Association between tactile over-responsivity and vegetable consumption early in the introduction of solid foods and its variation with age. *Maternal & child nutrition, 12*(4), 848-859.

65 Geisel, Theodor Seuss (1960). *Green eggs and ham*. Penguin Random House Beginner Books.

Favorite Resources

Here are some of my favorite feeding support resources. They come in the form of clinic and approaches, websites, books and online support.

Ages and Stages www.agesandstages.net
Feeding Your Baby and Toddler Right, 2018
Nobody Ever Told Me (or my Mother) That! (Everything from Bottles and Breathing to Healthy Speech Development, 2010
Diane Bahr, MS, CCC-SLP, CIMI

Baby Self Feeding: Solid Food Solutions to Create Lifelong, Healthy Eating Habits, 2016
Melanie Potock, MA, CCC, SLP and Nancy Ripton

Baby Led Weaning: The Essential Guide to Introducing Solid Foods and Helping Your Baby Grow up a Healthy and Confident Eater, 2008
Gill Rapley, PhD and Tracey Murkett

Chicago Feeding Group
www.chicagofeedinggroup.org

Conquering Picky Eating for Teens and Adults, 2018
Katya Rowell, MD and Jenny McGlothlin, MS, CCC-SLP
www.extremepickyeating.com

Ellyn Satter Institute
Child of Mine, 2000
Ellyn Satter, RD, MS, MSSW
www.ellynsatterinstitute.org

Emotionally Aware Feeding
Helping Children Develop a Positive Relationship With Food, 2016

Jo Cormack, MA, Therapist and Feeding Specialist
www. jocormack.com

Feeding Matters
www.feedingmatters.com

Food Chaining: The Proven 6 Step Plan to Stop Picky Eating, Solve Feeding Problems and Expand Your Child's Diet, 2007
By Cheri Fraker, Laura Walbert, Mark, Fishbein and Sibyl Cox
(Facebook) Preemietalk Cheri Fraker, CCC-SLP, CLC and Laura Walbert, CCC-SLP, CLC

Grasshopper Story
https://youtu.be/V675_yjFQRE Grasshopper story

Helping Your Child with Extreme Picky Eating: Step-by-Step Guide for Overcoming Selective Eating, Food Aversion, and Feeding Disorders 2015
Katya Rowell, MD and Jenny McGlothlin, MS, CCC-SLP
www.extremepickyeating.com

Homemade Blended Formula Handbook 2007
Marsha Dunn Klein, OTR/L, MED and Suzanne Evans Morris, PhD

Love Me, Feed Me: The Adoptive Parent's Guide to Ending the Worry about Weight, Picky Eating, Power Struggles and More. 2012
Katja Rowell, MD
and Helping Your Child with Extreme Picky Eating: Step-by-Step Guide for Overcoming Selective Eating, Food Aversion, and Feeding Disorders Katja Rowell with Jennifer McGlothlin
www.thefeedingdoctor.com
www.extremepickyeatinghelp.com

Mealtime Connections
www.mealtimeconections.com

Mealtime Notions
Marsha Dunn Klein OTR/L, MED, FAOTA
Get Permission Workshops
www.mealtimenotions.com

New Visions
Suzanne Evans Morris, PhD, CCC-SLP
New Visions
www.new-vis.com

Pediatric Feeding Association
www.pedsfeeds.com

Pediatric Feeding News
Krisi Brackett, MS, SLP-CCC
When Your Child Can't Eat or Won't Eat
www.pediatricfeedingnews.com

Prefeeding Skills, Second Edition, 2000
Suzanne Evans Morris, PhD and Marsha Dunn Klein,OTR/L, MEd

SOFFI® Supporting Oral Feeding in Fragile Infants
Erin Sundseth Ross, Ph.D., CCC-SLP
www.feedingfundamentals.com

SOS Approach (Sequential Oral Sensory)to Feeding
Dr. Kay Toomey, Pediatric Psychologist
Developer, SOS Approach to Feeding program
www.sosapproach.com

Thrive with Spectrum Pediatrics
Jennifer Berry, MS, OTR/L, Owner, Thrive with Spectrum Pediatrics
Heidi Moreland, MS, CCC-SLP,CLC, Clinical Coordinator Thrive with Spectrum
Pediatrics
www.thrivewithspectrum.com
www.spectrumpediatrics.com

Index

Printed in the United States
By Bookmasters